DEATH AND THE PEARL MAIDEN

INTERVENTIONS:
NEW STUDIES IN MEDIEVAL CULTURE
Ethan Knapp, Series Editor

DEATH AND THE PEARL MAIDEN

~

Plague, Poetry, England

DAVID K. COLEY

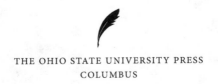

THE OHIO STATE UNIVERSITY PRESS
COLUMBUS

Copyright © 2019 by The Ohio State University.
Library of Congress Cataloging-in-Publication Data
Names: Coley, David K., author.
Title: Death and the Pearl maiden : plague, poetry, England / David K. Coley.
Other titles: Interventions: new studies in medieval culture.
Description: Columbus : The Ohio State University Press, [2019] | Series: Interventions: new
    studies in medieval culture | Includes bibliographical references and index.
Identifiers: LCCN 2018044681 | ISBN 9780814213902 (cloth ; alk. paper) | ISBN 0814213901
    (cloth ; alk. paper)
Subjects: LCSH: Pearl (Middle English poem)—Criticism, Textual. | Plague in literature.
    | Plague—England—London. | English poetry—Middle English, 1100–1500—History
    and criticism.
Classification: LCC PR2111 .C55 2019 | DDC 821/.1—dc23
LC record available at https://lccn.loc.gov/2018044681

Cover design by Laurence J. Nozik
Text design by Juliet Williams
Type set in Adobe Minion Pro

For Theresa Coletti, *a frende ful fyin*

CONTENTS

~

List of Illustrations   viii

Acknowledgments   ix

A Note on the Text   xi

INTRODUCTION   Forgotten History   1

PART 1 · PLAGUE IN THE *PEARL* MANUSCRIPT: SYMPTOM AND RESPONSE

CHAPTER 1   Trauma, Witness, and Representation in *Cleanness*   29

CHAPTER 2   *Pearl* and the Language of Plague   56

PART 2 · BEYOND THE SYMPTOMATIC: CONSIDERING THE PLAGUE IN FOURTEENTH-CENTURY ENGLAND

CHAPTER 3   Flight and Enclosure in *Patience*   93

CHAPTER 4   Sex, Death, and Social Change in *Sir Gawain and the Green Knight*   126

CONCLUSION   A Pestilence Whispered   167

Bibliography   193

Index   211

ILLUSTRATIONS

FIGURE 2.1 The Covering of Christ's Loins; Christ's Side Pierced, from the *Holkham Bible* 57

FIGURE 2.2 The New Heaven and the New Earth; Christ Returns; the Last Trump Sounds, from the *Holkham Bible* 58

FIGURE 2.3 Matthias Grüenwald, Crucifixion, Saints, and Entombment, from the *Isenheim Altarpiece* 60

FIGURE 2.4 Matthias Grüenwald, The Resurrection of Christ, from the *Isenheim Altarpiece* 61

FIGURE 4.1 Josse Lieferinxe, Saint Sebastian Interceding for the Plague Stricken 152

FIGURE 4.2 Scenes from the Life of St. Sebastian: The Saint Healing a Woman from the Plague 153

FIGURE 4.3 The Triumph of Death 153

FIGURE 4.4 Giovanni di Paolo, The Triumph of Death (Death Assailing a Young Man) 154

FIGURE 4.5 Master of the Playing Cards (attributed), Saint Sebastian 154

FIGURE 4.6 Il Sodoma, The Martyrdom of Saint Sebastian 155

ACKNOWLEDGMENTS

THIS BOOK has been the project of nearly a decade. I first presented on plague and the Cotton Nero A.x poems in 2010, and so I have by now benefitted from the insight of more people than I can recall, let alone thank adequately in these acknowledgements. If I'm to make a go of gratitude, however, I need to start with my friend and colleague Matthew Hussey, who has been an inexhaustible source of knowledge and good humor since these ideas first started to take shape. Matt read the first draft of *Death and the Pearl Maiden* in its entirety, and his thoughtful responses, as well as his help with my somewhat shaky Latin, have been instrumental. Ronda Arab has also been a trusted reader as I developed this book, and I am genuinely grateful for her thorough readings of several of its chapters. Thanks also to Christine Kim, whose insights into trauma and memory have been fundamental to my thinking; Diana Solomon, for reading and commenting generously on several sections; and Anne Higgins for helping to convince me, early in my career at Simon Fraser University, that the Black Death was something worth looking into. And my sincere thanks to three of my former graduate students: Brenna Duperron and Maude Vachon-Roy, both of whom taught me every bit as much as I might have taught them, and Yusuf Varachia, who, despite his assertions to the contrary, brings a great deal to the table.

I have presented work from this project at the Medieval Academy of the Pacific, the Medieval Academy of America, the New Chaucer Society, the Sewanee Medieval Colloquium, and, of course, at Kalamazoo. I am grateful to the organizers of these scholarly gatherings for providing space for me to explore my arguments, and I am indebted to those who offered thoughtful critical responses. My thanks also to Alex Cook for inviting me to give a lecture on *Sir Gawain and the Green Knight* at the University of Alabama, which allowed me to develop several of the ideas that would eventually crystallize into chapter 4. Finally, this work has benefitted from the input, sometimes casual and sometimes concerted, of many scholars and friends. Among them, I would like to give particular mention to Lynn Staley, Richard Godden, Siân Echard, Alexandra Gillespie, Frank Grady, Elizabeth Scala, Patricia Ingham, David Matthews, Arthur Bahr, and Jeffrey Cohen.

Early versions of chapters 1 and 2 appeared in *Exemplaria* and *Studies in the Age of Chaucer,* respectively. I am grateful to the anonymous readers for those journals, as well as to their editors for pressing my arguments and prose. I also want to offer my sincere thanks to Sarah Stanbury and to the remaining anonymous readers for the Ohio State University Press, whose incisive reviews of (and challenges to) my manuscript have made this a more effective book. Ethan Knapp has been a supportive and responsive editor, and I owe him an enormous debt of gratitude for encouraging my scholarship and for steering me toward the Interventions Series.

Finally, thank you to my wife, Kimberly, and to our daughters, Johanna and Alison. The three of you have made my world a better place, and I am humbled by your patience, love, and support.

I dedicate this book to Theresa Coletti. It is impossible for me to overstate the impact that you have had as a teacher, a mentor, a colleague, and a friend. Thank you.

A NOTE ON THE TEXT

~

I HAVE, wherever possible, attempted to quote plague texts in their original languages. Translations of Latin, Castilian, Catalan, as well as simple French and Italian passages are my own unless otherwise noted. For all other languages, I have relied on published translations, which are cited in the notes. There are a few instances where I have not been able to access original language texts; in those cases, I have used modern English alone.

Rosemary Horrox's sourcebook, *The Black Death,* has been an invaluable resource over the course of my exploration of the plague. In particular, I have often used it as a starting point for tracking down treatises, in both print and manuscript form. I want here to acknowledge Professor Horrox's meticulously edited volume, which has done much to open the field of plague studies to a wider range of scholars, and also to acknowledge my debt to her scholarship.

INTRODUCTION

Forgotten History

*It gives me no pleasure to go raking over all these
tribulations, and I propose to make no mention of
whatever may be suitably passed over in silence.*

—GIOVANNI BOCCACCIO, *DECAMERON*[1]

THERE IS A certain irony in Boccaccio's proposal to pass over in the *Decameron's* now celebrated plague narrative whatever might remain unspoken. Putatively informed by Boccaccio's own witness to the 1348 pestilence in Florence, the introduction to the *Decameron* has become not only a literary benchmark in studies of the pandemic but a historical one as well, providing a description of the plague-ravaged city that exceeds, as the work's most prominent twentieth-century editor has argued, "*sensi allegorici e metaforici e allusivi per ancorare saldamente alla realtà, alla 'storia'*" [allegorical, metaphorical, and allusive meanings in order to anchor solidly to reality, to "history"].[2] This claim for the historiographical *realtà* of the *Decameron*—its status as an eyewitness account of an event that swept away as much as 60 percent of the population of Europe, North Africa, and the Middle East[3]—has become something of a critical commonplace, and Boccaccio's description is now regularly treated as a de facto historical narrative, one frequently included in academic

---

1. "*A me medesimo increst andarmi tanto tra tante miserie ravolgendo: per che, volendo omai lasciare star quella parte di quelle che io acconciamente posso schifare.*" Boccaccio, *Decameron*, 20 (Waldman, 14).

2. Branca, *Boccaccio medievale e nuovi studi sul "Decameron,"* 34.

3. Benedictow, *The Black Death 1346–53*, 383. The precise mortality rate for the Black Death in both England and mainland Europe remains a topic of scholarly debate. The rough figure of sixty percent is from Benedictow's exhaustive study of the pandemic and currently stands as the best estimate of the disease's mortality rate.

sourcebooks and in medical surveys of the Black Death.[4] Clear-eyed and verisimilar, the introduction to the *Decameron* appears to be a rare moment in which a historical event—in this case a deeply traumatic one—leaves an unambiguous trace of itself on the literary page.

As recent discussions in medieval studies have demonstrated, however, the response of literature to history—the witness that literature provides within history—is never a straightforward one. It is, at this point, impossible to state flatly that texts such as the *Decameron,* Guillaume de Machaut's *Jugement dou Roy de Navarre,* or William Langland's *Piers Plowman* stand as "accurate indices of the world from which they arise and upon which they reflect," and it is equally difficult to claim, without careful qualification, that such texts "bear a privileged relation to their historical moment" or allow readers a glimpse of "the historically real."[5] Such tenets of New Historicist thought propose a more immediate and straightforward relationship between the historical and the literary than often exists. Indeed, literary critics have increasingly recognized that the space between history and text is always, as Ardis Butterfield writes, a "delicate area of negotiation" and that even a work like Boccaccio's, which seems to offer readers an encounter with the past marked by phenomenological concreteness and historiographical verisimilitude, mediates history through a prismatic range of social, psychological, cultural, and literary filters.[6] History is always apprehended in the literary through a nexus of contingencies, unacknowledged desires, and half-understandings, occluded by the same language that promises to reveal it and exposed by words and phrases that may seem initially to offer little revelation. To Branca's insistence that we read Boccaccio's pestilential introduction as anchored *"saldamente alla realtà"* then, we might add David Wallace's somewhat more complicated assessment of the *Decameron*'s relationship to its historical moment, a moment in which the plague existed in a past so recent that it might barely be called past at all: "History acquires pathos, as Boccaccio contemplates it, by virtue of [the] difference between the objective knowledge and relative security of *now* and the claustrophobic subjectivity of *then.* It is only through the power of such *imaginative retrospection* that the plague becomes fully visible or intelligible."[7] In this respect, it is useful to recall that even if Boccaccio was an eyewitness to the plague, the "imaginative retrospection" that renders it "fully visible" in

---

4. See, for instance, Steel, "Plague Writing: From Boccaccio to Camus," and Marafioti, "Post-*Decameron* Plague Treatises." The description is also included in Horrox, *The Black Death,* and Aberth, *The Black Death,* two recent sourcebooks for the pandemic.

5. Patterson, *Negotiating the Past,* 74, 62.

6. Butterfield, "Pastoral and the Politics of Plague," 4.

7. Wallace, *Boccaccio: Decameron, Landmarks of World Literature,* 19.

his work is informed by earlier depictions of epidemic disease from classical authorities like Lucretius, Thucydides, and Ovid.[8] Even Boccaccio's searing evocation of the Black Death, then, is already bookish, already mediated by the writing of the past, tangled in a process of literary becoming.

If such an approach suggests to us how the allusive and the fictive might read as the historiographical, it also asks, by the same token, that we recognize the presence of history in literary texts that seem to eschew overt historiography. As D. Vance Smith writes, readers of the past must "grapple with the problem of discussing texts and events . . . that are not fit subjects for practices of deliberate memory"; they must "[think] about how things get forgotten, and how they can be remembered."[9] Such forgotten histories (Smith calls them "irregular histories") exist within literature as surely as do the sorts of overt histories that we perceive in the introduction to Boccaccio's *Decameron*.

Seeking those histories, remembering them, perhaps even prizing them from their texts, is the impulse that drives *Death and the Pearl Maiden*. It is likewise an impulse that has driven much recent work in medieval literary studies. Elizabeth Scala opens her monograph on absent narratives by asserting, "The primary function of the medievalist is to locate missing stories," and while Scala's focus is explicitly on the structural and textual features that animate medieval narrative, her attention to "not simply what the [text] says but also to what it cannot know it is saying" gestures toward the historical and textual silences that always exist as part of the medieval literary tradition, as well as the critical desire to account for them.[10] Similarly, Patricia Clare Ingham's analysis of traumatic voicing in *Troilus and Criseyde* considers how Chaucer's *litel tragedye* gives voice to "the traumatic rhythms upon which realist history depends but about which it can rarely speak." Literature itself, in Ingham's (and perhaps Chaucer's) understanding, becomes "a frail representational mode" that nonetheless embodies, even as it reanimates, a cultural and historical memory troubled by moments of profound trauma.[11] Such critical work—and here Scala and Ingham stand in for many critics of the last few decades—ultimately reinforces a key observation made by Aranye Fraden-

---

8. The now canonical survey of these sources is Getto, "*La peste del* Decameron *e il problema della fonte Lucreziana.*" See also Gittes, *Boccaccio's Naked Muse.* Charles de Paolo, *Epidemic Disease and Human Understanding*, further reminds us that "no compelling evidence exists that Boccaccio was on the scene" (63) in Florence to witness the event he describes.

9. Smith, "Irregular Histories," 171.

10. Scala, *Absent Narratives*, 1, 5.

11. Ingham, "Chaucer's Haunted Aesthetics," 228. More recently Lynn Arner has highlighted the "incoherence and fragmentation of the consciousness of the late medieval English nonruling classes," suggesting how literature might not only absent particular histories but willfully obscure them. See Arner, *Chaucer, Gower, and the Vernacular Rising*, 6–7.

burg, who invites us to see the past as fractured and densely layered, teeming with unexpressed and unknowable memories and possibilities. "Past times do not know themselves, or their pasts or their futures, in fullness, free of desire," Fradenburg writes, an assertion that holds as true for literary texts as it does for the patrons, poets, and scribes who created them.[12] It is, moreover, an assertion that implicates both medieval writers and the modern publics who engage with their writing, one that asks us to account for and address the blind spots inherent in medieval literary works and in our own contemporary critical methods.

This book proposes to take seriously both Smith's invitation to consider the amnesias and mnemonic lacunae of the past and Fradenburg's insistence on the always compromised state of historical memory as it addresses a problem that has long vexed readers of late medieval English literature, namely that one of the great historical ruptures of the European Middle Ages, perhaps *the* signal historical event of the late medieval period, seems to exist as a forgotten history in the corpus of fourteenth-century Middle English literature, a body of work as daring, experimental, and socially engaged as any in English literary history. That event, of course, is the pandemic that Boccaccio, writing in the Italian vernacular, describes passing through Florence "*non altramenti che faccia il fuoco alle cose secche o unte quando molto gli sono avvicinate*" [just as fire catches on to any dry or greasy object placed too close to it][13] and that Machaut, writing in French, personifies as an uncaged beast, "*Pleinne de forsen et de rage, . . . / Si gloute et si familleuse / Que ne se pooit säouler / Pour riens que peüst engouler*" [Full of rage and anger . . . / So gluttonous and so famished / That he could not be satisfied / By anything that he could consume].[14] The Black Death and its recurrences passed through England as well, and the English mortality rate of 62.5 percent comports with similar figures from Europe, North Africa, Western Asia, and the Arabian Peninsula.[15] All told, England contributed around 3.5 million deaths to the 50 million estimated in Europe alone.[16] And yet, within postplague English literature generally and, more particularly, within the efflorescence of vernacular English literature that marks the second half of the fourteenth century, the plague's presence

---

12. Fradenburg, *Sacrifice Your Love*, 63–64.

13. Boccaccio, *Decameron*, 13 (Waldman, 7–8).

14. Machaut, *The Judgment of the King of Navarre*, 16, trans. on 17 (ll. 356–62).

15. Benedictow, *The Black Death*, 368, 383.

16. Benedictow, 382–83. Benedictow puts the population of England before the plague at approximately 6 million and the population of Europe at roughly 80 million, figures that draw the respective losses of 3.5 million and 50 million into even sharper perspective. The loss of life engendered by the plague, even in a period not highly regarded for its long lifespans, is astounding.

is surprisingly subdued. References to it are not entirely absent. Chaucer and Langland refer respectively to the "Deeth / That in this contree al the peple sleeth" [Death, that in this country slays all the people] and to the "pokkes and pestilences [that] muche peple shente" [poxes and plagues that brought about the death of many people], while poems such as *Wynnere and Wastour* allude broadly to the social consequences of the cataclysm.[17] Compared to the incandescent descriptions of the disease emerging from mainland Europe, however, the English response seems, at best, understated, and at worst, cowed. In one telling assessment, Siegfried Wenzel writes, "In vain does one look for a parallel from an English quill to the long and moving descriptions of the Black Death given by Boccaccio and by Machaut, or to the anguished outcry in one of Petrarch's letters."[18] It is an evaluation that echoes earlier complaints about Chaucer's "timid" references to the pandemic, and it underscores the lingering critical puzzlement—one that I hope to show is founded as much on critical and methodological failings as it is on literary ones—that late medieval English poetry seems, unlike many of its Continental counterparts, to have cast the plague experience "barely a glance."[19]

To explore this distinction and, more broadly, to investigate how the history of the medieval plague experience might be simultaneously forgotten and remembered in late medieval English literature, I consider in this study a single group of Middle English poems, the works uniquely preserved in what is now British Library MS Cotton Nero A.x, article 3. On their face, these four late fourteenth-century poems—*Pearl*, an elegy on the loss of a young girl and an allegory of Christian soteriology; *Cleanness*, a series of violent Old Testament exempla inveighing against sexual and spiritual *fylþe*; *Patience*, a faithful if somewhat embellished retelling of the Book of Jonah; and *Sir Gawain and the Green Knight*, an enigmatic Arthurian romance—would seem to have little to recommend them for such a project. None outwardly refers to the disease or openly discusses its social aftermath, much less offers the vivid images of the "*grans monciaus / Trouvoit on dames, jouvenciaus, / Juenes, viels, et de toutes guises . . . tous mors de boces*" [great heaps of women, youths, / Boys, old people, those of all stations . . . all of them dead from the buboes]

---

17. Langland, *Piers Plowman*, 724 (B.20.98); Chaucer, *The Riverside Chaucer*, 199 (*CT* 6.675–76). Henceforth, all quotations from Langland's and Chaucer's works will be cited parenthetically by line number.

18. Wenzel, "Pestilence and Middle English Literature," 131–32.

19. Shrewsbury, *A History of Bubonic Plague in the British Isles*, 42; Tuchman, *A Distant Mirror*, 105. Such assessments may be dated, but they still hold important critical currency. As recently as 2008, Katherine H. Terrell cites Wenzel's assessment of the plague's impact in order to discount any connection between the disease and *Pearl*, a reading that my study strenuously resists. See Terrell, "Rethinking the 'Corse in Clot,'" 433–34n9.

found in Continental works.[20] Nor do the poems as a group promise the kind of prophylactic response articulated by the hundred tales of the *Decameron*, stories recounted by Boccaccio's *brigata* with the explicit purpose of diverting the mind, and thus protecting the body, from plague. I want to suggest here, however, the more subtle ways that the poems of the *Pearl* manuscript *might* articulate the traces of the Black Death and its complex cultural aftermath, how they can be seen to offer a literary witness defined less by verisimilitude and directness than by oblique referentiality, linguistic play, and allusive embodiment. If these four poems speak in witness to the medieval pandemic, their voice emerges not simply as a direct response to the disease but as an unspoken symptom, not only as a conscious reaction to the personal and cultural upheavals catalyzed by the plague but also as an unconscious indicium. It is a voice that has remained largely unrecognized and unheard; however, as I hope to show, it is finally a voice no less powerful for its quiescence.

In articulating how the poems of the *Pearl* manuscript might stand as forgotten witnesses to the Black Death's unforgotten trauma, I am consciously responding to Smith's suggestion that "new kinds of history can be written by looking at the edges of memory," that history within literature exists not only in the overtly historiographical but also in the "shadowy events at the margins of texts," in elusive moments that simultaneously defy and instantiate the historical itself.[21] As such, my theoretical approach will be eclectic, drawing at various points from epidemiology, psychoanalysis, sociology, philology, and art history, as well as from a range of medieval historiographical and literary texts. If a single theoretical insight undergirds this project, however, it is the recognition that the human response to traumatic events exists as a negotiation between acknowledgement and suppression, between the need to speak events that are too terrible to ignore and the desire to deny events that are too painful to speak. Judith Herman states, "The ordinary response to atrocities is to banish them from consciousness"; however, she also acknowledges that the consciousness of trauma, whether understood as an individual consciousness or a cultural one, can never be entirely stifled, that the need to speak the unspeakable always stands in powerful opposition to the urge toward silence.[22] In this way, trauma "both records and effaces its own past," rendering itself unspeakable even as it leaves legible traces behind.[23] This key paradox— trauma as a text that simultaneously inscribes and effaces itself—is registered in *Death and the Pearl Maiden*, a study that reads the Black Death both as an

---

20. Machaut, *The Judgement of the King of Navarre*, 18–19 (ll. 370–74 [trans. ll. 371–74]).
21. Smith, "Irregular Histories," 171.
22. Herman, *Trauma and Recovery*, 1.
23. Caruth, "After the End: Psychoanalysis in the Ashes of History," 36.

unspeakable horror and as a unavoidable truth. The presence of the disease may be muted by posttraumatic inarticulacy and by critical misprision, but it is a presence nonetheless, and one that urgently demands to be given voice.

That the pandemic should be regarded as a traumatic event can hardly be denied: the sheer loss of life that it caused, compounded by the physical, emotional, and economic stress that it precipitated, rank it among the greatest disasters in human history.[24] By foregrounding the pandemic as a deep cultural trauma, this study will suggest how the idiosyncratic poems of the *Pearl* manuscript, each one "sengeley in synglure" [singular in its uniqueness] among Middle English verse, suggest the literary response to the Black Death so often seen as lacking, in both vigor and eloquence, in Middle English poetry.[25] It will also use these poems to posit a still underrecognized pestilential discourse in late medieval English literature, and it will consider why, in contrast to the overt engagement of Continental writers like Boccaccio, late medieval English poets might have offered such an insistently quiet witness to the defining event of their historical moment.

Such an argument is, I acknowledge, speculative by its very nature. As a study that focuses on one apparent absence (references to plague in the *Pearl*-group) in order to build a case about a larger and more puzzling one (engagement with the pandemic in fourteenth-century English poetry), *Death and the Pearl Maiden* necessarily relies on patterns of suggestion and implication, on cultural and textual context, on semantic and narrative parallel, even on informed conjecture to articulate and develop its arguments. Moreover, while this book offers significant historical and literary data to support its proposition that the plague is a presence in these four poems, such data do not, indeed cannot, crystallize into hard fact. Because the hard fact is that *Pearl, Cleanness, Patience,* and *Sir Gawain and the Green Knight* never mention the Black Death, not even in the fleeting ways that Chaucer and Langland do, not even once. And yet, if this study cannot provide conclusive proof that the poems of MS Cotton Nero A.x are in any straightforward way "about" the plague, the evidence it compiles and the arguments it offers raise important possibilities about the intersection of plague and literature in fourteenth-century England, not only for the works of a single unique manuscript but for Middle English poetry as a whole.

---

24. See Lerner, "The Black Death and Western European Eschatological Mentalities," 533.

25. All quotations from the poems of MS Cotton Nero A.x are from *The Poems of the Pearl Manuscript*. Henceforth, they will be cited parenthetically in the text by line number and, where necessary, by abbreviated title. The quotation above is from *Pearl*, l. 8.

THE BLACK DEATH:
EVOLVING PERSPECTIVES ON A MEDIEVAL PLAGUE

The biological culprit of the pandemic we now call the Black Death remained a point of contention into the twenty-first century, but in 2011, it was concretely determined to be *Yersinia pestis,* the same bacillus discovered by Alexandre Yersin in 1894 and named as the cause of the pandemic that struck China and India in the late nineteenth century.[26] Unlike the identity of the bacillus, the linked vectors that first brought the medieval plague to the Black Sea port of Kaffa—the immediate locus from which it moved into the Mediterranean basin and began its transit through the Middle East, Northern Africa, and Europe—are still uncertain and remain the subject of ongoing interdisciplinary investigation. The geographical origin of the disease has been traced with relative confidence to the Tibet-Qinghai Plateau; the pandemic itself seems to have been triggered by slight climate fluctuations in the region, changes that caused first an expansion in wild rodent colonies and then, in a Malthusian correction, a rapid population collapse.[27] As colony numbers declined, the density of plague-carrying fleas per rodent increased dramatically, forcing greater numbers of fleas to find alternative mammalian hosts, including domesticated animals and livestock such as camels, sheep, and goats.[28] Dislodged from their stable foci in rodent colonies and increasingly integrated with nomadic and interconnected human populations, infected fleas moved slowly overland across sparsely populated Western Asia, traveling via human paths and wildlife routes in a process that may have taken more

---

26. The term "Black Death" first appears in a nineteenth-century children's history, Penrose (Mrs. Markham), *A History of England,* 128. It also serves as the title of Hecker, *Der Schwarze Tod im vierzehnten Jahrhundert,* translated by B. G. Babbington into English as *The Black Death in the Fourteenth Century.* It is likely that the term was in common use before the publications of these works, however.

The identity of the Black Death microbe as *Y. pestis* was confirmed through molecular analysis of human remains at a Smithfield plague cemetery. See Bos et al., "A Draft Genome of *Yersinia pestis* from Victims of the Black Death"; Cui et al., "Historical Variations in Mutation Rate in an Epidemic Pathogen"; Green, "Taking 'Pandemic' Seriously." Benedictow provides an overview of the controversy surrounding the identification before the discoveries of 2011 in *What Disease was Plague?,* especially 3–69. Even with the confirmation of the bacterial cause, scholars still struggle to account for the plague's virulence in the Middle Ages. DeWitte suggests that the fourteenth-century pandemic capitalized on a general decline in health in the later Middle Ages. See DeWitte, "Setting the Stage for Medieval Plague." Researchers have also suggested the possibility of transmission through human body lice rather than fleas. See Dean et al. "Human Ectoparasites and the Spread of Plague."

27. Green, "Taking 'Pandemic' Seriously," 29–31; Schmid et al., "Climate-Driven Introduction of the Black Death," 3022.

28. Schmid et al., "Climate-Driven Introduction of the Black Death," 3020.

than a decade.[29] Eventually, the plague's track seems to have coalesced along the braided commercial networks of the Silk Road, facilitating its westward overland motion.[30] It reached Kaffa in late 1346, and the population density within the fortified port, coupled with the ready supply of animal and human hosts lingering on departing Venetian and Genoese trading vessels, rendered the city a pestilential powder keg.[31] In a matter of months, the plague would spread over water to most of the major trading ports in the Mediterranean. From those initial nodes—Constantinople, Alexandria, Dubrovnik, Split, Venice, Messina, Tunis, Pisa, Genoa, Marseilles—it would metastasize quickly along established trade arteries, moving inland by river and then fanning out through local and regional patterns of social and economic contact.[32]

Biologically, plague infection manifests in the human body in four distinct forms, each with a different presentation and each contributing to the pandemic's radial progress outward from the Mediterranean.[33] The best known is *bubonic plague*, which occurs when an infective flea bites a human host and

---

29. Schmid et al., 3022–23.

30. The story of the Black Death's path(s) from the Tibet-Qinghai Plateau is evolving, and this particular narrative may tell only one portion of it. Robert Hymes has recently posited that the disease also coincided with Mongolian incursions into the territories of Xia (modern Gansu) in North-Central China, perhaps moving from there to population centers in the east (Hymes, "Epilogue: A Hypothesis on the East Asian Beginnings"). For the movement and impact of the disease in the Islamicate world, see Dols, *The Black Death in the Middle East*. Monica Green, moreover, has powerfully argued that we should "broaden our narratives of the Second Pandemic to include sub-Saharan African and, by implication, the Indian Ocean basin" ("Taking Pandemic Seriously," 38), speculating that the disease may have traveled to Africa via transoceanic trade. In an opinion article released while this book was in its copyediting stage, she has further argued against a straightforward China-to-Crimea trajectory, stating, "Our current understanding of *Y. pestis* genetics and 14th-century history would make such a transmission scenario impossible" ("On Learning How to Teach the Black Death," 22).

31. Some medieval sources, including Gabriele de' Mussis's influential *Historia de Morbo*, suggest that the plague's foothold in Kaffa was established when a Mongol military force, which had besieged the port, catapulted diseased bodies into the town in order to infect Genoese and Venetian merchants (de' Mussis, *Historia de Morbo*, 48–49). While this spurious narrative is repeated in some modern studies (such as Ziegler, *The Black Death*, 15–16), it has been rightfully questioned by other historians who see Gabriele de' Mussis's blame of "infidels" as motivated by xenophobia and religious self-interest (Benedictow, *The Black Death*, 52). There is, frankly, little evidence for the account's validity and still less reason to perpetuate it further as historical fact.

32. The path of the plague from the Mediterranean outward is well-documented. Again, I follow Benedictow, *The Black Death*, especially pages 57–122.

33. The first of these three modes of transmission, *bubonic, pneumonic*, and *septicemic*, are those most commonly associated with the medieval plague pandemic. My descriptions of them follow largely from those provided by both the Centers for Disease Control and the National Institutes of Health, though I have also consulted Benedictow, *The Black Death*, 25–31, and Herlihy, *The Black Death and the Transformation of the West*, 17–38.

regurgitates plague bacteria into the bite wound, bacteria which rapidly multiply within the lymphatic system. The bubonic form aligns most closely with Boccaccio's famous description in the *Decameron*:

> *Ma nascevano nel cominciamento d'essa a' maschi e alle femine parimente o nella anguinaia o sotto le ditella certe enfiature, delle quali alcune crescevano come una comunal mela, altre come uno uovo, e alcune più e alcun'altre meno, le quali i volgari nominavan gavoccioli. E dalle due parti del corpo predette infra brieve spazio cominciò il già detto gavocciolo mortifero indifferentemente in ogni parte di quello a nascere e a venire: e da questo appresso s'incominciò la qualità della predetta infermità a permutare in macchie nere o livide, le quali nelle braccia e per le cosce e in ciascuna altra parte del corpo apparivano a molti, a cui grandi e rade e a cui minute e spesse.*[34]

[Its first sign here in both men and women was a swelling in the groin or beneath the armpit, growing sometimes in the shape of a simple apple, sometimes in that of an egg, more or less; a bubo was the name commonly given to such a swelling. Before long this deadly bubo would begin to spread indifferently from these points to crop up all over; the symptoms would develop then into the dark or livid patches that many people found appearing on their arms or thighs or elsewhere; these were large and well separated in some cases, while in others, they were a crowd of tiny spots.]

The buboes, or *gavoccioli,* which give bubonic plague its name, most often develop in the lymphatic clusters nearest the infected flea bite, emerging painfully in the neck, armpit, or groin. They represent the body's last line of defense against *Y. pestis* entering the circulatory system and developing into *septicemic plague,* a blood infection that causes subcutaneous hemorrhages (likely Boccaccio's "*macchie nere o livide*" [dark or livid patches]), clotting, necrosis, and eventually death.

Nether bubonic nor septicemic plague is easily transmissible from person to person. *Pneumonic plague,* which occurs when plague bacteria infect the lungs, *is* transmissible however, and it thus stands as the most contagious form of the disease. Individuals with pneumonic plague develop respiratory symptoms akin to those of pneumonia, including a persistent cough and the production of bloody or watery sputum. In fourteenth-century descriptions of the disease, such as Gabriele de' Mussis's *Historia de Morbo,* the pneumonic presentation is likely responsible for images of plague victims "*sputum ex ore*

---

34. Boccaccio, *Decameron,* 12 (Waldman, 7).

sanguineum" [spitting blood from the mouth], as well as for the rapid contagion noted by many medieval commenters.[35] Finally, *Y. pestis* can be spread
to humans through the meat of infected animals, presenting as *gastrointensti-
nal plague*. Such a mode of transmission is comparatively rare and not readily described in medieval sources, but twentieth- and twenty first-century
outbreaks of plague in Jordan, Afghanistan, and Libya (from infected camel
meat) and in Ecuador and Peru (from infected guinea pig meat) remind us
that gastrointestinal infection should be acknowledged as a possible mode of
transmission during the medieval pandemic, especially, as Michelle Ziegler
notes, during periods of shortage or famine.[36] Whether or not gastrointestinal
plague was a major factor in the development of the medieval pandemic, it
remains clear is that the disease was able to move in a variety of more or less
virulent forms as it tracked from port to city to town to manor house, moving steadily across Continental Europe, the Islamicate world, and eventually
the British Isles.

The Black Death first struck England in the summer of 1348, arriving at the
southern seaport of Melcombe (now Weymouth) on a trading ship returning
from Bordeaux. The fragmentary *Chronicle of the Grey Friars of Lynn* recounts
the event in straightforward terms:

Isto anno apud Melcoumbe in comitatu Dorsate parum ante festum nat'sancti
Iohannis Baptiste, due scaphe, quarum una erat de Bristollia, applicuerunt,
in quibus naute de Vasconia venientes quadam inaudita pestilencia epi-
demia nominata infecti, homines illius ville de Melcoumbe primo in Anglia
inficiebant.[37]

[In that year near Melcombe in the county of Dorset, a little before the feast
of Saint John the Baptist, two boats, one of them from Bristol, landed. In
them, the sailors coming from Gascony were infected with an unheard-of
epidemic of pestilence. The people of the town of Melcombe were the first
in England to be infected.]

From this first point of contact, the disease traveled much as it had through
the rest of Europe, journeying quickly from port to port over water and crawl-

---

35. Gabriele de' Mussis, *Historia de Morbo*, 55.
36. Ziegler, "The Black Death and the Future of the Plague," 266–67.
37. "A Fourteenth-Century Chronicle from the Grey Friars of Lynn," 274. The brief chronicle covers the years 1340–77. The annals seem to have been written year by year rather than
all at once, and they occupy two previously unused folios of a mid-fourteenth-century commonplace book.

ing more slowly over land. In the autumn of 1348, it reached the port of Bristol in the west and quickly spread up the River Severn to Gloucester; it also traveled up the Thames to London and from there percolated through England's Southeast.[38] At roughly the same time, the plague landed in the cities of Drogheda, Howth, and Dublin, and from those loci it advanced westward across Ireland.[39] By the beginning of 1349, the disease had moved by land as far north as East Anglia and the Southern Midlands, and it had traveled by ship to the Lincolnshire port of Grimsby, about sixty miles south of York.[40] By the end of the year, it engulfed all of England, Wales, Ireland, and parts of the Scottish Lowlands,[41] and in 1350 it raked across Scotland, spreading even to the Hebrides in the northwest and to the remote islands of Orkney and Shetland.[42]

The pestilence subsided in the British Isles by the end of 1350, but as the fourteenth century wore on, it became clear that the initial cataclysmic event was to be only the first of a recurring series of epidemics, a chain of traumatic aftershocks that would continue, in varying capacities, for several hundred years.[43] The environmental and biological triggers for subsequent outbreaks, like those of the initial outbreak, remain unclear, and while it has traditionally been assumed that the plague found a stable foothold in Europe among native populations of black and brown rats (*Rattus rattus* and *Rattus norvegicus*), recent findings have called this assumption into question.[44] Some zoological

---

38. Benedictow, *The Black Death*, 130–34. Benedictow's assessment of the movement of the disease through Southern England is corroborated by Ziegler, *The Black Death*, especially at 122–24, 151–60. I have relied most heavily on Benedictow and Zeigler to inform my chronology of the plague's advance through the British Isles but have also considered the chronology presented in Shrewsbury, *A History of Bubonic Plague*.

39. Zeigler, *The Black Death*, 194–98.

40. Benedictow, *The Black Death*, 138, 139–40; Zeigler, *The Black Death*, 178–79, corroborates this pattern of spread.

41. Chronicle accounts and other historical sources show that 1349 was the year that the Black Death effectively colonized the entirety of Britain south of Scotland. Months and sometimes precise dates of outbreaks in individual jurisdictions are recorded in Benedictow, *The Black Death*, 133–45; Zeigler, *The Black Death*, 161–86; and Shrewsbury, *A History of Bubonic Plague*, 53–125.

42. Philip Zeigler suggests that Scotland's lower population density meant that the Black Death affected the country comparatively lightly, at least by the standards set in England (*The Black Death*, 199–201). Benedictow finds it "virtually impossible to discuss the matter at all" due to a lack of historical source material (*Black Death*, 145), but an Icelandic annal cited in his study describes the presence of the disease even in Scotland's far Northwestern islands (154).

43. The last recognized major plague outbreak in England was 1679, while the last major outbreak in Continental Europe (Marseille) was in 1720. See Green, "Editor's Introduction," *Pandemic Disease in the Medieval World*, 14.

44. Indeed, despite the traditional understanding of the rat as the key vector for the spread of the Black Death (and here I acknowledge that I may have furthered this understanding by having a rat peeking out from the cover of this book), the role of rats in the plague's spread

research, for instance, has suggested that the climate-driven process that first pushed the plague outward from the Tibet-Qinghai Plateau may itself have been a recurring phenomenon, precipitating wave after wave of the ongoing pandemic.[45] Whatever the environmental or demographic trigger, the first of these cyclical aftershocks came to England in 1361, when a second national epidemic, sometimes known as the Gray Death, swept across the country. Though it seems to have taken a similar geographical trajectory as the first epidemic, the second plague was notable for its heightened effect on children and adolescents. The Northern English *Anonimalle* chronicler, one among several historical chroniclers who cited this pattern of mortality, refers to the epidemic as "*la mortalite des enfauntz*" [the mortality of children] and laments that in it a "*graunt noumbre des enfauntz furent devyes et a Deu comandes*" [a great number of children were killed as God ordained].[46] A third national epidemic followed, spreading through most of England in 1369; fourth and fifth epidemics unfolded in a series of sporadic bursts between 1374 and 1379 and again between 1390 and 1393.[47] These later epidemics, which, like the Gray Death, often disproportionately affected the young, were less global than the first two waves, but they were nonetheless fearsome. Moreover, the progression that they articulate—from the apocalyptic shape of the first outbreak, to the overwhelming Children's Plague, to the irregular but still powerful cycles of the 1370s, '80s, and '90s—would continue through the closing decades of the Middle Ages and beyond. The disease's terrifying cyclical persistence over many generations ensured that medically, physically, and psychologically, the plague was never only in the past in medieval England. It was always— and still remains today—a future, a bleak harbinger of mortality that existed simultaneously as traumatic memory and as terrible portent.

THE POEMS OF THE *PEARL* MANUSCRIPT: DATE, PROVENANCE, AND AUTHORSHIP

The four poems that form the nucleus of this study—*Pearl, Cleanness, Patience,* and *Sir Gawain and the Green Knight*—were written during this pestilential

---

may have been overstated and the role of other vectors understated. See especially Schmid et al., "Climate-Driven Introduction of the Black Death"; Green, "Editor's Introduction," *Pandemic Disease in the Medieval World,* 12; "Taking 'Pandemic' Seriously," 32–33.

45. Schmid et al., "Climate-Driven Introduction of the Black Death," 3022–23.

46. *The Anonimalle Chronicle,* 50. For the dates of the epidemic and further historical citations for its strong effect on children, see Rawcliffe, *Urban Bodies,* 362. Shrewsbury, *A History of the Bubonic Plague,* gives the slightly earlier date range of 1360–61 for the second epidemic but also remarks that it was particularly fatal to the young (127–30).

47. Rawcliffe, *Urban Bodies,* 362–63; Horrox, *The Black Death,* 88–92.

period, and while it remains impossible to fix the composition date of each work firmly, the preponderance of evidence points to the late fourteenth century, certainly after the pandemic's first wave and likely during the epidemics of the 1370s and 1390s. The manuscript suggests a rough *terminus ad quem* for all four poems. Based on paleography, illustrations, and border decorations, Cotton Nero A.x was most likely completed around or just after 1400, and since it is a copy of at least one earlier exemplar, the poems were probably composed a decade or two earlier, in the late fourteenth century.[48] Internal evidence from *Sir Gawain and the Green Knight* has also tended to confirm a late Ricardian date—based on language and poetics, Tolkien and Gordon argue that it was probably written near the end of the century[49]—though a few critics push the likely composition closer to midcentury, nearer the 1361 Children's Plague or even before.[50] Meanwhile, Susanna Greer Fein's analysis of the twelve-line stanza form reveals 1375–85 to be likely years for the composition of *Pearl*, a range that has been slightly extended by important historical analyses by John Bowers and H. L. Spencer.[51] Fewer analyses have been performed on *Cleanness* and *Patience*; however, those that have been have tended to confirm a mid- to late-fourteenth-century date.[52]

I want to note one recent effort to fix the date of *Pearl* in relation to the medieval plague pandemic. Basing his conclusions on an article by Jean-Paul Freidl and Ian Kirby, which posits that the historical original for the Pearl Maiden died in the pestilence, Andrew Breeze suggests that the poem was likely completed during or shortly after the fifth epidemic of 1390. He further speculates that such connections would be strengthened by attributing the poem's authorship to the Staffordshire aristocrat John Stanley, particularly if it could be determined "if Stanley had a daughter called Margaret, who died in infancy."[53] Such readings are exciting, and insofar as they insinuate the pres-

48. See Wright, *English Vernacular*, 15 [last quarter of the fourteenth century]; Doyle, "English Books in and out of Court," 166–67 [second half of the fourteenth century]; Fredell, "The *Pearl*-Poet Manuscript in York," 32 ["near or after 1400"].

49. Tolkien and Gordon, *Sir Gawain and the Green Knight*, xxv. See also Miller, "The Date and Occasion of *Sir Gawain and the Green Knight*." For a dissenting view and a Herician dating, see Stephens, "The 'Pentangle Hypothesis.'"

50. Cooke, "A Restored Dating," 44; Cooke and Boulton, "A Poem for Henry of Grosmont."

51. Fein, "Twelve-Line Stanza Forms," 395; Bowers, *The Politics of Pearl*, 23; Spencer, "*Pearl*: 'God's Law' and 'Man's Law,'" 319.

52. See, for instance, Anderson's standalone edition of *Patience*, 20–22.

53. Breeze, "*Pearl* and the Plague of 1390–1393," 340. Breeze's speculation that Staffordshire aristocrat Sir John Stanley is the author or patron of *Pearl* relates to two earlier studies: Breeze, "Sir John Stanley (c. 1350–1414) and the *Gawain*-Poet"; Mathew, *The Court of Richard II*, 166. See also Freidl and Kirby, "The Life, Death, and Life of the *Pearl*-Maiden." I will return to Freidl and Kirby's work in chapter 2 of this book.

ence of the plague within the Cotton Nero A.x manuscript, they are consonant with the aims of this study. Freidl and Kirby in particular note several of the linguistic markers in *Pearl* that I develop at length here, and their suggestion that a specific historical original of the Pearl Maiden was likely a victim of the disease, like Breeze's suggestion that the poem can be dated to within a three-year window based on the timing of outbreaks, is a compelling and seductive one.[54] Yet both of these conclusions rely on a more or less immediate and fully conscious response of a specific poem to a specific event, a relationship between literature and history that is, I suggest, less historical than it is topical.

Because they are predicated first on the recognition that traumatic history is *not* always immediately accessible for coherent witness—be it in the form of verisimilar narrative representation, overt memorialization, or conscious lament—the readings that I propose in *Death and the Pearl Maiden* neither depend upon nor presume the presence of point-to-point historical originals for the events and figures that they describe, nor do they assume that the poems themselves are grounded in the immediate and self-aware responses that many New Historicist studies assume as the de facto mode of historiographical response. Profound trauma, as Lauren Berlant reminds us, renders "a scene of impact beyond the eloquence of history," and thus responses to trauma can express in ways that are deferred, submerged, deflected, or unrecognized—in ways that are resistant to transparent narrative representation.[55] Silence and inarticulacy, as much as speech and narrative, emerge from trauma; in many respects, such inarticulacy finally speaks to the fractured past with a power that equals or even exceeds more overt poetic evocations of it. The response to the pestilence suggested in the Cotton Nero A.x poems—a response that ranges from the subtle to the allusive to the submerged to the unconscious—is never, or never *only,* as straightforward as such seemingly concrete relationships would imply.

If the date of the poems has proven a point of ongoing debate, the geographical provenance of the works has, until relatively recently, appeared settled. Details in landscape and geography, especially from *Sir Gawain and the Green Knight,* have long been used to assign the works to the Northwest Midlands, and dialectical markers have further encouraged critics to pinpoint the poems' language to "a very small area in either SE Cheshire or just over the border in NE Staffordshire."[56] The assignment of this precise location gained

---

54. Freidl and Kirby, "The Life, Death, and Life of the *Pearl*-Maiden," 395.

55. Berlant, "Trauma and Ineloquence," 43.

56. McIntosh, "A New Approach to Middle English Dialectology," 5. In his 1940 edition of *Sir Gawain and the Green Knight,* for instance, Israel Gollancz concludes that the poem's "geographical knowledge of the North-West Midlands and its realistic wintry landscape . . . is

traction with Michael Bennett's historical study of medieval Cheshire and Lancashire—"the little world . . . in which the author of *Sir Gawain and the Green Knight* and his patrons were rooted"[57]—and it has continued to inform studies linking the Cotton Nero A.x poems to "a Cheshire literary culture existing very solidly on the outskirts of the royal court."[58] New scholarship, however, has put pressure on the Northwest Midlands provenance of the Cotton Nero A.x poems, dislodging them from a cultural milieu that has, until recently, seemed certain.[59] While the global scale of the medieval plague pandemic in some ways overrides specific questions of geographic provenance in this study, we should nonetheless recognize that many of the assumptions arising from the poems' putative Cheshire origin, assumptions still often treated as fact, should be met with a renewed sense of caution.

Beyond date and provenance, the prize questions remaining for these poems have to do with authorship: do the four works share a common author, and, if so, who is it? Barring unexpected discoveries, we must be content with a high degree of uncertainty for both questions, particularly the latter. Most attempts to identify the author have focused on perceived acrostics and cryptograms, and they run to the tendentious;[60] determinations of authorship based on provenance, date, literary evidence, and even numerology have proven little more conclusive.[61] More fruitful than the question of authorial identity, at least to my mind, is the question of common authorship, and while certainty

---

obviously due to the West Midland poet himself," while Tolkien and Gordon follow Gollancz in citing the "local knowledge shown by the author" to determine a Northwest Midlands identity for the poem. See Gollancz, *Sir Gawain and the Green Knight*, xxxi; Tolkien and Gordon, *Sir Gawain and the Green Knight*, xxvi; Elliott, "Landscape and Geography."

    This geography is reconfirmed in the *Linguistic Atlas of Late Medieval English*, which again locates the poems in Cheshire based on their specific "linguistic profile." See McIntosh, Samuels, and Benskin, *A Linguistic Atlas of Late Middle English*. MS Cotton Nero A.x is discussed in linguistic profile 26.

    57. Bennett, *Community, Class and Careerism*, 7.

    58. Bowers, *The Politics of Pearl*, 15–16. See also Chism, *Alliterative Revivals*, 77–81; Schiff, *Revivalist Fantasy*, 79–83.

    59. Putter and Stokes, "The *Linguistic* Atlas and the Dialect of the *Gawain* Poems," 470; Fredell, "The *Pearl*-Poet Manuscript in York," 13–14.

    60. Some readers have found the name "Massey" embedded in these ways, and thus John Massey of Cotton, Cheshire; John Massey of Sale, Cheshire; and William Massey of Lancaster have been proposed as possible authors. Evidence for and against the Massey acrostic is compiled in Andrew, "Theories of Authorship," 29–31.

    61. See, for instance, Breeze, "Sir John Stanley," 15–30; Bennett, "*Sir Gawain and the Green Knight* and the Literary Achievement of the North-West Midlands," 63–89. Never one to mince words, Derek Pearsall writes, "These attributions are based on such naive and improbable assumptions concerning what constitutes evidence as to bring the study of attribution into disrepute." See Pearsall, "The Alliterative Revival: Origins and Social Backgrounds," 52.

still remains impossible, the four poems of Cotton Nero A.x express broadly similar concerns, bear remarkably close linguistic and structural affinities, and speak to one another in evocative and important ways.[62] Such an assessment smacks of subjectivity, but the fact remains that the four poems were compiled early into the single, carefully illustrated manuscript that now preserves them, a manuscript additionally unique for consisting solely of alliterative works.[63] Whether this compilation bespeaks a single authorial genius, a school of poets working together, or the efforts of an early compiler, the poems are richer for their intersectionality. I consider them in this study with the assumption that their mutual presence within the manuscript is intentional and important. In making this decision, I am bolstered by the "blatantly interpretive questions" that Christine Chism first posed regarding the works of the so-called Alliterative Revival: "Do these poems share common interests? Do the worlds they create resonate with each other? Can we balance fidelity to their 'features of extreme detail' with an observance of larger generic affiliations? What can these tell us about the interests of the writers and the cultural work of the writing?"[64] Whatever we can or cannot determine about the identity of the author, the poems remain bound together, both physically and culturally. By treating them as such, this study allows for synthetic interpretive connections to emerge among them.

The shimmering uncertainty that surrounds the poems—the essential unknowability of their authorial, temporal, and geographical origins—is important to their still-developing critical tradition, and it is similarly important to my own decision to turn to them in my consideration of the medieval plague pandemic. That is not to say that I've focused on these poems because arguments about them are "unprovable" in an empirical sense; rather, it is to acknowledge that these four works are informed not only by the many cultural and theoretical frames that have been brought to them but also by what Arthur Bahr might call their "manifold singularity, the way in which [their] unique physical survival (singularity) imbues the poem[s] with wide-ranging (manifold) forms of interpretive potential [they] would not otherwise have."[65] Bahr writes specifically about *Pearl* here, and I have taken liberties with his argument (and his prose) in applying it to the other poems of the manuscript; however, the textual and literary "uniqueness" that Bahr recognizes in *Pearl*, as well as the interpretive potential that such uniqueness promises, extends to all four of the poems equally. Despite the density of the critical tradition

---

62. See Borroff, "Narrative Artistry in *St. Erkenwald* and the *Gawain*-Group."
63. Edwards, "The Manuscript," 197.
64. Chism, *Alliterative Revivals*, 19–20.
65. Bahr, "The Manifold Singularity of *Pearl*," 729.

surrounding them, despite the convincing and occasionally moving readings that have emerged from them, the works continue to resist closure and hermeneutic sterility, and they stridently disallow "our interpretations to become calcified into conventional wisdom."[66] Equally important, the poems themselves emerge from their historical moment precisely as textual revenants, chance survivors of the cataclysms of the late Middle Ages and of the centuries that followed. Through the fourteenth-century pestilence itself, through the sporadic violence surrounding the Lancastrian ascension and the sustained destruction linked to the Dissolution of the Monasteries, through the Ashburnham House library fire of 1731 and the more common but no less destructive exigencies of time, age, and environment, the single manuscript that has carried *Pearl, Cleanness, Patience,* and *Sir Gawain and the Green Knight* into the modern age enacts as a textual artifact the stubborn, fragile witness that its poems alternately interrogate and provide in their own literary narratives.

THE BLACK DEATH IN MIDDLE ENGLISH LITERATURE: SURVEY AND PROPOSAL

René Girard writes, "The Plague is found everywhere in literature . . . from pure fantasy to the most positive and scientific accounts. It is older than literature—much older, really, since it is present in myth and ritual in the entire world."[67] This assertion stands in sharp contrast to Wenzel's more historically specific claim: "In England the medieval plague experience has left a relatively small impact on works of the imagination, if any at all."[68] Critical assessments of the plague in English literature have navigated close to either the Scylla of Girard's ubiquity (as in Ernest B. Gilman's decision, in a discussion of plague writing in seventeenth-century England, to regard "all literary texts written during plague times as plague texts"[69]) or the Charybdis of Wenzel's denial (as in Katherine Terrell's assertion that "there seems to be no particular reason to assume that the plague is the main source of either the [*Pearl*] poet's or the narrator's anxieties about death"[70]). If the relative paucity of scholarship on the subject can be taken as negative evidence, most readers who have

---

66. Bahr, 730.

67. Girard, "The Plague in Literature and Myth," 833.

68. Wenzel, "Pestilence and Middle English Literature," 149. Tellingly, Girard includes no medieval English writers in his survey, moving from the Italian Boccaccio to the English Defoe without mentioning Chaucer, Langland, or any other medieval English poets. For this absence, see Girard, "The Plague in Literature and Myth," 833–34.

69. Gilman, *Plague Writing in Early Modern England,* 48.

70. Terrell, "Rethinking the 'Corse in Clot,'" 433–34n9.

focused on medieval England tend toward the latter. To wit, within the diverse and increasingly rich body of criticism on the Cotton Nero A.x poems, only the two short articles I have already mentioned, by Freidl and Kirby and by Breeze, posit the presence of the plague within *Pearl*, a scholarly marginalization representative of criticism on fourteenth-century English literature as a whole.[71]

This assertion should not be taken to imply that there is *no* scholarship linking the plague to Middle English literature; such work does exist, and it is frequently illuminating. Within the body of literary criticism dealing with the English pandemic, the clear majority has focused on Chaucer. Peter Beidler's reading of "The Pardoner's Tale" in particular makes the claim that "we [cannot] understand the Pardoner or his *exemplum* if we overlook either the plague backdrop which Chaucer provided for the story or the evidence toward the plague," and Beidler urges us to think broadly about how the lived experience of the disease may have affected Chaucer's body of work.[72] Criticism following Beidler's work has affirmed the importance of the plague in "The Pardoner's Tale"; indeed, with its direct reference to the death itself—"he hath a thousand slayn this pestilence" [he has slain a thousand people, this pestilence] (*CT* 6.679)—the tale has become the most common English literary touchstone for tracing the impact of the Black Death.[73] More recent studies have also considered "The Knight's Tale" in pestilential terms, locating references to contagion in the work's visual discourses and recognizing spatial and mnemonic hallmarks of the disease within the tale.[74] Despite these provocative readings, however, few critics have moved from analyses of individual tales to a consideration of the *Canterbury Tales* as a whole. One notable exception is Celia Lewis, who argues that Chaucer's final unfinished work "reflects a widespread fourteenth- and fifteenth-century preoccupation with morality," which she sees as engendered by the plague.[75] Like Boccaccio's explicitly pestilential

---

71. This statement excludes my own two articles on the subject, both of which are revised and integrated into this monograph: Coley, "Remembering Lot's Wife / Lot's Wife Remembering" and "*Pearl* and the Narrative of Pestilence."

72. Beidler, "The Plague and Chaucer's Pardoner," 264–65.

73. Byron Grigsby, for instance, follows Beidler closely in linking the perceived moral causes of the Black Death to the Pardoner's "moral tale" (6.460). See Grigsby, *Pestilence in Medieval and Early Modern English Literature*, 117–22. See also Snell, "Chaucer's Pardoner's Tale and Pestilence in Late Medieval Literature," which asserts the relevance of the disease to the tale even as it remarks that "the general attitude toward the Black Death and later plagues in England seems to have been rather low keyed" (12).

74. See respectively Fumo, "The Pestilential Gaze"; Smith, "Plague, Panic Space, and the Tragic Medieval Household."

75. Lewis, "Framing Fiction with Death," 141. Lewis also responds specifically to Wenzel's denial of the impact of the Black Death in a way consonant with the aims of my own study:

Decameron, Lewis argues, *The Canterbury Tales* celebrates the potential of fiction to ward off death, even as it also recognizes the limitations of storytelling as prophylaxis and the concomitant need for spiritual comfort in the face of such vast mortality.[76]

Aside from *The Canterbury Tales, The Book of the Duchess* has also occasionally been read against the aftermath of the pandemic. Written as an elegy for John of Gaunt's wife Blanche, who died of the disease in 1368, the work renders a lament for the Duchess of Lancaster without ever naming the sickness that killed her, a paradigm that offers tantalizing parallels (which I will develop later in this study) to *Pearl.* Norman Hinton first identified the importance of the pandemic to the work in 1967, and his work has been powerfully developed by both Ardis Butterfield and D. Vance Smith, both of whom focus on crises of representation that evoke, as Smith puts it, "memory in a time of plague."[77] Similar arguments have been made by Sealy Gilles about *Troilus and Criseyde,* a poem that translates the lovesickness of Boccaccio's preplague *Il Filostrato* into "a world shaped by another, far more lethal disease."[78]

The already limited discussion of the plague in Middle English literature flags further when we move away from Chaucer, even in critical responses to William Langland, who overtly mentions the pestilence at several key points in *Piers Plowman.* In the prologue to his thrice-written poem, Langland alludes in broad terms to the economic consequences of the Black Death, particularly excoriating priests for abandoning parishes that "weren pouere siþ þe pestilence tyme" [were poor since the plague time] (B.Pro.84) to take up lucrative positions in London. His jeremiad is ventriloquized by Dame Study, who complains that "freres and faitours han founde [vp] swiche questions / To plese wiþ proude men syn þe pestilence tyme" [friars and deceivers have invented such theological problems to please proud men since the time of the pestilence] (B. 10.71–72), and by Reason, who tells Will that "pestilences were for pure synne" [pestilences were purely for sin] (B.5.13), drawing a link between disease and morality consonant with contemporary understandings of the plague's root and dispersion. The Black Death is most powerfully evoked in the poem's apocalyptic final passus, where Kynde, working on behalf of Conscience, assails the denizens of Unity with "kene soores / As pokkes and pestilences" [sharp sores, such as poxes and plagues] (B.20.98) to

---

"If the impact of sequential plagues on imaginative literature seems to us, as Siegfried Wenzel suggests, 'sparse,' perhaps we should reassess our evaluative terms" (148).

76. See also Sandidge, "Attitudes toward Old Age."

77. Smith, "Plague, Panic Space, and the Tragic Medieval Household," 389. Hinton, "The Black Death and the Book of the Duchess"; Butterfield, "Pastoral and the Politics of Plague," 27.

78. Gilles, "Love and Disease in Chaucer's *Troilus and Criseyde,* 184, 158.

spur them to repentance. Many, Langland writes, "swowned and swelted for sorwe of [deþes] dyntes" [swooned and expired for sorrow of death's blows] (B.20.105).

As Wenzel notes, these few lines near the conclusion of the poem stand as "the most brilliant poetic expression of the plague experience that remains from medieval England," the only one to approach the descriptions emerging from Mainland Europe.[79] Nonetheless, most critics considering the Black Death in *Piers Plowman* have done so in terms of historical context rather than poetic content. David Aers, for instance, reads the social and religious crises staged in Langland's work against the economic changes catalyzed by the plague,[80] while Wendy Scase and Justine Rydzeski both detail how Langland's social outlook was largely shaped by the cultural and demographic shifts occasioned by the disease.[81] *Piers Plowman*, then, is most commonly apprehended as a work steeped less in the pestilence itself than in the "essentially traditional and moralistic character which distinguishes late medieval English literature from its Continental counterparts," a poem that ultimately responds not to the disease but to the social ills and dubious opportunities that emerged in its wake.[82]

Finally, sustained considerations of the pestilence in medieval drama are, as in Middle English poetry, thin on the ground. In the York play of Pharaoh and Moses, the biblical plague of the firstborn is reinterpreted as a "grete pestelence / [that] is like ful lange to last" [great plague that is likely to last a long time], a change that Richard Beadle calls "a striking alteration to the canonical source" and one that offered the play's late medieval audience "a moment of remembrance for survivors of the Black Death and those born in the succeeding generation."[83] Again though, this exception ultimately proves the rule: the pestilence is mainly regarded, even in the civically and socially engaged genre

---

79. Wenzel, "Pestilence and Middle English Literature," 133.

80. Aers, *Faith, Ethics, and Church*, especially chapter 3, "Justice and Wage-Labor after the Black Death," 59. See also Simpson, Piers Plowman: *An Introduction*, 31–32, 74.

81. Scase, *Piers Plowman and the New Anti-Clericalism*, 144; Rydzeski, *Radical Nostalgia in the Age of* Piers Plowman, 56.

82. Wenzel, "Pestilence and Middle English Literature," 150–51. One notable exception to this rule is Byron Grigsby, who draws from several plague tracts and sermons to suggest how Langland "operates within a plague discourse informed by both medicine and theology . . . and blames the medical and ecclesiastical communities for failing to protect the physical and moral health of society." See Grigsby, "Plague Medicine in Langland's *Piers Plowman*," 200. Grigsby expands his argument in *Pestilence in Medieval and Early Modern Literature*, 102–17.

83. "Pharoah and Moses," in *The York Corpus Christi Plays*, 69–80 (ll. 345–46); Beadle, "The York Corpus Christi Play," 99. See also Grigsby, *Pestilence in Medieval and Early Modern Literature*, 122–24.

of cycle drama, as existing at the margins of the text. And while some critics have registered the theatrical possibilities of the pestilence in the early modern period, studies of English drama in the Middle Ages have not considered how the medieval stage might have offered a space for evoking, interrogating, exploiting, or even repelling the plague epidemics of the fourteenth century.[84]

Using Cotton Nero A.x as a test case, *Death and the Pearl Maiden* ultimately seeks both a corrective to the critical marginalization of the plague in studies of Middle English literature and, perhaps paradoxically, a rationale for that marginalization. More immediately, it proposes that the works of the *Pearl*-Poet can be recognized as witnesses to the trauma of the Black Death and its recurrences, that these works—like Boccaccio's *Decameron*, Machaut's *Jugement*, Petrarch's *Epistolæ*, Gabriele de' Mussis's *Historia de Morbo*, and Michele da Piazza's *Cronaca*—are both suffused with the plague and offer a distinguishable literary response to it. Chapter 1, "Trauma, Witness, and Representation in *Cleanness*," begins this project by considering the possibility of an unwitting mediation of the disease, one that exists beyond what Smith might call the "practices of deliberate memory."[85] Focusing on the second poem of the *Pearl* manuscript, the chapter considers *Cleanness*'s string of biblical calamities in the terms proposed by modern studies of trauma, reading them not only in the robustly didactic terms of the poem itself but also as symptomatic of posttraumatic repetition. Considered in this context, the poem, most often noted for its abject violence and disturbing homophobia, emerges as a surprisingly delicate meditation on loss and survival, a work that divides its focus between the wrenching dramas of divine retribution that structure its narrative and the no less crucial episodes of human persistence that inform a quiet counternarrative to it. *Cleanness* thus evokes an unspoken lament that implicitly resists its otherwise inflexible Christological telos. Fragmented and structurally riven, the poem further testifies to the importance and the danger of witnessing, even—and perhaps especially—within the moralizing schema implied by its own aggressive didacticism. Equally significant, it implicates its readers in the same struggles of representation that it limns in its compulsively repetitive exempla, a compulsion that scans as a symptom of posttraumatic ineloquence. *Cleanness* thus becomes the very figure it repeatedly describes within its linked narratives: a mute but legible witness to a profound cultural trauma, a reminder of the inscrutability of history itself.

The second chapter, "*Pearl* and the Language of Plague," further explores the presence of a pestilential discourse in the four poems; however, it raises

---

84. See MacKay, *Persecution, Plague, and Fire*, especially 94–102.
85. Smith, "Irregular Histories," 171.

the possibility of a more intentional response than the symptomatic evocations predominating in *Cleanness*. Beginning with *Pearl*'s signature punning
and semantic play, the chapter suggests that the poem develops and incul-
cates a pestilential lexicon through its concatenating terms, polyvalent images,
and ever-shifting metaphors, one that aligns with a broader English lexicon
of disease. It then moves beyond this narrowly topical approach to consider
Pearl as not only evoking the plague but also becoming a pestilential object
itself, embodying the physical marks of the disease even as it inscribes the
flawless transcendence of its Christian soteriology. The stark oppositions that
Pearl initially implies between perfection and flaw, child and parent, quick
and dead, and (as evidenced by so many critical responses) elegy and allegory become the grounds for the poem's somewhat austere consolation; taken
together, they articulate a response to a deeply felt individual loss, but they
also, more covertly, gesture toward a larger cultural collapse, toward an England that perceived itself veering dangerously close to the "meruelous merez"
[marvelous seas] (*Pe.* 1166) separating this world from the next. A formally
brilliant work written for a courtly audience, the *Pearl* described in this chapter emerges as a private poem with a surprisingly public voice. Its understated
and hesitant evocation of the plague experience, moreover, further suggests
the complex response of the Cotton Nero A.x poems to the pandemic: hybrid
and paradoxical, oscillating between unconscious embodiment and unassum-
ing reply.

Taken together, these analyses of *Cleanness* and *Pearl*, which constitute
part 1 of this study, articulate two somewhat contradictory models of reading: the first recognizes the presence of the Black Death as an unconscious
and even unintended symptom of the poems' cultural environment; the second locates a conscious if ciphered response to the pandemic in the works.
The chapters that comprise part 2 develop these models to investigate specific
cultural and social contexts associated with plague in medieval England. The
third chapter, "Flight and Enclosure in *Patience*," considers two customary
reactions to the disease and entertains the idea that *Patience* develops its core
exemplum—the story of the reluctant prophet Jonah—within the context of
individual and communal responses to encroaching epidemics. Drawing from
modern developments in social psychology as well as medieval documentary
sources, chapter 3 shows *Patience* moving away from the eschatological absolutes of *Pearl* and the apocalyptic repetitions of *Cleanness*, and it suggests how
the poem's psychologically resonant depiction of Jonah may draw from contingent behaviors arising from situations of profound threat. In this respect,
Patience is, as one critic has noted, directed toward "those who must work
within history," a poetic and discursive distinction with important ramifica-

tions for both poet and audience.[86] And while *Patience* still bears the same courtly hallmarks as *Pearl* and *Cleanness*, it evinces in the pestilential contexts of flight and enclosure in both a recognition of the struggles of the clerical class during times of plague and, more radically, an embrace of England's poor, who suffered disproportionately the effects of the disease.

Patience's late swerve toward the intersection of disease and poverty reveals an unexpected engagement with broad social and economic concerns, an impulse that we might even term "Langlandian." That impulse carries into the final poem of the manuscript, a bewildering Arthurian romance that stages, through the troubled progress of its errant knight protagonist, several key cultural and economic fractures within fourteenth-century England. Informed by recent historical studies on economic and social opportunities that emerged in the wake of the plague, particularly for women of the artisan and aristocratic classes, chapter 4, "Sex, Death, and Social Change in *Sir Gawain and the Green Knight*," regards the distinct gender dynamics of Hautdesert and Camelot as separated not only by distance but also by time. Indeed, *Sir Gawain and the Green Knight* defines Bertilak's court most powerfully through the very social and economic shifts catalyzed by the postplague demographic collapse. Not simply a margin to Camelot's center or a province to Camelot's capital, Hautdesert also exists as the tomorrow to Camelot's today or, more speculatively, the postplague "fynisment" [end] of a doomed preplague "forme" [beginning] (*Gaw.* 499). By focusing on this de facto temporal disjunction, chapter 4 considers how *Sir Gawain and the Green Knight* might speak to cultural efforts at recovery, as well as to the novel but fragile opportunities that emerged in the wake of the Black Death. More darkly, it also suggests the virulently misogynistic backlash against those opportunities, a reactionary impulse embodied by Arthur's stratified patriarchal court and Gawain's infamous outburst against the "wyles of wymmen" [wiles of women] (*Gaw.* 2415). Chapter 4 will thus argue that *Sir Gawain and the Green Knight* pushes even more firmly than *Patience* into the specific cultural milieu of postplague England, and it will further suggest how the poem might be seen to bring the crisis of the Black Death into conversation with a mythical British past, subtly mapping it onto the *translatio imperii* and giving (admittedly ambivalent) voice to processes of cultural change and conservative resistance catalyzed by the disease.

The final chapter of this study circles back to the question addressed at its beginning: why does the English literary response to the pestilence appear so subdued in comparison to plague writing from the European continent? The conclusion does not articulate an overarching "silver bullet" answer to

---

86. Prior, *The Fayre Formez of the Pearl Poet*, 146.

that question. No such single answer exists. Rather, it suggests a constellation of loosely affiliated causes that inhere to medieval English texts themselves, as well as to our critical apprehension of them. These linguistic, historical, economic, religious, and psychological factors contribute to the outline of English literary engagement with the plague, shaping an idiosyncratic English response to the pandemic and, moreover, hampering our ability as contemporary readers to recognize that response for what it is. Acknowledging and understanding how such factors were coterminous with the explosion of vernacular English writing in the late fourteenth century, as well as confronting our own critical reception of the pestilence in Middle English poetry, allows for an important reconsideration of the impact of the Black Death on medieval English literature, and it further suggests the need to rewrite our prevailing narratives of England's literary response to a transformative cultural trauma.

PART 1

Plague in the *Pearl* Manuscript

Symptom and Response

CHAPTER 1

Trauma, Witness, and Representation in *Cleanness*

It is thus known to all Christians that because of sin the pestilence
and all other vengeances of God arise: first in heaven God wrought
vengeance when the angel Lucifer fell; second in paradise when Adam
was expelled; third in the whole world when all His various works
were drowned in a cataclysm, except for those that were saved in
Noah's Ark; fourth when Sodom and Gomorrah were engulfed in an
infernal river; fifth when Lot's wife was turned into a statue of salt.

—"A NOTABILITE OF THE SCRIPTURE WHAT
CAUSITH THE PESTILENCE"[1]

"LOSS," DAVID ENG and David Kazanjian write, "is inseparable from what
remains, for what is lost is known only by what remains of it, by how these
remains are produced, read, and sustained."[2] Proposed as a response to the terrible losses of the twentieth century, Eng and Kazanjian's assertion also resonates powerfully with the second poem of the Cotton Nero A.x manuscript,
a work that articulates the losses of its Old Testament episodes through the
grisliest of remains: the bodies of doomed antediluvians who "fellen in fere
and faþmed togeder" [came together and embraced one another] (*Cl.* 399) in
the rising waters; the smoldering landscape left behind after the obliteration
of Sodom and Gomorrah; dismembered "wombes" [wombs] (1250) and "boweles" [bowels] (1251) scattered about the fallen Jerusalem; the battered corpse

---

1. "*Notum sic omnibus Cristianis quod propter peccata orituo pestilencia et omnis alia vindicta dei unde: in celo fecit deus primam vindictam quando decidit angelus Lucifer; secundo in
Paradiso quando expulsus fuit Adam; tercio in universa terra quando omnia opera umencia
diversa fuerunt in cathaclismo, preterito illo quibus salvata fuerunt in Archa Noye; quarto quando
Sodoma et Gomorra demersa fuerunt flumino infernali; quinto quando uxor Loth versa sunt in
statuam salis.*" "A Notabilite of the Scripture What Causith the Pestilence," in BL Sloane MS
965, folio 143r., punctuated for sense.

2. Eng and Kazanjian, "Mourning Remains," 2.

of the Babylonian king, "feryed out bi þe fete and fowle dispysed" [dragged out by the feet and foully abused] (1790). These bodily remains have led one prominent critic to call *Cleanness* "the most frightening poem in Middle English in its invocation of God's anger" and another to regard it as "a terrifying panorama of mass destruction."[3] In their brutality, however, these same remains also obscure a surprisingly subtle and nuanced engagement with loss. Indeed, even as *Cleanness* answers the question "What remains?" by revealing a tangle of broken bodies and bricks, it also focuses upon the few who emerge from their biblical calamities to negotiate such losses: Noah and his family, who step from the Ark onto uncertain new ground; Abraham, who surveys the devastated Jordan Plain and the pit of the Dead Sea; Daniel, who survives the destruction of Jerusalem only to prophesy the sack of Babylon. Such figures suggest that *Cleanness* is concerned not only with the violent ruptures that traumatize its narrative but also with the linked teloi that give its narrative an anxious continuity, the Christological arc that culminates in the Incarnation and the arc of human community itself, in which generation begets generation and biblical history blends into human history. *Cleanness* turns its gaze upon the survivors of trauma as well as upon the dead, pointing not only toward the fractured bodies of those killed but also toward the fractured psyches of those left to bury and remember them.

Most studies of *Cleanness* reinforce a reading grounded in the poem's own didactic and moralistic terms, one in which the three core episodes— the Flood, the Destruction of Sodom and Gomorrah, and the linked events that culminate in Belshazzar's feast—serve as negative exempla for the virtue extolled in the opening line, *clannesse*.[4] Without denying *Cleanness*'s investment in moral and religious instruction, this chapter strives to complicate that default critical position by reading the poem as a work informed by and fundamentally engaged with the issue of human trauma, a work that tempers its

---

3. Respectively, Watson, "The *Gawain*-Poet as a Vernacular Theologian," 306; Wallace, "*Cleanness* and the Terms of Terror," 93.

4. Among these studies, see Kittendorf, "Cleanness and the Fourteenth Century *Artes Praedicandi*"; Glenn, "Dislocation of *Kynde* in the Middle English *Cleanness*"; Brzezinski, "Conscience and Covenant: The Sermon Structure of *Cleanness*"; Twomey, "The Sin of Untrawþe in *Cleanness*; Calabrese and Eliason, "The Rhetorics of Sexual Pleasure and Intolerance"; Frantzen, "The Disclosure of Sodomy in *Cleanness*"; Keiser, *Courtly Desire and Medieval Homophobia*. Two notable exceptions to this rule are Citrome, "Medicine as Metaphor in the Middle English *Cleanness*," and Reading, "'Ritual Sacrifice and Feasting.'" Citrome discerns the interpenetrating discourses of surgery and medicine as providing a metaphorical vocabulary for the poem, while Reading understands *Cleanness*'s exempla as connected by a common concern with "the hierarchical relationship between man and God" (275), a relationship that the poem repeatedly reinscribes through images of ritual sacrifice and feasting.

intense concern over physical and spiritual sin with a sustained meditation on loss and the related issues of traumatic witness and representation. Stridently moralistic in tone, *Cleanness* couples its descriptions of divine vengeance with the dramas of survival that follow. It dwells mournfully on the losses of the past even as it looks toward the salvation implicit in Christ's Incarnation, exploring in its central exempla the stubborn fact of human recovery in the face of great loss, as well as the concomitant vestiges of loss that punctuate human recovery. As it focuses at once on the bodies of the dead, the terror of the doomed, and the suffering of the living, *Cleanness* emerges as a poem that speaks to both the necessity and the danger of standing witness, a poem that negotiates the problem of traumatic representation at a site still contested by contemporary trauma theorists. It becomes, moreover, a poem that insistently subverts its own didactic narrative in order to implicate readers in the same fraught paradigms of representation that it stages in its exempla.

Having established the terms of *Cleanness*'s engagement with traumatic response, this chapter then considers how the poem might enact the strategies of witness it develops in its exempla to stand as literary witness to the Black Death, an ongoing traumatic event that, as D. Vance Smith writes, "exceeds the resources of representational practice—and the ability of the memory to make sense of it."[5] On the one hand, such a proposition may seem axiomatic: the recurring waves of pestilence that harrowed England in the second half of the fourteenth century necessarily constitute an aspect of the poem's textual and cultural environment. On the other hand, *Cleanness*, like so many other late fourteenth-century Middle English works, never directly addresses the trauma of the Black Death, nor does it provide the powerful descriptions of the disease prominent in some Continental works. Instead, like Chaucer's *Book of the Duchess*, *Cleanness* shudders "with a sense of unnamed and unnamable fears," invoking the trauma of the plague indirectly through a semantically dense and richly allusive biblical matrix.[6] The textual and historical evidence that I present to suggest *Cleanness*'s engagement with the plague thus occupies the forbidding space between the self-evident and the speculative. Nonetheless, I posit that the particular mode in which *Cleanness* articulates *what remains*— the way that it reads, sustains, and reinscribes the traumas of the past—subtly mediates the interactions among traumatic event, human witness, and textual representation; among plague, survivor, and poem.

---

5. Smith, "Plague, Panic Space, and the Tragic Medieval Household," 383–84.
6. Butterfield, "Pastoral and the Politics of Plague," 22.

LOT'S WIFE REMEMBERING:
THE WITNESS IN THE TEXT

Trauma, in the words of Lauren Berlant, is "an overwhelming event, a scene
of impact beyond the eloquence of history, the literal, unsymbolizable
mark of pure violence, or its opposite, violence congealed in an intensified
representation."[7] For survivors, traumatic events frequently remain unavailable to consciousness, revealing their impact belatedly, sometimes in fragments, often through compulsive behaviors that unwittingly (if recognizably)
reenact the events themselves. As Judith Herman asserts, "The ordinary
response to atrocities is to banish them from consciousness. Certain viola-
tions of the social compact are too terrible to utter aloud: this is the meaning of the word *unspeakable*." With equal conviction, however, Herman states
that "atrocities . . . refuse to be buried," and she notes how victims of trauma
frequently engage in behaviors that unconsciously and repeatedly allow them
to relive the suppressed traumatic event.[8] Considered in these terms, the traumatic response exists as a negotiation between the need to deny events too
terrible to acknowledge and the need to acknowledge events too terrible to
deny. Unknowable and unspeakable, even (or especially) to those who have
lived through it, trauma conceals its own history and, thus, resists memorialization through linguistic or literary means.

The unspeakable nature of trauma complicates the question of what
remains. The physical, psychic, and textual vestiges of traumatic events are
often scattered and fragmented, suppressed by survivors, misapprehended,
forgotten. How can the impact of an event be articulated if that event is
unspeakable? How can the remains and losses of an unknown and unknowable trauma be witnessed or expressed? Shoshana Felman and Dori Laub suggest that in such cases literature is uniquely positioned to offer testimony,
becoming "a witness, and perhaps the only witness, to the crisis within history
which precisely cannot be articulated, witnessed in the given categories of
history itself."[9] And yet, precisely how that witness emerges within literature
remains an open question.[10]

By its very magnitude, trauma can exceed or even precede consciousness,
revealing itself through the chronic nightmares and compulsive behaviors of
those who lived through it.[11] Nonetheless, as Cathy Caruth argues, though

---

7. Berlant, "Trauma and Ineloquence," 43.
8. Herman, *Trauma and Recovery*, 1.
9. Felman and Laub, *Testimony*, xviii.
10. A similar question is raised in McHugh, "The Aesthetics of Wounding," 118.
11. Caruth, *Unclaimed Experience*, 4.

often fragmented and submerged, the response to trauma is one of voice, of speech, "not just the unconscious act of the infliction of the injury and its inadvertent and unwished-for repetition, but the moving and sorrowful *voice* that cries out, a voice that is paradoxically released *through the wound*." The reflexivity of Caruth's paradigm—both voice from wound and voice as wound—suggests that trauma is represented in the same complex ways it is so often experienced, "in a language that is always somehow literary: a language that defies, even as it claims, our understanding."[12] But as Patricia Clare Ingham has shown, paradigms of traumatic representation remain unsettled. In particular, Ingham points to an ongoing debate between Caruth and Ruth Leys over "where we might locate the compensatory 'truth' of trauma: in the unambiguous, accurate, expressive witness to a historical event . . . or in the mimetic repetitions that express the pain of the suffering subject."[13] Unlike Caruth, Leys neatly (if somewhat artificially) distinguishes the traumatic experience from its representation, and she attacks the idea of a "literary" traumatic voice as "[collapsing] distinctions between victims and perpetrators, or simply between victims and others."[14] Instead of understanding trauma as engendering a mimetic identification with the event that "[makes] the traumatic scene unavailable for a certain kind of recollection,"[15] Leys privileges an antimimetic paradigm, in which trauma is experienced "in a mode that allows [victims] to remain spectators, who can see and represent to themselves what is happening."[16] Such a model offers a heuristic solution to the problems of lost memory, fragmented representation, and compulsive repetition raised by mimetic identification with the traumatic event, a means of circumventing or even undoing the psychological and representational issues caused by trauma.

---

12. Caruth, 2, 5.

13. Ingham, "Chaucer's Haunted Aesthetics," 230.

14. Leys, *Trauma: A Genealogy*, 8.

15. Leys, 8–9.

16. Leys and Goldman, "Navigating the Genealogies of Trauma," 658. Leys uses the term "mimesis" and "antimimesis" in a manner contrary to the expectations of most literary scholars, who tend to think of mimesis in the Platonic/Aristotelian terms theorized by Erich Auerbach. In Leys's usage, mimesis does not refer to the representation of reality through literature; rather it refers to an emotional, psychic, and even bodily reenactment of the traumatic event on the part of the victim, a consuming identification with the trauma that works to frustrate coherent narrative representation. Conversely, the antimimetic model that Leys favors sees trauma as a distinct and external event, one which engenders suffering and emotional responses from its victims but that does not induce a physical or psychic identification. Historically straightforward narrative is thus (somewhat counterintuitively) aligned with the antimimetic model of traumatic response. See Leys, *Trauma: A Genealogy*, 10; Ingham, "Chaucer's Haunted Aesthetics," 229.

Following Ingham's pathbreaking work on Chaucer's *Troilus and Criseyde*, I engage the debate between Caruth and Leys to consider *Cleanness* as a work that explores traumatic witness, as well as the issue of traumatic representation, a work that reveals the exigencies of the human response to trauma and that ultimately becomes symptomatic of such a response itself. While *Cleanness*'s clear, scripturally based narrative of past traumas hints at an antimimetic paradigm, the compulsive imagistic and semantic repetitions that both characterize the poem and define key figures of witness within it point toward a fraught mimetic identification with trauma, as do the relationships that the poem articulates between victims of biblical traumas and those individuals authorized to represent and interpret them. Cleanness operates at the intersection of the mimetic and the antimimetic, anticipating (and revealing the limitations of) both models as it explores the human response to a series of apocalyptic cataclysms.

Paramount among *Cleanness*'s figures of witness is the complicated (and not entirely sympathetic) figure of Lot's wife. Introduced as a foil to her properly hospitable husband, Lot's wife is vilified for her disobedience and lack of social decorum, condemned for turning toward the destruction of Sodom in defiance of God's command, and excoriated for salting the food of the angels in defiance of Lot. Her fate, putatively the result of those "two fautes . . . founde in mistrauþe" [two faults . . . found in unfaithfulness] (996), follows as poetic justice for her sins, and her posthumous humiliation is assured when, following her transformation into a pillar of salt, "alle lyst on hir lik þat arn on launde bestes" [all of the beasts of the land are like to lick her] (1000). Nonetheless, the poet softens his scorn for Lot's wife at the instant of her punishment, juxtaposing her decision to look at the destruction of Sodom with the willful blindness of Lot and his daughters:

> Bot þe balleful burde, þat neuer bode keped,
> Blusched byhynden her bak þat bale for to herkken.
> Hit watz lusty Lothes wyf þat ouer her lyfte schulder
> Ones ho bluschet to þe burȝe, bot bod ho no lenger
> Þat ho nas stadde a stiffe ston, a stalworth image,
> Al so salt as ani se—and so ho ȝet standez.
> Þay slypped bi and syȝe hir not þat wern hir samen-feres,
> Tyl þay in Segor wern sette, and sayned our Lorde.
> (979–86)

[But the baleful woman, who never heeded God's command, glanced behind her back to attend to the sorrow. It was Lot's lusty wife who glanced once toward the city over her left shoulder; but not a moment later, she stood there a stiff stone, a stalwart statue, as salty as any sea—and so she still stands. Those who were her companions slipped by and did not see her until they were in Segor and blessed by our Lord.]

Crucial here is the use of the word "herkken" to describe the impetus for Lot's wife's fateful backward glance, a term that means to listen attentively, take heed, or harken.[17] Though she looks back over her left shoulder—a sinister gesture to be certain—Lot's wife does not turn just to gawk at the destruction of Sodom but to attend to it, to "herkken" the event just as Noah "herken[s] typyngez" [heeds the tidings] (458) of his dove after the Flood. Lot's wife is not, in other words, the biblical equivalent of a freeway rubbernecker. Though guilty of contravening God's command, she nonetheless emerges as both witness to and victim of a traumatic event, a woman who sees firsthand the destruction of the Cities of the Plain, who grieves their losses, and who is made to share in their ruin.

In their respective reactions to the destruction of Sodom, Lot and his wife anticipate Judith Herman's précis of the traumatic condition: the "conflict between the will to deny horrible events and the will to proclaim them aloud."[18] Unfailingly obedient to God—obedient, that is, to the very figure who precipitates Sodom's annihilation—Lot forces himself to turn away from the "grete rowtes of renkkes withinne" [great crowds of people within] (969) and the "ʒomerly ʒarm of ʒellyng þer rysed" [miserable cries and yelling that rose from there] (971). He flees from the site of the traumatic event at "ay a hyʒe trot" [always a quick run] (976), refusing even to look at his own wife as she is transformed into a salt statue. In Lot, then, the poet registers the urge to avoid the discomfort and psychological danger of facing the traumatic event, a powerful human will to ignorance that, in this case, is also mandated by God.[19] Lot's wife, by contrast, resists God's edict to avert her eyes, turning toward Sodom in an effort to witness the same human suffering that Lot refuses to see. In her punishment, Lot's wife registers the mutual annihilation and preservation to which the historical witness is subject, as well as the paradoxical conflation of knowledge and silence recognized as a symptom of the trau-

---

17. *MED*, s.v. "herken" v.

18. Herman, *Trauma and Recovery*, 1.

19. Studies of political and cultural traumas, as well as studies of such traumas as domestic abuse, rape, and childhood abuse, reveal a persistent pattern in which the agents and structures responsible for the trauma work tirelessly to encourage, even to mandate, the amnesia that follows the traumatic event. (See Herman, *Trauma and Recovery*, 8.) We might imagine God, whose vengeance is made manifest in the destruction of Sodom, as filling such a role here.

matic experience. Indeed, the contradictory properties of the Dead Sea itself—
a body of water whose salinity both prevents the growth of "gresse [and] wod"
[grass and tree] (1028) and preserves those bodies "schowued þerinne . . .
to dayes of ende" [shoved into it . . . until the end of days] (1029–32)—are
repeated in Lot's wife, a figure simultaneously stripped of life and created as a
permanent reminder of the traumatic event she turned to see.[20] Mineral and
mnemonic, her eyes fixed always on the absent Sodom, Lot's wife becomes the
central figure of witness in *Cleanness*: a physical reminder of the Cities of the
Plain and a powerful example of the dangers of attending to traumatic events.

As a figure of witness, Lot's wife also anticipates a key issue on which
contemporary debates over traumatic representation and expression hinge. A
close physical analogue for the otherworldly mineral landscape of the Dead
Sea, she literally becomes the traumatic event that she witnesses, reiterat-
ing the destruction of Sodom and Gomorrah in her body's transformation
from flesh into salt. Lot's wife thus embodies the mimetic response to trauma
described by Caruth, revealing how "the experience of a trauma repeats itself,
exactly and unremittingly, through the unknowing acts of the survivor and
against [her] very will."[21] Moreover, as she is made physically to incarnate
the Dead Sea, Lot's wife implicitly repudiates the idea that "the subject [of
trauma] remains aloof from the traumatic experience, in the sense that [she]
remains a spectator of the scene, which [she] can therefore see and represent to [herself]."[22] On the contrary, her active investment in the destruction
of Sodom—her transgressive act of looking back and her bodily sympathy
with the destruction—binds Lot's wife to the trauma and determines how
she represents it. Because of her mimetic identification with the destruction
of Sodom, Lot's wife is unable to provide the clear narrative representation
promised by the antimimetic paradigm. Instead, she channels the traumatic
event as a silent, non-narrative memento whose significance can only be constructed from without. Lot's wife's voice is neither unambiguous nor verisimilar; it is the product of a consuming alignment with the traumatic wound,

---

20. The relationship between God's punishment and Lot's wife's decision to dwell on the
past is further suggested in St. Augustine's *Writings against the Manicheans* as well as in *The
City of God*. In the former, Augustine argues that "Lot's wife was the type of a different class of
men—of those namely who, when called by the grace of God, look back, instead of, like Paul,
forgetting the things that are behind and looking forward to the things that are before" (*Manicheans*, 288). In the latter work, Augustine posits that Lot's wife "became a sign warning us that
no one who has set foot on the path of redemption should yearn for what he has left behind"
(*City of God*, 402).

21. Caruth, *Unclaimed Experience*, 2.

22. Leys, *From Guilt to Shame*, 9.

a voice that emerges out of stasis, inarticulateness, silence—out of the self-abnegation of the trauma itself.

But is such a voice even a voice? The experience of mimetic identification provides a frame through which to understand Lot's wife's reaction to the destruction of Sodom, but Caruth's suggestion that trauma is the "*voice . . . paradoxically released *through the wound*" begs the question of what constitutes a voice in the first place, what constitutes a linguistic or literary witness.[23] Perhaps by physically and silently embodying the trauma, Lot's wife more accurately offers a text than produces a voice, a representation that demands to be read and glossed but that cannot speak for itself. Within *Cleanness*, the silenced figure of Lot's wife "speaks" only insofar as she is accorded a significance from without, only insofar as her remains are read by those able and privileged to speak for her. To employ terms articulated by Gayatri Spivak and usefully deployed by Ingham, Lot's wife offers a representation of her trauma in the sense of *Darstellung* rather than in the sense of *Vertretung*—a "representation as 're-presentation,' as in art or philosophy" rather than "representation as 'speaking for,' as in politics."[24] She represents the destruction of Sodom as a portrait of the event and of its victims; she is not empowered to speak on their behalf.[25]

The separation of *Darstellung* (representation-as-portrait) and *Vertretung* (representation-as-proxy) is important to *Cleanness*, not least because it provides a structural means for the poem to isolate the mute figures of witness that punctuate its core exempla and to circumscribe them in ways that advance its central didactic agenda. A poem that presents "a history lesson about how God has evolved a covenant with humankind through a process . . . of trial and error," *Cleanness* necessarily insists upon the Christological force of its collective Old Testament narratives.[26] Noah and his family repeople the Earth after the Flood; Abraham and Sara are promised a son; Lot and his daughters beget the Moabites and the Ammonites; Daniel receives a vision of

---

23. Caruth, *Unclaimed Experience,* 2.

24. Spivak, "Can the Subaltern Speak?" 275. See also Ingham, "Chaucer's Haunted Aesthetics," 227.

25. In this respect, Dori Laub's understanding of the figure of the witness is particularly evocative. A psychotherapist and Holocaust survivor, Laub recognizes three distinct levels of witnessing in his own experience: "The level of being a witness to oneself; the level of being a witness to the testimonies of others; and the level of being a witness to the process of witnessing itself" (75). The witness, then, may function doubly as text and reader—both as one who has experienced the traumatic event and as one who reads and testifies to the truth witnessed by another, a truth written upon memory and body and text. See Felman and Laub, *Testimony,* 75.

26. Watson, "The *Gawain*-Poet as a Vernacular Theologian," 308.

Christ's Incarnation and ministry after the fall of Babylon.[27] These prophetic figures remain, wax, and multiply after their respective biblical catastrophes, pointing always toward the moment "when [Christ] borne watz in Beþlehem þe ryche" [When Christ was born in rich Bethlehem] (1073). They frame the remains of their associated traumas to comport with the didactic impulse that informs *Cleanness*'s central narrative line. Thus, even as Lot's wife recasts the salty remains of Sodom and Gomorrah in her body, she is never empowered to read those remains or to articulate the metonymic significance of her own mineral form.

Those tasks fall instead to Abraham, who surveys the aftermath of God's wrath from a comfortable distance:

> He sende toward Sodomas þe sy3t of his y3en,
> Þat euer hade ben an erde of erþe þe swettest,
> As aparaunt to paradis, þat plantted þe Dry3tyn;
> Nov is hit plunged in a pit like of pich fylled.
> Suche a roþun of a reche ros fro þe blake,
> Askez vpe in þe arye and vsellez þer flowen,
> As a fornes ful of flot þat vpon fyr boyles
> When bry3t brennande brondez ar bet þeranvnder.
> Þis watz a uengaunce violent þat voyded þise places,
> Þat foundered hatz so fayr a folk and þe folde sonkken.
> (1005–14)

[He sends the sight of his eyes toward Sodom, which had always been one of the sweetest regions on earth, heir to the paradise which was created by God; now it is plunged into a pit filled with pitch. Such a redness of smoke rose from the black pit, ashes up in the air, flowing like a furnace full of scum that boils over the fire when bright burning coals are kindled beneath it. It was a violent vengeance that destroyed these places, that engulfed so fair a people and submerged the land.]

The carnage that greets Abraham in the valley—the smoldering remains of Sodom submerged in the Dead Sea—is the same carnage that Lot's wife is for-

---

27. The salient biblical references are respectively Genesis 8.15–17, 18.10, 19.36–38, and Daniel 6.21–27. While both God's exhortation to Noah to repopulate the earth (*Cl.* 521–22) and his promise to Abraham and Sara (648–52) are explicitly reiterated in *Cleanness*, Lot's procreative incest with his daughters and Daniel's vision of Christ are present only in the presumed scriptural knowledge of the reader. For a discussion of Lot and incest in *Cleanness*, see Calabrese and Eliason, "The Rhetorics of Sexual Pleasure and Intolerance," 270–71; for Daniel as visionary, see Potkay, "*Cleanness*'s Fecund and Barren Speech Acts," 104.

bidden to see. That Abraham can send "toward Sodomas þe syȝt of his yȝen" [the sight of his eyes toward Sodom] without meeting her same fate (and that we as readers are invited to witness the trauma only through his eyes) implies several key differences between the figures. First, Abraham is both temporally and spatially removed from the traumatic event, turning to see it only after it has occurred. While Lot's wife witnesses the trauma *in medias res,* Abraham sees not the burning buildings and collapsing towers but the sea that covers them, not the holocaust itself but its smoldering aftermath. Second, unlike Lot's wife, that "wrech, so wod . . . [who] wrathed oure Lorde" [mad wretch . . . who angered out Lord] (828), Abraham is a figure selected by God "to be chef chyldryn fader, / Þat so folk schal falle fro to flete alle þe worlde" [to be the chief father of children, from whom people will descend to fill the whole world] (684–85), a "burne blessed" [blessed man] (686). In the gendered logic of the poem, then, it is the patriarch and not the pillar of salt who finally narrates the trauma, the paternal figure who moralizes the Dead Sea and its ashen fruits into "teches and tokenes to trow vpon ȝet . . . þat oure Fader forþrede for fylþe of þose ledes" [signs and tokens to think upon still . . . that our Father carried out because of the filth of those people] (1049–51). In *Cleanness*, Abraham's representation (*Vertretung*) belatedly frames the trauma that Lot's wife represents (in the sense of *Darstellung*) with such immediacy, packaging and reconstructing it in the service of the poem's stringent Christian didacticism. The unambiguous narrative associated with the antimimetic response is thus never articulated directly by the traumatic witness herself in *Cleanness;* rather, it is constructed *post hoc* by those authorized to interpret and to articulate on her behalf.

Nonetheless, even as *Cleanness* exerts a careful control over the representations of its biblical traumas and their silent (silenced) witnesses, it also repeatedly calls attention to those biblical cataclysms precisely as traumatic events, acts of destruction that exceed both the sins that precipitate them and the narrative frames meant to justify them. The Flood, the annihilation of Sodom and Gomorrah, the sack of Jerusalem and the fall of Babylon—the losses stemming from these events are made vivid to the reader in the desperate antediluvians carrying their babies to higher ground, in the once beautiful cities of Sodom and Gomorrah swallowed by the stinking Dead Sea, in the carnage of Jerusalem's women and children and the butchery of Babylon's sleeping citizens. By dwelling upon the emotional and physical excess of these catastrophes, the poem unsettles its explicitly Christological contours and reveals an impulse toward memorial preservation *without* the promise of redemption, an implicit counternarrative of memory and loss made urgent by the divinely sanctioned cruelty of the traumas themselves. This insistent counternarrative subverts *Cleanness*'s didactic thrust, offering a mnemonic counterweight to the forward momentum of the poem and frustrating its "authorized" narratives of recovery and incremental progress.

Again, we can consider both Lot's wife and the Dead Sea in these terms. Although poignantly recognized as "aparaunt to paradis, þat plantted þe Dry3tyn" as [heir to the paradise that was created by God] (1007), Sodom and Gomorrah are more frequently rendered in language that Michael Calabrese and Eric Eliason call a "rhetoric of revulsion," emphasizing the "smod" [filth] (711), "scharpe schame" [sharp shame] (850), and "spitous fylþe" [disgraceful filth] (845) of the Cities of the Plain and their inhabitants.[28] Such rhetoric is markedly homophobic in tenor, but equally important, it is also uncannily persistent, outlasting the destruction of the cities to reemerge in the Dead Sea itself. This linguistic and sensual continuity—the "smelle" [smell] and "smach" [flavor] (1019) of the Dead Sea that carries over from the "3estande sor3e" [yeasty filth] (846) of Sodom—offers an object lesson in the stubborn recalcitrance of memory, the persistence not only of the *fylþe* that God tries repeatedly to efface but also of the past itself. Indeed, by recapitulating in its salty waters the very aspects of Sodom and Gomorrah that most "scorned natwre" [scorned nature] (709), the Dead Sea paradoxically preserves what God sought to destroy, a site marked both by infertility and a defiance of *kynde,* where lead floats and feathers sink and where "schal neuer grene þeron growe, gresse ne wod nawþer" [green will never grow, nor grass nor tree neither] (1028). Lot's wife, too, is destroyed in a way that preserves both of her defining sins: a salt statue looking defiantly over her left shoulder. While Lot and his daughters escape Sodom, and while Abraham surveys the shattered plain knowing that Sara will "consayue and a sun bere" [conceive and bear a son] (649), the Dead Sea and Lot's wife persist, fixing the past in a static, non-narrative, backward stare and reminding us not of the bright future promised by Christ but of the losses provoked by God's costly attempts to cleanse the world of *fylþe.* We cannot look at the Dead Sea and the pillar of salt without recognizing the loss of the Cities of the Plain, of both their putative sinfulness and their Edenic beauty. In their textual presence, the mute witnesses to Sodom's destruction unsettle the moralized representation of the trauma provided by Abraham, exceeding his narrative with their own copious *Darstellung* and empowering the poem's readers to provide a *Vertretung* of their own. In this way, the voice stripped from Lot's wife is placed in the mouth of the reader. Cleanness, then, reveals the insufficiency and contingency of any single "authorized" narrative

---

28. Calabrese and Eliason, "The Rhetorics of Sexual Pleasure and Intolerance," 264.

of the traumatic event and, in so doing, invites a critical reassessment of the prescribed, didactic narrative intended to justify it.

NARRATIVE AND COUNTERNARRATIVE, PROPHECY AND LAMENT

Lot's wife is the preeminent figure of traumatic witness in *Cleanness,* but the division that the poem forces between narrative and counternarrative structures its two other Old Testament exempla and defines its ruminations on biblical history and human trauma. Told by God to "waxez now and wendez forth and worþez to monye, / Multeplyez on þis molde, and menske yow bytyde" [grow now and go forth and become many; multiply on this earth, and honor befall you] (521–22), Noah and his menagerie emerge from the Ark with their eyes fixed firmly on the future, not mourning what was lost in the Flood but appealing to what will grow and become many. To this end, God's command, "multeplyez on þis molde," is followed immediately by images of "sede" [seed] and "heruest" [harvest] (523), "somer" [somer] and "wynter" [witner] (525)— images of seasonal growth that emphasize the circular patterns of germination and fecundity that must prevail after the cataclysm. Significantly, just as Abraham emerges to witness only the aftermath of Sodom's destruction, Noah and his family experience the Flood only in its aftereffects, in the soggy new Earth that they have been chosen to replenish.[29] Nonetheless, it is Noah, "a wy3e . . . ful redy and ful ry3twys" [a man . . . full ready and fully righteous] (293–94), who frames God's act of destruction with his survival and thus imputes the didactic *Vertretung* of the trauma itself.

While the figure of Lot's wife has no exact counterpart in the exemplum of the Flood, the poet provides a representation (*Darstellung*) of the traumatic event that evinces a surprising degree of sympathy for its victims, the very men and women God has deemed unworthy to live. Indeed, by "[locking] us out of the ark, which is figured as a closed, water-tight casket, and [leaving] us to share the fate of drowning Creation," the author of *Cleanness* ensures that the same human suffering so carefully hidden from Noah is made painfully visible to the reader.[30]

---

29. As Sarah Stanbury points out, the sole human survivors of the flood "are enclosed in their ark, an inviolate sanctuary" from which they "have no view of the Judgment." See Stanbury, "Space and Visual Hermeneutics in the *Gawain-Poet*," 483.

30. Wallace, "*Cleanness* and the Terms of Terror," 93.

And alle cryed for care to þe Kyng of heuen,
Recouerer of þe Creator þay cryed vchone,
Þat amounted þe mase His mercy watz passed,
And alle His pyté departed fro peple þat He hated.
Bi þat þe flod to her fete floȝed and waxed,
Þen vche a segge seȝ wel þat synk hym byhoued.
Frendez fellen in fere and faþmed togeder,
To dryȝ her delful destyné and dyȝen alle samen;
Luf lokez to luf and his leue takez,
For to ende alle at onez and for euer twynne.
(393–402)

[And all cried for mercy to the King of heaven; each one of them cried for rescue from the Creator, but their amazement only showed that His mercy had passed, and all His pity for the people He hated had departed. By the time the flood had waxed and flowed to their feet, then each person saw well that he must drown. Friends came together and embraced one another, to suffer their doleful fate and to die together; love looks to love and takes his leave, to end their lives at the same moment and to part forever.]

Several critics have noted how the poem evokes our sympathy for the antediluvians in these lines, presenting them simultaneously as deserving of God's scorn and as unfairly victimized by an inflexible divine order.[31] I would argue that *Cleanness* places a *greater* emphasis on the senselessness and cruelty of the Flood than it does on the Flood's putative necessity. Indeed, in the piteous suffering of the Flood's victims, their tender farewells and their huddled resignation to their own deaths, the poem emphasizes the terrible human toll of God's wrath while simultaneously calling into question its justification. For this reason, it is difficult to read the Flood in *Cleanness* simply as a cautionary tale against succumbing to "fylþe in fleschlych dedez" [filth in deeds of the flesh] (265) or even as a tragic but necessary step in God's evolving covenant with humankind. As with the destruction of Sodom, the portrait representation of the traumatic event overwhelms its authorized narrative, and it is in this excess that we are confronted with the antediluvians' own apprehension of "her delful destyne" [their doleful destiny] (400), a startling recognition of traumatic loss that the poet will not allow to be silenced by the rising waters. Noah and his family may provide the justification for the Flood and the prom-

---

31. See, for example, Calabrese and Eliason, "The Rhetorics of Sexual Pleasure and Intolerance," 253; Reading, "Ritual Sacrifice and Feasting," 282.

ise of the new Earth; however, in the rationale-defying trauma of the event (an event that Noah himself is never allowed to see) the reader is forced to recognize the catastrophe's human dimensions. The counternarrative that we are encouraged to create from such a recognition—a counternarrative that engages the full physical and emotional horror of the destruction of the antediluvian world—resists the didactic narrative that Noah so carefully frames.[32]

A somewhat different variation of this pattern emerges in the destruction of Jerusalem and the sack of Babylon, a pair of linked traumatic events that foregrounds issues of mimesis and antimimesis. As with its treatment of the Flood and the Cities of the Plain, *Cleanness* insists upon the human costs of both disasters. In its account of the destruction of Jerusalem in particular, the poem amplifies the understated violence of its biblical source, relating how the conquering Babylonians "baþed barnes in blod and her brayn spylled" [bathed children in their own blood and spilled their brains] (1248) and lingering over the "wombes tocoruen" [sliced-open wombs] and "boweles outborst" [burst out bowels] (1250–51) of the city's slaughtered women. When Babylon falls to the Persians, *Cleanness* again plays the exemplum for pathos, describing how "segges slepande were slayne er þay slyppe myȝt" [people were slain sleeping, before they might escape] (1785) and offering a lament for "þat londe lost for þe lordes synne" [the land that was lost for the lord's sin] (1796). Here too, the representation of human suffering overwhelms the exemplum's didactic impulse, bringing into focus the losses caused by God's judgment while raising uncomfortable questions about their justification. Our pity for the victims forces us to consider the destruction of Jerusalem and the sack of Babylon not only as lessons in piety but also—and perhaps primarily—as human trag-

---

32. In addition to the doomed (and effectively silenced) antediluvians, it is worth briefly considering the Ark itself as another silent witness to the flood. A safe but ultimately infertile enclosure, the Ark is not an agent of the Earth's regeneration but rather a catalyst for it, an inert floating storehouse filled with necessarily quick material. Emptied of its vital cargo after the waters recede and stranded on Mount Ararat, it becomes a lifeless, static memento of a past washed clean. Significantly, the figure of the *arca sapientiae*, the ark of wisdom, was a common model for memory during the Middle Ages. As Mary Carruthers explains in *The Book of Memory*, "One's memory is the ideal product of a medieval education, laid out in organized *loci* . . . that makes it a construction, an *aedificatio*. As something to be built, the trained memory is an *arca* in the sense understood by the biblical object called Noah's Ark" (51). The Ark's multiple chambers—the respective halls, recesses, divisions, bowers, and pens that the poem extrapolates from its biblical source—are metaphorically the divisions by which memory was organized in the Middle Ages, the metaphysical structures that made the trained mind effective as a "compartmentalized, thoroughly filed, labelled, and addressed mental storage-chest" (54). Alternately described as a "mancioun" (309) and a "cofer" (310), two other medieval paradigms for human memory, Noah's Ark is thus figured not only as the repository for animals that will repopulate the earth but also as a mnemonic object that reaches beyond the devastation of the Flood, a memory of what has been lost.

edies.[33] Thus, *Cleanness* once again generates in its linked traumatic events a pair of contradictory impulses: a carefully framed didactic narrative that reads the past trauma as both lesson for and portent of a better future, and a subversive counternarrative that registers the same trauma as a site of devastating human loss.

The figure most responsible for framing the didactic narrative is, of course, Daniel, a survivor of Nebuchadnezzar's destruction of Jerusalem and a man recognized, even by the corrupt Babylonian court, as "prophete of þat prouince and pryce of þe worlde" [prophet of the province and the worthiest of the world] (1614). Commanded by Belshazzar to interpret the words *Mane, Techal, Phares* carved into the temple wall, Daniel not only presents Babylon's destruction by the Persians as a *fait accompli* but also provides a justification for the impending sack of the city, citing God's displeasure at Belshazzar's profanation of Solomon's sacred vessels. Addressing the king, Daniel says,

Bot ay hatz hofen þy hert agaynes þe hyȝe Dryȝtyn,
With bobaunce and with blasfamye bost at Hym kest,
And now His vessayles avyled in vanyté vnclene,
Þat in His hows Hym to honour were heuened of fyrst.
(1711–14)

[But always you heaved up your heart against the high God; with pride and blasphemy you cast your boasts at Him. And now, His vessels, which were once used to exalt and honor Him in His house, are defiled in unclean vanity.]

The rationale for the destruction of Babylon is less carnally inflected than the rationale for the earlier cataclysms. Nonetheless, Daniel's prophetic interpretation of the temple wall's "runisch sauez" [mysterious words] (1545) performs work analogous to Abraham's belated consideration of Sodom and Gomorrah, in which the obliterated cities are reconstructed as "tokenes to trow vpon" [tokens to think upon] (1049). Indeed, because his narrative of Babylon's fall precedes the event itself, Daniel takes an even more active role in framing the trauma, prereading it into a familiar schema of human sin and divine punishment. More significant still, Daniel's ability to provide a lucid narrative of the imminent cataclysm stands in stark contrast to Belshazzar's inability to read the mysterious signs. As with Lot's wife, Belshazzar's close identification

---

33. As Reading notes in "Ritual Sacrifice and Feasting," the victims are made to appear "undeserving of [their] disproportionately severe fate" (293).

with the impending disaster renders the king mute, unable to comprehend the words that spell his fate. Only Daniel, whose separation from the sack of Babylon is regularly reinforced by his identity as a Jew, can read and construct the straightforward narrative associated with antimimesis.

The prophetic mode of Daniel's narrative thus allows the poet to separate the mimetic response of the victim from the historically legible narrative of trauma itself; however, that narrative's position prior to the traumatic event also highlights the doubleness of the exemplum: the poem presents the sack of Babylon by the Persians as a sequel to the destruction of Jerusalem by the Babylonians, an event in which Daniel figures not as interpreter of signs but as "catel [given] to þe kyng" [chattel given to the king] (1296). Situated between the two halves of this double trauma, the prophecy takes on a twofold significance, for while it clearly points toward the impending fall of Babylon, it also inscribes an implicit shadow narrative of the earlier conquest, a trauma that Daniel never openly addresses. Indeed, Zedechiah's "abominaciones of idolatrye" [abominations of idolatry] (1173), which precipitate the sack of Jerusalem, are repeated in Belshazzar's worship of "fals fantummes of fendes, formed with handes" [false phantasms of devils, made by the hands of men] (1341), while the Babylonian soldiers who "baþed barnes in blod and her brayn spylled" [bathed children in their own blood and spilled their brains] (1247–48) are likewise repeated when "Baltazar in his bed [is] beten to deþe, / Þat boþe his blod and his brayn blende on þe cloþes" [Belshazzar is beaten to death in his bed so that his blood and his brains blended on the bedclothes] (1787–88). In the context of these careful interconnections, Daniel's extensive focus on Nebuchadnezzar, who is Belshazzar's father and the instrument of God's destruction of Jerusalem, becomes particularly significant. Although Daniel enumerates Belshazzar's sins and offers a cogent narrative of Babylon's impending fall, he devotes the lengthy beginning of his prophecy to the doomed king's father, describing Nebuchadnezzar's faith, sinful pride, madness, and eventual reconciliation to God.[34] Only after this long excursus does Daniel turn to Belshazzar and the imminent collapse of his kingdom. The energy that drives Daniel's prophecy, then, derives always from Daniel's memory of Belshazzar's father and predecessor. Both destroyer and progenitor, Nebuchadnezzar binds the trauma of the past to the trauma of the future, while his overarching presence in the prophecy ensures that Daniel's brazen vision of the future resonates as a still unspoken lament for the past.

---

34. In the Book of Daniel, the prophet briefly discusses Nebuchadnezzar in his interpretation of the writing on the wall (Daniel 5:18–21). *Cleanness* greatly exaggerates that discussion so that it occupies two-thirds (*Cl.* 1642–1707) of the total prophecy, leaving only one-third (1708–40) directly concerned with Belshazzar.

This double-exemplum largely eschews the "rhetoric of revulsion" so prominent in the Flood and the destruction of Sodom and Gomorrah, and in doing so, it breaks with the earlier two biblical stories. But even as the exemplum tempers such rhetoric, its compulsive repetition of a central traumatic event suggests how the poem both investigates and participates in the patterns of displacement and repetition associated with severe trauma.[35] Freud posits that "the dreams of patients suffering from traumatic neuroses lead them back with . . . regularity to the situation in which the trauma occurred," recurring behavior that reveals a subconscious effort "to conjure up what has been forgotten and repressed" and to "master the [traumatic] stimulus retrospectively."[36] This foundational argument is central to the insights of contemporary theorists, who continue to articulate the ways that "trauma as experience is 'in' the repetition of an early event in a later event—an early event for which one was not prepared to feel anxiety and a later event that somehow recalls the early one and triggers a traumatic response."[37] In *Cleanness*, the traumas of the destruction of Jerusalem and the sack of Babylon mimic in their plurality the compulsive will toward repetition common among survivors of trauma. Taken together, they also suggest how the profound losses of a traumatic event can remain unspoken by their own witnesses but still be comprehensible to others. For Daniel, a survivor of the destruction of Jerusalem charged to foretell the destruction of Babylon, the unarticulated trauma of the past becomes legible in his prophetic narrative of the future. Though we might initially associate the lucid prediction of Babylon's fall with the antimimetic response (and thus with the authorized *Vertretung* of the kingdom's conquest), the prophecy that Daniel offers equally reveals his mimetic identification with the destruction of Jerusalem and suggests the unspoken and unspeakable narrative of that earlier event. Daniel reads the fall of Babylon in the handwriting on the temple wall; it is for us to read the fall of Jerusalem in the words of Daniel's prophetic speech.

REMEMBERING LOT'S WIFE:
THE TEXT AS TRAUMATIC WITNESS

The mimetic identification with the destruction of Jerusalem that Daniel exhibits in his prophecy is suggestive for *Cleanness*'s exploration of the human response to trauma and the fraught voice of the traumatic witness. In the

---

35. Berlant, "Trauma and Ineloquence," 43.
36. Freud, "Beyond the Pleasure Principle," 32.
37. La Capra, "Trauma, Absence, Loss," 725.

aggregate, moreover, the poem's three Old Testament exempla produce a pattern of violence, survival, silence, witness, and memory that reiterates, in its compulsive repetition, a key pattern that trauma theorists recognize in survivors, as well as in modern and postmodern literature written out of trauma. With this pattern in mind, I want to move from theoretical to speculative and consider the possibility that *Cleanness* may be not only a poem *about* trauma but also a poem emerging *from* trauma, a work that enacts in its own form the responses it explores within its exempla. By drawing its readers into the process of constructing the counternarratives implied by such figures of witness as Daniel and Lot's wife, *Cleanness* limns a model for its own reading, a hermeneutic through which to apprehend its symptomatic response to trauma and to excavate the primal traumatic scene that the poem buries within its exempla.

Might the late medieval plague pandemic be that central trauma? Certainly, in both scope and consequence, the Black Death and its aftershocks constitute a profound cultural and social rupture, one that catalyzed frequently painful changes not only to the civic and religious institutions of England but also, and more acutely, to the social, interpersonal, and familial bonds of those who lived through it. Moreover, as I discussed earlier, the plague was not a single event but rather a powerfully and demonstrably cyclical series. After its initial outbreak in England in 1348, the disease struck again in 1361 with the so-called Children's Plague and then, repeatedly, in lesser but still powerful outbreaks into the fifteenth century. The pattern that such repetitions rendered within England was not unlike the pattern of traumatic events inscribed within *Cleanness* itself: the world-consuming Flood; the regional annihilation of Sodom and Gommorah; the local but devastating events of Jerusalem and Babylon. In this respect, it is suggestive that one fifteenth-century English scientific text, now catalogued in the British Library as Sloane MS 965, advises that the pestilence is of a piece with the very cataclysms that *Cleanness* narrates, from the Fall to the destruction of the Cities of the Plain.

Notum sic omnibus Cristianis quod propter peccata orituo pestilencia et omnis alia vindicta dei unde: in celo fecit deus primam vindictam quando decidit angelus Lucifer; secundo in Paradiso quando expulsus fuit Adam; tercio in universa terra quando omnia opera umencia diversa fuerunt in cathaclismo, preterito illo quibus salvata fuerunt in Archa Noye; quarto quando Sodoma et Gomorra demersa fuerunt flumino infernali; quinto quando uxor Loth versa sunt in statuam salis.[38]

---

38. Sloane MS 965, folio 143r., punctuated for sense.

[It is thus known to all Christians that because of sin the pestilence and all other vengeances of God arise: first in heaven God wrought vengeance when the angel Lucifer fell; second in paradise when Adam was expelled; third in the whole world when all His various works were drowned in a cataclysm, except for those that were saved in Noah's Ark; fourth when Sodom and Gomorrah were engulfed in an infernal river; fifth when Lot's wife was turned into a statue of salt.]

That this Latin work, part of a compendium containing an English translation of John of Burgundy's fourteenth-century plague treatise, so closely tracks the Old Testament exempla presented in *Cleanness* implies that while the disease is not addressed directly in the Middle English poem, it nonetheless simmers behind it as a cultural analogue, shadowing its language, its structure, and even the specific episodes around which it is organized. *Cleanness* might thus be said to emerge from and to subtly reinscribe a textual and cultural environment in which the consequences of the first totalizing waves of the plague were still unfolding and in which increasingly localized recurrences remained a constant threat.

Sloane MS 965 offers a tantalizing parallel to *Cleanness*, but it is hardly the only medieval description of the plague to do so. The Flood above all is a common touchstone for fourteenth-century historiographers discussing the Black Death; so too, albeit to a lesser degree, is the destruction of Sodom and Gomorrah. The Louth Park chronicler, for instance, laments, "*Tantaque pestilentia ante hec tempora non est visa nec audita, nec scripture commendata. Creditur enim multitudinem hominum tam copiosam aquis diluvii quod in diebus Noe evenit, interceptam non fuisse*" [So great a plague (as the Black Death) had not been seen or heard or committed to writing. Indeed, it is believed that such a large multitude of people were not killed in the waters of the Flood that happened in the age of Noah].[39] The *Historia de Novitatibus Paduae et Lombardie* also invokes the Flood, though it finds the destruction wrought by the plague to be more inescapable and more final than God's earlier act of vengeance: "*Deus enim tempore Noe tantas animas vix consumpsit, cui possibile est humanum genus etiam de lapidibus restaurare*" [In the time of Noah, God did not in fact consume *all* souls, by which it was possible to rebuild the human race from the stones].[40] Other Continental works, such as Symonis de Covino's allegorical *De Judicio Solis*, propose that the plague "*processit a*

---

39. *Chronicon Abbatie de Parco Lude*, 38.
40. Guillelmi de Cortusiis, *Chronica de Novitatibus Padue et Lombardie*, 121.

Deo propter peccata generis humani sicut fuit tempore diluvii" [proceeded from God on account of the sins of the human race, as it was in the time of the Flood],[41] while within England itself, a 1375 sermon by Thomas Brinton challenges those who view the pestilence as an astrological event by asking, "*qualis planeta regnauit tempore Noe, quando exceptis octo animabus Deus totum mundum per diluuium submergebat, nisi planeta malicie et peccati*" [what kind of planet reigned at the time of Noah, when, except for eight souls, God submerged the whole world, if not the planet of malice and sin?].[42]

Within the context of these broad exemplary parallels, lexical parallels between *Cleanness*'s exempla and contemporary plague writing can also be detected. The terms used to describe the first two biblical calamities in particular, terms drawn from discourses of medicine and surgery, resonate strongly with diagnostic and scientific tracts on the pestilence, as well as, we must imagine, the observations of those who watched neighbors, friends, and family members die of the disease.[43] Consider *Cleanness*'s description of the rising waters of the Flood:

> Þen bolned þe abyme, and bonkez con ryse,
> Waltes out vch walle-heued in ful wode stremez;
> Watz no brymme þat abod vnbrosten bylyue;
> Þe mukel lauande loghe to þe lyfte rered.
> Mony clustered clowde clef alle in clowtez;
> Torent vch a rayn-ryfte and rusched to þe vrþe,
> Fon neuer in forty dayez.
> (*Cl.* 363–69)

[Then the abyss swelled forth, and the banks begin to rise; every spring gushes forth in angry streams. There was truly no bank that remained unbroken. The great cleansing flood reared up to the sky. Many clustered clouds split into pieces; each rain-rift tore open and rushed to the earth, never ceasing for forty days.]

The word *bolned* in particular, which means "swelled" or "distended," comports strongly with language used to describe symptoms of pestilence, with the "hardenesse and *bolnynge* of þe flesche" [hardness and swelling of the flesh] that occurs with plague infections of the lymph nodes, as well as other disfig-

---

41. Symonis de Covino, "De Judicio Solis in Conviviis in Saturni," 207.

42. Brinton, *The Sermons of Thomas Brinton*, 323.

43. See Citrome, "Medicine as Metaphor in the Middle English *Cleanness*."

uring diseases such as leprosy.[44] Medieval medical texts, such as the writings of John of Arderne, use the verb *bolnen* to describe the swelling of any number of ulcerous sores—the "bolnyng3 of diuerse spice3 and schape3" [swellings of various kinds and shapes].[45] More pointedly still, the fifteenth-century *Life of Saint Cuthbert,* a hagiography of an seventh-century bishop who survived one outbreak of pestilence and died in a second, describes a "bolnyng" carbuncle "ware [pus] out ran" [that oozed pus] and remarks that a bubo on the saint's leg "so bremly *bolned*" [swelled so terribly] that the saint could not move it.[46] Similarly, the word *clowtez,* which can mean "patches" or "blotches," appears in medieval medical texts to signify blemishes or lesions, as when Guy de Chauliac prescribes a poultice of tartar, rainwater, and other curatives to treat "bleynes, clowtes and frakenes" [pustules, blotches and blemishes] of the face and body.[47] Thus—and particularly in light of the Flood's currency in contemporary discourses of the plague—*Cleanness*'s image of the sea *bolnyng* into "ful wode stremez" [angry streams] and fed by *clowtez* of clouds begins to appear as a festering canker, a suppurating bubo consuming the antediluvians then for their *unkynde* acts.

Like the drowning of the antediluvian world, the destruction of the Cities of the Plain also evokes symptoms of the fourteenth-century plague pandemic. Indeed, if the language of disease and pestilence emerges in *Cleanness*'s first exemplum, it is drawn into still sharper relief by the poet's rendering of Sodom and Gomorrah. The Dead Sea in particular appears as an open sore on the earth, a festering bubo where the Cities of the Plain used to be:

> Þer þe fyue citées wern set nov is a see called,
> Þat ay is drouy and dym, and ded in hit kynde,
> Blo, blubrande, and blak, vnblyþe to ne3e;
> As a stynkande stanc þat stryed synne,
> Þat euer of smelle and of smach smart is to fele.
> Forþy þe derk Dede See hit is demed euermore,
> For hit dedez of deþe duren þere 3et;
>
> . . .

---

44. Guy de Chauliac, *The Cyrurgie of Guy de Chauliac,* 380. Guy establishes the medical use of the word in the second book of his *Cyrurgie,* noting, "It sufficeth to a cirurgien to knowe þat a posteme, a swellynge, a *bolnynge,* an ingrossacioun, an outsemynge, a lyftynge vp, a growyng out ben names as it were signyfieng þe same þing" (74).

45. John of Arderne, *Treatises of Fistula in Ano,* 57.

46. *The Life of Saint Cuthbert,* 32 (l. 1071), 102 (l. 3492).

47. Guy de Chauliac, *The Cyrurgie of Guy de Chauliac,* 633.

And suche is alle þe soyle by þat se halues,
Þat fel fretes þe flesch and festres bones.
(1015–21, 1039–40)

[Where the five cities once stood is now a sea, turbulent and dark and dead
in its nature, ashen, burbling and black, dismal to approach, like a stinking
pool that destroyed sin and that is always foul with its stench and sharp fla-
vor. Therefore, it is forever named the dark Dead Sea, because the deeds of
death endure there still. . . . And the soil on the shore of that sea is such that
it rots the flesh and festers bones.]

The language describing the Dead Sea in this passage parallels the poet's earlier description of Sodom: the "vnclene" [unlcean] (710) city that "stynkes /
Of þe brych" [stinks of vomit and sin] (847–48) becomes a lake, a "stynkande
stanc" [stinking pool] (1018). But while Sodom is also mentioned as "aparaunt
to paradis" [heir to paradise] (1007), the Dead Sea has most in common with
the ulcerated sores that so frequently heralded the onset of the plague—the
"*macchie nere o livide*" [dark or livid patches] that Boccaccio observes on the
bodies of his plague stricken Florentines.[48] Guy de Chauliac's description of
a "festred cancre [as] an vlcer or festre apperinge rownde, horrible and stink-
ynge . . . hauing wan and blo coloure, and derk" [festering canker, like an ulcer
or abscess, appearing round and horrible and stinking . . . and having a wan,
ashen, and dark color] accords with *Cleanness*'s description of the Dead Sea
as a "blo . . . stynkande stanc" [ashy stinking pool] that "festres bones" [fes-
ters bones].[49] Moreover, Guy's description of plague "bubones" as "vlceres of
þe extremytees . . . , bocches . . . , carbuncles . . . , and felons" [ulcers of the
extremities . . . , pustules . . . , carbuncles . . . , and suppurating sores] recalls
how the Dead Sea's soil "fretes þe flesch" [rots the flesh] (1040).[50] *Cleanness*'s
description of the Dead Sea also resonates with John of Arderne's description
of "vlcere3 . . . , which floweþ out blode, and . . . yuel carbuncle3 þat ar called
pestilenciale3" [ulcers . . . , which give out blood, and . . . evil carbuncles that
are called plague sores][51]; more generally, the image of the festering, reeking
sea comports with common images of plague buboes, which were thought to

---

48. Boccaccio, *Decameron*, 12 (Waldman, 7).
49. Guy de Chauliac, *The Cyrurgie of Guy de Chauliac*, 299.
50. Guy de Chauliac, 157–58.
   51. John of Arderne, *Treatises of Fistula in Ano*, 81. Citrome in "Medicine and Metaphor"
sees similar details in Arderne's treatise, which deals specifically with anal fistuale, as support-
ing an "anal pathology" (269) in Cleanness.

be contagious because the "the reke or smoke of suche sores is venemous and corruptith the ayer" [the reek or vapor from such sores is venomous and corrupts the air].[52]

Such linguistic and narrative parallels can, of course, only suggest how the poem might offer an implicit response to the pestilence. With more certainty, however, they ask us to consider why, if *Cleanness* does draw from contemporary discourses about the plague, it never acknowledges its engagement with this trauma of biblical proportions. Indeed, unlike the witness provided by some Continental works, which explicitly and graphically depicts the horrors of the disease, and unlike that of Anglo-Latin chronicle writing, which is rendered in gasping narrative cliché,[53] the witness I am positing for *Cleanness* is a tacit or even unwitting one, not a full-throated lament but a series of referential exempla whose imagery and language evoke the language of the pestilence. In this respect however, *Cleanness* has much in common with almost all fourteenth-century Middle English poetry, a body of work that, as Ardis Butterfield notes of Chaucer's *Book of the Duchess,* tends to suppress any direct mention of the disease "in favor of a more generalized and abstract allusion to death."[54]

One way we can begin to intuit *Cleanness*'s purchase in the Black Death (and, indeed, the relationship between the disease and the remaining poems of MS Cotton Nero A.x) is by recognizing the poem as symptomatic of the trauma itself, by apprehending it in the same terms of traumatic response and witness that the poem develops within its own narrative structures and in such figures as Daniel and Lot's wife. To this end, we might recognize the anxious repetition of the traumatic scene that *Cleanness* enacts—Flood, Sodom and Gomorrah, Jerusalem, Babylon—as indicative of the mimetic repetitions evinced by the survivors of its biblical exempla. Perhaps such repetition reveals an unstated or even unrecognized impulse behind the poem itself, an urge to master in its accounts of past biblical traumas an ongoing trauma regularly conceived of in biblical terms. Indeed, *Cleanness*'s cyclical narrative

---

52. *A Litil Boke the Whiche Traytied Many Gode Thinges for the Pestilence,* 3 verso.

53. We might, for example, consider the statement of Oxfordshire chronicler Geoffrey le Baker, who describes how "[vulgus] *innumerum, et religiosorum atque aliorum clericorum multitudo soli Deo nota, migravere*" [innumerable common people and a multitude of religious as well as other clerics only known to god departed], or the *Brut* chronicler, who recalls that "whan þis pestilens was cesid & endid, as God wolde, vnneþes þe x. parte of þe peple was left alyve" [when the pestilence had ceased and ended as God would, only a tenth of the population was left alive]. See Geoffrey le Baker, *Chronicon Galfridi le Baker de Swynebroke,* 99; *The Brut,* 303. On the "therapeutic cliché" as a symptom of post-traumatic inarticulateness, see Berlant, "Trauma and Ineloquence," 48–52.

54. Butterfield, "Pastoral and the Politics of Plague," 22.

of destruction and recovery provides a literary framework upon which the recurring trauma of the Black Death might be repeatedly reimagined, reread, and even transmuted into something akin to biblical truth. As such, the poem is akin to those emblems of memory that punctuate its narrative, emerging as both witness and text. A literary artifact whose oblique response to a contemporary trauma is revealed through a direct focus on biblical disasters that perplex and resist assimilation into the stream of human history, *Cleanness* implies the losses of the plague by openly disclosing the losses of those events most frequently employed to describe the disease's putative causes and apocalyptic effects. So, too, does it embody in its poetic form the repetitions and reiterations recognized by contemporary theorists as posttraumatic symptoms. As a poem in which "the act of writing [is] tied up with the act of bearing witness," *Cleanness* may, I want to suggest, be considered a plague poem.[55] It might not be a work that can respond directly to the pestilence—it might not even *intend* to respond to the pestilence—and yet, it is also a work upon which that unspeakable event is, if not spoken, at least made legible: a pillar of salt, a windowless ark, three words carved on a temple wall.

I do not want to argue here that *Cleanness* addresses the plague to the exclusion of its generally recognized didactic focus on sexual and spiritual purity, nor do I claim that the poem is *about* the plague in any absolute or outward facing way. If a response to the pestilence is woven into the poem's exemplary and imagistic fabric, such a response just as readily advances the poet's investment in a stringent Christian moralism as it evokes the horrors of the Black Death. Nonetheless, it may ultimately be through this tacit but persistent mode of witness—a tacitness that stands in sharp contrast both to the poem's overt violence and didacticism—that *Cleanness* most powerfully articulates the experience of trauma, as well as the medieval plague experience more broadly.

At the outset of this chapter, I proposed that we might begin to answer the question "What is lost?" in *Cleanness* by considering the bricks and bodies that remain after God's destructions, as well as those few shattered souls left living after his anger has passed. Were we to consider that same question with regard to the Black Death, we might also begin with bodies, the most immediate physical reminders of a disease whose mortality rate, some scholars estimate, was as high as 62.5 percent.[56] This tremendous loss of human life

---

55. Felman and Laub, *Testimony*, 2.

56. Benedictow, *The Black Death*, 383. As I have already noted, the precise mortality rate for the Black Death in both England and mainland Europe remains a topic of scholarly debate. The figure of 62.5 percent is from Benedictow's exhaustive study and, to my mind, is the best estimation for the mortality rate in England and Europe as a whole. Earlier scholars have some-

is clearly what Boccaccio registers when he describes the streets of Florence littered with the corpses of plague victims and what Petrarch laments when he asks of his lost friends, "*Quod fulmen ista consumpsit? Quis terræ motus evertit? Quæ tempestas demersit? Quæ abyssus absorbuit?*" [What lightning consumed them? What earthquake overthrew them? What tempest drowned them? What abyss swallowed them?][57] It is also what chronicle writers register when they describe the countless men, women, and children taken by the Black Death—so many that, as Thomas Walsingham recounts, "*villæ olim hominibus refertissimæ suis destitutæ sunt colonis, & adeo crebra pestis inualuit, ut uix uiui potuerunt mortuos sepelire*" [villages formerly crowded with people were destitute of their inhabitants, and the pestilence grew to such a degree that the living were hardly able to bury the dead].[58] If these texts, which speak conventionally if movingly of the deaths caused by the plague, stand witness to the 62.5 percent of the population killed, perhaps *Cleanness* quietly stands witness to the 37.5 percent who survived, to those left behind to remember, forget, grieve, interpret, and carry on from the trauma of the Black Death, even as they continued to live in its shadow.

Suggesting the inadequacy of literature to represent the signal trauma of the twentieth century, Theodor Adorno has famously contended, "To write poetry after Auschwitz is barbaric."[59] For English writers living through the defining trauma of the fourteenth century, was writing poetry after the Black Death similarly barbaric? On the one hand, this reading of *Cleanness* implies that it was. If the poem truly does submerge a response to the plague deep within its biblical narratives, it can even be understood as retreating from the barbarism of representing the pestilence overtly, giving only indirect expression to the traumatic event.[60] On the other hand, the poem shows the need for literature to provide a lasting witness to events that might otherwise remain unspoken, the need for poetry to disclose aspects of trauma that other forms of written witness cannot or will not reveal. In its peculiar combination of unforgiving cruelty and surprising tenderness, *Cleanness* thus participates in

---

times determined more conservative figures for plague mortality; Philip Ziegler, for example, offers a very low estimate of 23 percent in *The Black Death*, 230.

57. Petrarch, *Epistolæ de rebus familiaribus et variæ*, 442.

58. Walsingham, *Historia breuis Thomæ Walsingham*, 185.

59. Adorno, *Prisms*, 34.

60. This studied misdirection is a strategy that we will see further displayed in *Pearl*, where an elegy for a single young girl gestures toward a much broader lament. Also suggestive here is Langland's tortured "autobiographical passage" in the *Piers Plowman* (C.5.1–108) in which Will agonizes with Conscience and Reason over the propriety of writing poetry in a world beset by grave physical and spiritual need.

what we might think of as a necessary barbarism, one that reveals how poetry can (and sometimes must) recall events too painful to remember. Moreover, it suggests how literature articulates and embodies the strategies by which survivors struggle to remember the impact of past trauma, even as they strive to move forward from the site of profound human loss.

CHAPTER 2

Pearl and the Language of Plague

O father, why have you deserted me?
O children, whom I raised with much sweat
and labor, why have you fled?

—GABRIELE DE' MUSSIS, *HISTORIA DE MORBO*[1]

THE LAVISHLY ILLUSTRATED book now known as the *Holkham Bible* was produced in London between 1327 and 1340, four or five decades before *Pearl* was written and at least eight years before the first appearance of the plague in England. In its scope and its structure, the *Holkham Bible* is a product of the typological sensibility that informed medieval Christianity as a whole; it dwells first on several scriptural and apocryphal episodes from the Book of Genesis and then turns to the "fulfillment" of those episodes in the life of Christ, the Passion, and the Apocalypse. Among the more arresting of its images, the illustrations comprising the Passion sequence stand out for their "stylized gruesome, gritty realism," as well as for their emotional intensity and their unflinching focus on the bodily pain suffered by Christ (see figure 2.1).[2] By presenting his pale skin covered with dark spots and oozing wounds, the *Holkham Bible* succeeds in offering both a startling realization of Christ's Passion and a grisly if inadvertent portent of things to come: Christ resembles nothing so much as the doomed Florentines that Giovanni Boccaccio would later describe covered in the "*macchie nere o livide*" [dark or livid patches] of the plague.[3] While the blood that drips from his stigmata and wounded side is a vibrant red, the patches and spots covering Christ's *corpus* are a mottled blue-black, equally appropriate to the pestilence as they are to the Passion.

---

1. "*O pater cur me deseris. . . . O, filij, quos sudore et laboribus multis educauj cur fugitis.*" Gabriele de' Mussis, *Historia de Morbo*, 53.
2. *Holkham Bible*, 2.
3. Boccaccio, *Decameron*, 12 (Waldman, 7).

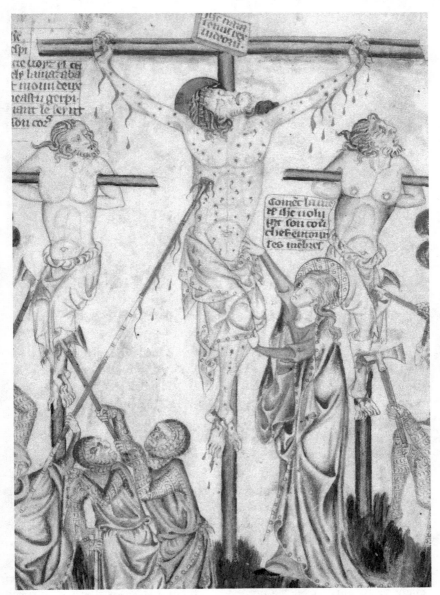

FIGURE 2.1. The Covering of Christ's Loins; Christ's Side Pierced, from the *Holkham Bible*. Used with permission from the British Library, London.

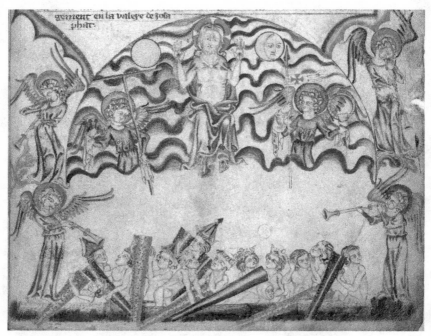

FIGURE 2.2. The New Heaven and the New Earth; Christ Returns; the Last Trump Sounds, from the *Holkham Bible.* Used with permission from the British Library, London.

When the *Holkham Bible* depicts Christ enthroned several folios later, the black spots are gone. Though red blood still flows from his five holy wounds, the resurrected Body is healed and radiant (see figure 2.2). Christ is transcendent here, a redeemed and redeeming figure "withouten spottez blake" [without black spots] (*Pe.* 945).

It will rightly be objected that I am playing fast and loose with chronology by linking the *Holkham Bible* to the pestilence. Nonetheless, I would argue that images like those presented in the manuscript—the spotted and bleeding Man of Sorrows transcended by the luminous Christ enthroned— are important to the cultural imaginary that comes to surround the disease not because such images are contemporaneous with the plague but rather because they precede it, providing a ready frame through which to understand both the sufferings of victims and the traumatic memories of survivors, a flexible cultural context into which the spots and boils of the disease might be assimilated. Such a process—such a response—is clearly on display in the monumental altarpiece painted by Matthias Grünewald for the Antonine Monks of Isenheim, a hospital order that cared for individuals suffering from plague and other disfiguring diseases such as ergotism and leprosy.[4] Supported by a predella depicting Christ's entombment and flanked by panels representing Saint Sebastian (plague saint par excellence) and Saint Anthony, the *Isenheim Altarpiece*'s Crucifixion features a spectacularly contorted Christ in visible agony, his flesh, like that of the *Holkham Bible*'s Christ, covered in the blue-black wounds of his buffeting (see figure 2.3). In its open position, Grünewald's polyptych likewise culminates in an image of the Ascension in which Christ's spotless body, free of the scourges of the Passion save the holy wounds, is inseparable from the nimbus of golden light surrounding it (see figure 2.4). But while the *Holkham Bible* was produced several years before the first outbreak of plague, the *Isenheim Altarpiece* was painted in its wake, commissioned by a religious order devoted to the care of those suffering with disease and crafted by a painter who, as Linda Nochlin notes, "must surely have mused over plague victims [and been] intrigued by their suppurating boils."[5] Grünewald's altarpiece so thoroughly integrates its religious imagery with representations of contemporary illness that for patients contemplating the painting, "disease must have been experienced as a composite testing ground of religious commitment," a trial whose most dangerous symptoms were not only the disfigurement, pain, and death arising from the illness itself but also the potential loss of faith attendant upon such human suffering.[6]

The images of Christ's Passion and Resurrection (see figure 2.4), which existed long before the first wave of pestilence, provide a working visual vocabulary for artists like Grünewald to engage at once with the cosmic mysteries of Christian soteriology and the traumatic realities of communicable disease. In their hands, the traditional iconography of Christ's Passion and the contemporary imagery of physical disease become mutually informing and mutually interpenetrating cultural discourses. In this chapter, I want to investigate the possibility that, in a similar manner, prevailing preplague discourses of mortality and resurrection—both the death and rebirth of the Christian faithful and the Passion and Ascension of Christ himself—provide a meaningful frame through which the *Pearl*-Poet interrogates, understands, and assimilates the pestilence. If, as I propose in the previous chapter, the Old Testament exempla developed in *Cleanness* make legible the unspeakable trauma of the Black Death, perhaps the narrative and imagistic lexis of Christian soteriology likewise functions as a vocabulary, a working lexicon for speaking the

---

4. See Hayum, *The Isenheim Altarpiece*, especially 16–20.

5. Nochlin, *Mathis at Colmar*, 33.

6. Hayum, *The Isenheim Altarpiece*, 30–31.

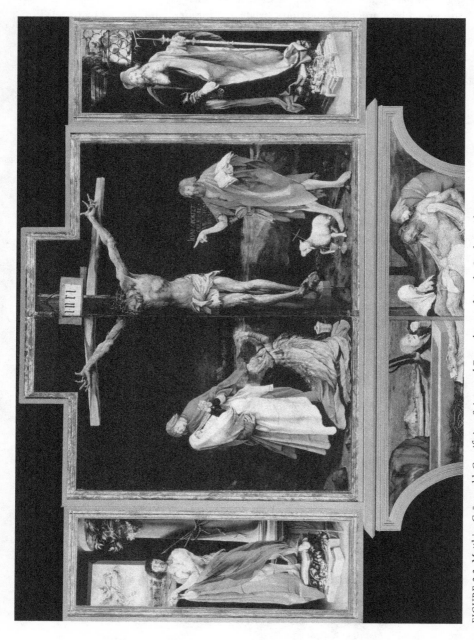

FIGURE 2.3. Matthias Grüenwald. Crucifixion, Saints, and Entombment, from the *Isenheim Altarpiece.* Used with permission from Erich Lessing / Art Resource, NY.

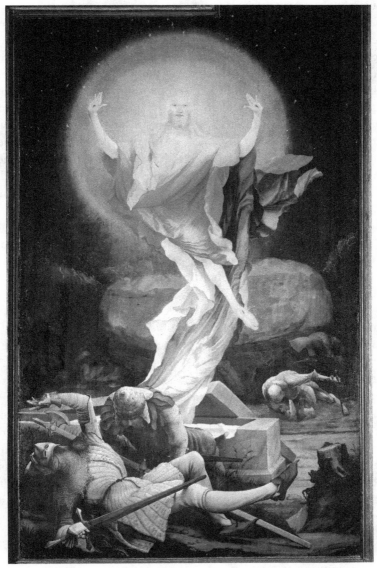

FIGURE 2.4. Matthias Grüenwald. The Resurrection of Christ, from the *Isenheim Altarpiece*. Used with permission from Erich Lessing / Art Resource, NY.

medieval pandemic, a means of relating and subduing the cultural and personal losses of the disease and, furthermore, of offering solace to the poet's courtly audience and public.[7]

Such a proposal is necessarily speculative. Like *Cleanness*, *Pearl* does not mention the disease that informed its immediate textual environment. Working within that speculative mode, however, I will consider how the poem folds the black spots and morbid swellings of the plague into its own paradoxically beautiful poetics, even how it becomes a pestilential object itself as it negotiates between the private pressures of its courtly milieu and the public demands of a global catastrophe. Indeed, as it reveals a simmering discomfort with its jewel-like transformation of death into a work of transcendent beauty, *Pearl*, like the *Isenheim Altarpiece,* marshals the "pre-existing languages" of Christian salvation and eschatology to contain and to transfigure the losses of the plague.[8] The poet thus mingles the cultural discourses surrounding the disease with the dominant elegiac and religious concerns of his poem. More important, he draws from the corporeal realities of the pestilence to vivify his spiritual allegory while simultaneously deploying the established vocabulary of Christian soteriology to inform a lament for one young girl, a lament that eventually reaches beyond the individual to mourn the losses suffered by an entire nation.

By focusing on both the discomfiting ethos of transformation that *Pearl* manifests and the carefully controlled pestilential lexicon that it manages, this chapter also continues to address the broader concern of this study, the puzzlingly muted response of Middle English poetry to the Black Death. As an allegory, an elegy, an apocalypse, a social commentary, and a courtly production—often all at once—*Pearl* is unusually well situated to register an event that resonated broadly across familial, social, civic, and spiritual lines. In fact, for a poem most frequently considered in the rarefied contexts of the court and sometimes regarded as an example of occasional verse, *Pearl* reveals a surprisingly generous civic scope, and it develops a voice that at times verges on the public.[9] Moreover, *Pearl* shares with *Cleanness* an impulse toward understanding the experience of trauma both within its narrative and through its struc-

---

7. See Middleton, "The Audience and Public of *Piers Plowman*." Most critics have described *Pearl*'s audience as a courtly one, including Bowers, *The Politics of* Pearl; Aers, "Christianity for Courtly Subjects."

8. Jenni Nuttall, in *The Creation of Lancastrian Kingship,* describes a "pre-existing language" as one in which "elements of the *langue,* namely particular topoi or metaphors, were found to be especially pertinent . . . because they were already available and readily understood" (27).

9. See Middleton, "The Idea of Public Poetry in the Reign of Richard II"; Staley, "*Pearl* and the Contingencies of Love and Piety."

ture, revealing the Dreamer's own struggle to define and articulate the evasive object of his loss and forcing the reader to share and recapitulate that struggle.[10] Physically, linguistically, and formally, traumatic loss in *Pearl* becomes an asymptote. The Dreamer nears but can never cross the river, implies but can never speak his trauma; likewise, the poem circles and approaches—but can never name—the traumatic loss at is core. In this way, the strategies used by the poet alternately to evoke and to suppress the pestilence in this intricate work suggest the understated yet powerful imprint of the Black Death in Middle English poetry as a whole. While they gesture toward the presence of an English literary response, they also articulate how the pestilence registers in Middle English poetry, both actively and, as in *Cleanness*, symptomatically. *Pearl* thus points toward several of the key cultural and linguistic factors that contribute to the seeming reticence of the Middle English response to the Black Death, factors that help to explain one of the key distinctions between postplague vernacular literature in England and its counterparts on the European continent.

THE LANGUAGE OF PLAGUE, THE PLAGUE AS POEM

More than any other poem of the later Middle Ages, *Pearl* revels in the pregnant ambiguity of the English vernacular, the potential for individual words and phrases—*pearl, py3t, prynces paye*—to sustain a multiplicity of metaphoric valences within diverse, sometimes contradictory fields of discourse. The poem does not explore this semantic potential through one-to-one equivalences but through the gradual accretion of mutually interpenetrating metaphors. The pearl, for example, always remains a pearl, even as it becomes a seed, a courtly maiden, a dead child, a daughter, the pure Christian soul, the Pearl of Price, the Lamb of God, the Kingdom of Heaven. The Jeweler is always a merchant hovering at the edges of aristocratic society, even as we come to recognize him as a dreamer, a mourner, a father, a penitent, and a visionary.[11] The individual metaphors that cling to these central terms never fully displace one another at the locus of the word itself. Instead they coexist within that locus, building upon one another in successive translucent layers and investing *Pearl* with what Sarah Stanbury calls a "set of metaphoric registers that with extraordinary facility rewrites the definitions of the poem's

---

10. For *Pearl*'s engagement with loss, see Stanbury, "Introduction," *Pearl*, 7; Edmondson, "The Shadow of the Object."

11. Barr, "The Jeweller's Tale," 60.

central terms."[12] Such palimpsestic multiplicity is supported by *Pearl*'s complex patterns of alliteration, rhyme, repetition, word variation, and concatenation—the hallmarks of the poem's astonishing formal design. Within *Pearl*'s poetic structure, key words recur and run up against suggestively inexact synonyms; phrases echo from stanza to stanza, gathering new significances and destabilizing established ones. Such structural and formal virtuosity is integral to the poem's hypersaturated language and thus integral to the most basic way that *Pearl* creates meaning.

On the most fundamental semantic level, then, *Pearl* immediately generates a palpable tension between the metaphoricity of its language and the literal, almost-physical lexicon in which its metaphors are rooted, the terrestrial pearls and spots and muck that it gradually reveals as the holy city, the immortal soul, and the filth of human sin. That same tension, too, is recast within the figure of the celestial Pearl Maiden, whose heavenly perfection is inextricable from, even predicated upon, the "corse in clot" [body in earth] (320) that the Dreamer mourns.[13] Finally, and crucially, the stubbornly literal basis of all metaphor is registered by the Dreamer himself, a figure who clings to the manifestly physical even when he is confronted with the transcendent otherworld of his vision. From her perspective in the "gostly" [spiritual] (185) realm, the Pearl Maiden may "halde þat jueler lyttle to prayse / Þat leuez wel þat he sez wyth yȝe" [hold little praise for that jeweler that believes only what he sees with his eye] (301–2), rebuking him for his literal-mindedness and his failure to apprehend the metaphorical terms of her teachings. In his chronic inability to disregard the earthly and fully embrace the transcendent, however, the Dreamer approximates the experience of *Pearl*'s readers.[14] Like him, we cannot entirely escape the physicality, and frequently the courtly materiality, that simmers beneath the poem's metaphorical language, nor can we entirely forget the bodies and blemishes that precede and underwrite the New Jerusalem and its spotless inhabitants. More important, we cannot forget that the poem's dazzling metaphors themselves are always grounded by their mundane linguistic referents, that the boundless significances of the pearl arise from the simple image of a gem lost in the mud, just as the beatific Pearl Maiden arises from the human body marred by "moul" [earth/muck] (23). The fleeting

---

12. Stanbury, "Introduction," *Pearl*, 4. See also Tomasch, "A *Pearl* Punnology."

13. Terell, in "Rethinking the 'Corse in Clot,'" writes, "The Dreamer's perception of the situation has been backward: he has been grieving that his precious pearl has been 'marred' by death, while in fact death has enabled her to become a fully incorruptible pearl" (441).

14. James Rhodes, in *Poetry Does Theology*, describes the interrogative power of the Dreamer's questions to "enlarge the scope of the debate and stretch the discourse of the Maiden to address the very real concerns that trouble him" (126). Also see Gustafson, "The Lay Gaze: *Pearl*, the Dreamer, and the Vernacular Reader."

access to the divine that *Pearl* grants its Dreamer, as well as the fleeting access to transcendence that it promises its readers, cannot be glimpsed without the germ of the terrestrial. Transcendence in *Pearl*—linguistic, poetic, and spiritual—is always anchored to the material, to the "fylþe oþer galle" [filth or gall] (1060) of the earth, to the spotty human body itself.

The persistent materiality of its metaphoricity is central to *Pearl's* layered allegorical and elegiac senses, as well as to the way the poem engages with the trauma of the pestilence. The opening stanza group itself, which concludes with the Dreamer falling "vpon a slepyng-slaȝt" [upon a deathly sleep] (59), implicates a semantic register in which words, phrases, and images evocative of the plague suffuse the poem's linguistic fabric.

> Allas! I leste hyr in on erbere;
> Þurȝ gresse to grounde hit fro me yot.
> I dewyne, fordolked of luf-daungere
> Of þat pryuy perle withouten spot.
> (9–12)

> [Alas! I lost her in a garden; it slipped away from me through the grass to the ground. I languish, wounded by lovesickness of that secret pearl without spot.]

The concatenating link word for the first stanza group, *spot,* has uniformly been read as both "flaw" and "place"; the pearl is "withouten *spot*" in that it is flawless and in that it has no earthly location. This latter meaning (which initially appears as subordinate to the first) is reinforced and expanded by the line that begins the second stanza, in which the most prominent sense of *spot* is "place": "Syþen in þat *spote* hit fro me sprange" [Since it sprang away from me in that spot] (13). These two primary meanings gather metaphoric richness as *spot* is continually recontextualized throughout the work: as the Dreamer mourns over the place where his pearl was lost, the *spot* becomes a grave as well as the earth itself; as the pearl is steadily revealed to be not just a gem but a being (a courtly maiden, a heavenly child, the Lamb of God), its physical spotlessness is twinned by moral and spiritual spotlessness.[15] But as Jean-Paul Freidl and Ian Kirby note, in addition to signifying "blemish" and "place" the word *spot* can also signify "any morbid eruption on the skin, a pimple; a leprous lesion," meanings that they suggest introduce the possibil-

---

15. See Tomasch, "A *Pearl* Punnology," 11–20. Tomasch follows the word *spot* as it develops throughout the poem, focusing on its meanings of "blemish" and "place," and analyzing "the changes rung on these two meanings, by use of *traductio, adnominatio,* and *expolitio*" (11).

ity of spots as plague lesions.[16] Not simply generic imperfections or locations on the ground, spots can also read as the material and corporeal symptoms of illness: the "spotte3 and filþe3 of þe skyn which giffeþ out watre and maketþ rednez" [spots and filths of the skin which give out fluids and make redness][17]; the "spotty defoulynge of þe playne skynne" [spotty corruption of the smooth skin][18]; the "black spotts of the face" [black spots of the face][19]; the "bocches" [pustules] and "felons" [suppurating sores] of the Black Death.[20]

Like the sense of *spot* as "location," the sense of *spot* as "bodily sore" is initially obscured by the more immediate definition of "flaw." In *Pearl*'s second stanza, however, the word repeats within semantic and imagistic contexts that allow the submerged meaning to develop, particularly for late fourteenth-century readers familiar with the physical symptoms of the pestilence.

> Syþen in þat *spote* hit fro me sprange
> . . .
> My breste in bale bot bolne and bele.
> 3et þo3t me neuer so swete a sange
> As stylle stounde let to me stele.
> Forsoþe þer fleten to me fele.
> To þenke hir color so clad in clot!
> O moul, þou marrez a myry juele,
> My priuy perle wythouten *spotte*.
> (12, 18–24)

[Since it sprang away from me in that spot . . . my breast swells and throbs with sorrow. And yet I thought there was never so sweet a song as the moment of stillness that stole over me. In truth, many such moments once came to me. But to think of her complexion so covered in clods! O earth, you mar a beautiful jewel, my secret pearl without spot.]

---

16. Freidl and Kirby, in "The Life, Death, and Life of the Pearl-Maiden," briefly sketch some of the overtones of *spot* and *moul* that I develop in detail here. They see these overtones reach their apex in the phrase quoted toward the opening of this chapter, "withouten spottez blake" [without black spots] (945). See also Breeze, "*Pearl* and the Plague of 1390–1393," which uses Freidl and Kirby's work to support an authorship claim. Quotations above are from *MED*, s.v. "spot" n. 1.

17. John of Arderne, *Treatises of Fistula in Ano*, 50.

18. Guy de Chauliac, *The Cyrurgie of Guy de Chauliac*, 390.

19. Whytlaw-Gray, "John Lelamour's Translation of Macer's Herbal in MS Sln.5," qtd. in *MED*.

20. Guy de Chauliac, *The Cyrurgie of Guy de Chauliac*, 157.

Where the first stanza emphasizes the pearl's physical perfection and intrinsic value as a jewel, the second more overtly develops the human aspects of the pearl, revealing her to be an absent maiden "clad in clot" [covered in clods] (22) and marred by "moul" [earth/muck] (23). Still a valuable but lost gem, the pearl hidden by earth now becomes (also) a body in the grave, that of a girl, we later learn, who was "nerre [to the Dreamer] þen aunte or nece" [closer (to the Dreamer) than an aunt or a niece] (233). The gradual metaphoric shift from *lapis* to *corpus* perplexes the semantic registers that the poem has already developed, providing new and troubling contexts for the pearl itself and forcing a similar shift in our understanding of the link word, *spot*. Specifically, the incarnation of the gem as the dead girl—as the body itself—allows *spot* to be perceived more readily as a physical sore. "Þat pryuy perle withouten *spot*" (12) thus scans as that special gem without flaw, that unseen pearl without place, and, more speculatively, that hidden body without the "spotteȝ and filþeȝ" of the plague.[21]

Further word play in the second stanza reinforces the nascent sense of *spot* as "physical sore." The word *moul*, usually glossed as "earth" or "muck," can also be defined as "spot or blemish" or "sore,"[22] as in Guy de Chauiac's *Cyrurgie*, which advises on the treatment "of mormol & saucefleume & cancrous . . . [and] of akþis & *moulis*" [of ulcers and saucephlegm and cancerous lesions . . . and of blemishes and sores].[23] In that respect, the Dreamer's lament, "O *moul*, þou marrez a myry juele" [O earth, you mar a beautiful jewel] (23), suggests that the pearl-as-body is marred by sores just as the pearl-as-jewel is marred by bits of muck, contradicting the Dreamer's earlier insistence that his pearl is "withouten spot" [without spot] (12). The paradox embodied in this contradiction—that the spotty and the spotless necessarily coexist within a single spot—is one that will eventually find its apotheosis in the "Jerusalem Lombe" [Lamb of Jerusalem] (841), whose own spotless form belies the "boffetez" [blows] (809) and "payne" [pain] (954) that he suffered in the earthly Jerusalem. The Dreamer likewise complains that, in his misery over his loss, "[his] breste in bale bot bolne and bele" [his breast swells and throbs with sorrow] (18). In the most immediate sense, the Dreamer is revealed here as suffering the physiological pain of his grief or, alternatively, the pangs of longing associated with his *fin' amor*–inflected "luf-daungere" [lovesickness] (11). As we saw in *Cleanness*, however, *bolnen* literally means to swell and is used in

---

21. John of Arderne, *Treatises of Fistula in Ano*, 50.

22. *MED*, s.v. "mōl" n. 3, (also mole, moile, moule). See again, Freidl and Kirby, "The Life, Death, and Life of the *Pearl*-Maiden," 395.

23. *A Middle English Version of the Introduction to Guy de Chauliac's "Chirurgia magna,"* 32.

medical texts to denote the physical symptoms associated with infection and disease.[24] *Belen*, too, a verb which means to become inflamed or to fester, is similarly suggestive of the bodily signs of the pestilence.[25]

The presence of so many words in *Pearl's* second stanza with so consistent a set of double (or triple) meanings—*spot, clot, moul, bolne, bele*—creates a linguistic field that persistently, if indirectly, evokes the symptoms of pestilence. By developing the rich *potentia* of such words, the poet exploits "pre-existing languages" of bodily decay and corruption, enriching *Pearl* with pestilential contexts already latent within the *langue*.[26] The lexical richness of *Pearl*—an example of the "ornamental verbal 'density'" so prized in Middle English alliterative poetry and a lingering textual marker of the poem's specific milieu of the English aristocratic court[27]—thus insinuates a pestilential semantic register into the poem's broader thematic concerns.

Indeed, as *Pearl* turns to the garden in stanza three—the *locus amoenus* that serves as the earthly *spot* for the Dreamer's vision—the discourse on mortality and rebirth is further interwoven with language suggestive of the pestilence.

> Þat spot of spysez mot nedez sprede,
> Þer such rychez to rot is runne,
> Blomez blayke and blwe and rede
> Þer schynez ful schyr agayn þe sunne.
> (25–28)

[That spot of spices needs to spread where such richness has run to rot; blooms of pale yellow and blue and red shine brightly there in the sun.]

From buried pearl to budding flower, the pattern of loss and rebirth promised in the earthly *erber* presages the loss and rebirth proposed by the poem's elegiac narrative as a whole: the death of "þat specyal spyce" [the special person] (254), the spots and "spicez" [spices/symptoms] (25) that cover her earthly body, and her rebirth as a "maskelez perle" [spotless pearl] (745) in heaven.[28]

---

24. Guy de Chauliac, *The Cyrurgie of Guy de Chauliac*, 380.

25. *MED*, s.v. "belen" v. The fifteenth-century *Life of Saint Cuthbert* relates how a plague sore on the saint's leg "so bremly *bolned* and *belyd*, þat [Cuthbert] myght noȝt wele it weld," a phrase that closely echoes *Pearl's* "My breste in bale bot bolne and bele" (13). *The Life of Saint Cuthbert*, 102 (ll. 3492–94)

26. See Nuttall, *The Creation of Lancastrian Kingship*, 27.

27. Hanna, "Alliterative Poetry," 493.

28. *MED*, s.v. "spīce" n.(2)1 ("a type or kind of person," "the human species"), n.(2)2 ("the symptoms [of a disease]"). For the traditional reading of these metaphors, see Martin, "Allegory

But these images of redemption and resurrection, which gesture in equal measure to the resurrection of a dead child as the Pearl Maiden and to the resurrection of Christ as the Lamb, are planted linguistically and figurally in the "corse in clot" [body in earth] (320), the material *spot* [location, blemish, flaw, plague sore] that "to rot is runne" [has run to rot] (26). Thus, the heavenly perfection imagined by the poem, the spotlessness insisted upon by the Dreamer and eventually realized in both Maiden and Lamb, is predicated upon a bodily imperfection figured within the poem as a running sore: a spot, a symptom, and perhaps, in the phrase "þat spot of spysez mot nedez sprede" [that spot of spices needs to spread] (25), a vector for the spread of disease itself. Like the clot marring the pearl and the "wounde ful wyde" [wound so wide] (1135) of Christ, the symptoms of plague exist behind *Pearl*'s metaphors, a corporeal antecedent to the perfection of resurrection and spotty seed for "spycez" (35)—spices, symptoms, and "þat specyal spyce," the Maiden herself.

The hint of contagion that clings to the phrase "þat spot of spysez mot nedez sprede" (25) is particularly suggestive in this regard. On the one hand, the implication that the disease—metonymically "þat spot"—must spread from "spysez" [people, symptoms, flowers] comports with the rapid onset and the physical progress of the plague, both of which are described by Boccaccio in the *Decameron*:

> appresso s'incominciò la qualità della predetta infermità a permutare in macchie nere o livide . . . che essa dagli infermi di quella per lo comunicare insieme s'avventava a' sani, non altramenti che faccia il fuoco alle cose secche o unte quando molto gli sono avvicinate.[29]

[The symptoms would develop then into dark or livid patches . . . transmitted from the sick to the healthy through normal intercourse, just as fire catches on to any dry or greasy object placed too close to it.]

Though hardly as overt as Boccaccio's livid patches, the "blomez blayke and blwe and rede" [blooms of pale yellow and blue and red] (27) of the Dreamer's garden nonetheless limn the physical marks of the pestilence, the same symp-

---

and Symbolism," 324. The sense of *spice* as "symptom," which has not yet been noted in readings of *Pearl*, is nonetheless common both in medieval medical texts, which describe "bolnyng3 of diuerse spice3 and schape3," and in popular literary works like the *Gesta Romanorum*, where the infected Jonathas eats an enchanted fruit and becomes "hole of all the *spice* of the lepre." See respectively, John of Arderne, *Treatises of Fistula in Ano*, 57; *Early English Versions of the Gesta Romanorum*, 189.

29. Boccaccio, *Decameron*, 12–13 (Waldman, 7–8).

toms frequently related in medical treatises and in visual representations of the disease.[30] Moreover, if the livid patches of the plague are recast in "wortez ful schyre and schene" (42) [flowers so bright and shining], they are distinctly recast in terms that emphasize their beauty and fecundity. The *erber,* then, figures the spotty body within the ground, but it is also a body grown beautiful over its own mortal remains, a body redeemed and radiant. Once again, then, *Pearl* emphasizes how the fertility of the garden and the physical degeneracy associated with plague can and must occupy the same *spot,* how the burgeoning "flor and fryte" [flower and fruit] (29) of the *erber* necessarily arise where the pearl "doun drof in moldez dunne" [sank down into the dun earth] (30).[31] As both *locus mortis* and *locus amoenus,* the garden brings together spotted and spotless, boil and bloom, and reveals their inseparability.

A number of additional details from the first stanza group support the possibility that the pestilence partly drives the poem's language and imagery, further suggesting its importance to both the death and rebirth of the Pearl child, as well as to the salvific theology developed by the vision. At the moment that he falls into his dream, *Pearl's* Dreamer declares,

> I felle vpon þat floury flaȝt,
> Suche odour to my hernez schot;
> I slode vpon a slepyng-slaȝte
> On þat precios perle withouten spot.
> (57–60)

[I fell down upon that flower-filled field, for such odor shot to my brains; I slid into a deathly sleep on that precious pearl without spot.]

While the sensual stimuli of the natural world frequently spur medieval dream visions, the poet's emphasis on "odour," which is coupled with the Dreamer's sudden "slepyng-slaȝte" or deathly sleep (literally "sleeping-slaughter"), is particularly evocative. Medieval treatises on the pestilence consistently recognize the disease as highly contagious, and though the probable modes of

---

30. For the identification of "blayke" as pale-yellow (rather than "black"), see Klein, "Six Colour Words in the *Pearl* Poet."

31. The adjective "schyr" [bright, shining, white] is interesting here as it appears several times in the final poem of the *Pearl* manuscript, *Sir Gawain and the Green Knight,* as a noun meaning "flesh" or "bright skin." Gawain exposes "þat schyre al bare" (2255–56)—the bare white skin of his neck—to the Green Knight's blade at the moment of his would-be decapitation, while Bertilak himself knits up "þe schyre" (1331) of the deer he kills on the first hunt. *Schyr's* alternate meaning of "skin"—a sense readily available within the *Pearl* manuscript—further suggests how the flowers function metaphorically as sores blooming upon bright, pale skin.

transmission would remain unclear until the late nineteenth-century, most medieval authorities surmised that the plague was carried by toxic vapors that penetrated the "spyrytuall membres princypal" [principal spiritual parts] of the body, "that is for to say þe herte, the liuer, & the braine" [that is to say the heart, the liver, and the brain].[32] The influential 1348 report of the Paris medical faculty ascribes the pestilence to "*vapores malos putridos et veneno-sos . . . a paludibus lacubus profundis vallibus . . . a mortuis corporibus non sepultis nec combustis quod pernecabilius esset*" [bad, putrid, and poisonous vapors . . . from swamps, lakes, and deep valleys . . . (and) from unburied or unburnt dead bodies, which are even more pernicious].[33] Other treatises blame the pestilence on "the corrupcion of the ayre" [corruption of the air][34] and deduce that the smell of decaying corpses and "the reke or smoke" [reek or vapor][35] is toxic. Still others, as Jamie Fumo notes, posit vision itself as a means of contagion and figure the eyes as "portals of malady."[36] Coupled with the ravishing sight of the garden, the sudden odor that penetrates the "hernez" [brains] (58) of the Dreamer and catapults him into a "slepyng-slaȝte" might read not just as the *de rigueur* stimulus for a dream vision but rather as a vector far more menacing, even as a moment of potential infection. Indeed, his proximity to the Pearl child's buried corpse brings the Dreamer dangerously close to a potential locus of contagion and speaks powerfully to the perceived threat of transmission.

As foul smells were considered to carry gaseous venoms and pestilential contagion, so good smells were commonly believed to mitigate or even prevent transmission. Boccaccio's image of terrified Florentines "*portando nelle mani chi fiori, chi erbe odorifere e chi diverse maniere di spezierie, quelle al naso ponendosi spesso, estimando essere ottima cosa il cerebro con cotali odori confortare*" [holding flowers to their noses or fragrant herbs, or spices of various kinds, in the belief that such aromas worked wonders for the brain] is perhaps the most dramatic example of this belief in fourteenth-century litera-

---

32. Moulton, *The Myrrour or Glasse of Helth*, C.ii.verso. While Moulton's treatise dates from the mid-sixteenth century, it is itself a close translation of John of Burgundy's influential treatise, usually dated to around 1365. For a close analysis of the relationship between the two texts, see Keiser, "Two Medieval Plague Treatises and Their Afterlife in Early Modern England." The medieval recognition of the plague's virulence is noted in Winslow, *Conquest of Epidemic Disease:* "It was the Black Death which at last taught the communicability of disease beyond any peradventure" (96).

33. "The Report of the Medical Faculty of Paris," 154.

34. Moulton, *The Myrrour or Glasse of Helth*, B.ii.recto.

35. *A Litil Boke the Whiche Traytied Many Gode Thinges for the Pestilence*, 3 verso.

36. Fumo, "The Pestilential Gaze," 91.

ture, but the idea was prevalent in England as well.[37] John Lydgate's fifteenth-century "Doctrine for Pestilence," which postdates *Pearl* by several decades, urges readers to

> Walk in gardeyns sote of their savour,
> Temperatly, and take also good keep,
> Gorge vpon gorge is cause of gret langour,
> And in especial flee meridian sleep.[38]

[walk in sweet smelling gardens with temperance, and also be moderate (overindulgence causes great languor), and especially avoid midday sleep.]

A poetic distillation of several earlier plague treatises, Lydgate's fifteenth-century poem is relevant to *Pearl* not only because it advises readers to avoid sleeping during the day (advice that *Pearl's* Dreamer is clearly unable to follow) but because it advocates using the garden to guard against pestilence. Indeed, it is notable that all the plants mentioned by name in *Pearl*—"gilofre, gyngure, and gromylyoun, / and pyonys" [gillyflower clove, ginger, gromwell, and peonies] (43–44)—had well-established medicinal applications in the Middle Ages. Peonies and gillyflowers in particular were used in satchels and scented amulets thought to keep illness at bay, while ginger, as one 1384 plague treatise notes, was prescribed for "the confortis of the herte, & the principall membres" [the comfort of the heart and the principle parts of the body].[39] As many critics have noted, the image of the garden alludes to "the natural process of corruption-generation and the spiritual process of death-resurrection" that echo the poem's meditations on mortality and salvation; however, the specific lexicon that the poet deploys, the punning hints of sores and buboes woven into the poem's semantic fabric, the medicinal value of the herbs mentioned, and the sheer sensuality of the perfumed garden additionally raise the

---

37. Boccaccio, *Decameron*, 15 (Waldman, 9).

38. Lydgate, "A Dietary, and a Doctrine for Pestilence," in *Minor Poems*, 703 (ll. 37–40).

39. *A Litil Boke the Whiche Traytied Many Gode Thinges for the Pestilence*, 6 recto, 5 recto. For clove pink (gillyflower) and peony amulets as prophylactics against disease, see Jones, "Herbs and the Medieval Surgeon," 175; Dendle, "Plants in the Early Medieval Cosmos," 52–53, both in *Health and Healing from the Medieval Garden*, ed. Dendle and Touwaide. Gromwell seems slightly less relevant to the plague in particular, though it appears in a variety of recipes for poultices and other medicinal concoctions. See, for example, the Middle English *Liber de Diversis Medicinis*, 44–46, where the plant is prescribed as a diuretic to restore humoral balance.

possibility that the "fayrre flayr" [fair scent] (46) mentioned in *Pearl* may draw energy from contemporary measures against infection.[40]

Thus, like the youths of Boccaccio's *brigata*, who abandon Florence for a pastoral retreat with "*ogni cosa di fiori quali nella stagione si potevano avere piena e di giunchi giuncata*" [flowers in season everywhere, and the floors strewn with rushes], *Pearl*'s grieving Dreamer occupies a physical space meant to keep pestilence at bay but that also hums with the presence of bodily contagion and the anxious desire for prevention.[41] Read in this light, the Dreamer's sojourn in "þat erber wlonk" [that lovely garden] (1171) partially recasts a key movement in Boccaccio's *Decameron*: the *brigata*'s progress from pestilential Florence to the healthful and moderating influences of the Tuscan hills, or what Glending Olson has termed "the movement from plague to pleasure."[42] While that movement, explicitly traced in the *Decameron*, is only obliquely outlined in *Pearl*, the poem's concluding image of social and sacramental integration, in which the Dreamer rejoins his community to receive "Krystez dere blessing . . . in þe forme of bred and wyn" [Christ's dear blessing . . . in the form of bread and wine] (1208–9), nonetheless suggests that his isolation in the garden, like the self-imposed isolation of Boccaccio's *brigata*, is a departure from his customary urban environment.[43] Unlike the *Decameron*, however, which locates its remedy for the plague firmly within a physical progress from city to country, *Pearl* looks beyond the garden itself and signals its investment in a progress that transcends the earthly. In that respect, *Pearl*'s *locus amoenus* is not an end unto itself but rather a means for the Dreamer to glimpse an Edenic otherworld, one that, as he relates, "bylde in me blys, abated my balez, / Fordidden my stresse, dystryed my paynez" [built joy within me, eased my sorrows, undid my stress and destroyed my pains] (123–24). The poem might thus be understood as extending the terrestrial movement from plague to pleasure that we see in the *Decameron* into a soteriological movement from plague to satisfaction, one that holds onto its investment in earthly prophylaxis even as it reveals the fulfillment and spiritual transcendence achieved only through death.

---

40. Vasta, "*Pearl*: Immortal Flowers and the Pearl's Decay," 520. See also Johnson, *The Voice of the Gawain-Poet*, especially 180–85; Finlayson, "*Pearl*: Landscape and Vision."

41. Boccaccio, *Decameron*, 27 (Waldman, 20). I will address issues of plague flight and enclosure in my consideration of *Patience* below.

42. Olson, *Literature as Recreation*, 166.

43. Felicity Riddy writes, in "Jewels in *Pearl*," "The high culture sustained by the luxury system is the product of exchange between craftsmen, merchants and aristocrats: between the court and the city. The narrating voice of pearl, shifting between jeweller and courtly lover, is an acknowledgement of this. . . . Jewellers were urban, because they depended on the wealthy clientèle which a large centre of trade could supply" (59–60).

Finally, I want to explore the possibility here that the specific season of the Dreamer's vision—"In Auguste in a hyȝ seysoun, / Quen corne is coruen wyth crokez kene" [In August, in the harvest season, when corn is cut down with sharp scythes] (39–40)—works with the garden setting to draw the pestilence into dialogue with the poem's dominant allegorical and elegiac concerns. Critics have most frequently regarded *Pearl*'s departure from the traditional vernal dream vision as a complement to the poem's narrative of mourning:[44] the poet mines the associations of death and rebirth that append to England's August harvest much as Keats does in his season of mists and mellow fruitfulness. Equally important, the fecundity of the harvest amplifies the images already developed in the poem as metaphors for Christian resurrection: the fleshly fruit enclosing the seed that engenders anew the "wortez ful schyre and schene" [flowers so bright and shining] (42); the material corpse in the ground that finds "gostly" [spiritual] (185) perfection as a denizen of the New Jerusalem. Lingering within these discourses, however, is the far less metaphorical death associated with the pestilence itself, which often peaked in the summer months when comparatively warm conditions seem to have enabled its rapid spread.[45] Chronicle evidence from the fourteenth and fifteenth centuries shows that later outbreaks occurred most frequently in the summer. In London, the devastating 1361 epidemic reached its most violent levels from May to July, and in 1375 plague mortality was at its highest in many parts of England in July and August,[46] a period when, as Thomas Walsingham reports, the weather "*fuere calores nimij*" [was extremely hot].[47] The 1389 and 1391 plague outbreaks were also at their most severe in July and August, while a 1393 outbreak in Essex reached its apex in September and October.[48] There were, of course, exceptions to this pattern; the plague could and did strike throughout the calendar year. However, the correlation between summertime and plaguetime invests *Pearl*'s late summer meditations on death and new life with a surprising currency, particularly for fourteenth-century readers wary of how the "crokez kene" [sharp scythes] (40) of the harvest sometimes presaged the onset of the pestilence. It is precisely the plague's cyclical appearance, both

---

44. For one of many, see Spearing, *The Gawain Poet*, 140.

45. This pattern has been repeatedly traced in modern studies of the pandemic, especially by Cohn, *The Black Death Transformed*; Benedictow, *The Black Death*; and more recently Campbell, "The Great Transition." For a counterargument see Crespo and Lawrenz, "Heterogeneous Immunological Landscapes and Medieval Plague," 245–48.

46. Cohn, *The Black Death Transformed*, 184–85.

47. Walsingham, *Historia breuis Thomæ Walsingham*, 185.

48. See Creighton, *A History of Epidemics in Britain*, 217–21. Recent epidemiological studies of medieval plague cycles confirm similar seasonal patterns on the continent, especially Cohn, *The Black Death Transformed*, 140–87.

seasonally and diachronically, that allows the disease such seamless entreé into the human and soteriological cycles that *Pearl* explores in its own cyclical form, cycles that both turn within and transcend human history.[49]

Darkly, the corporeal corruption of the pestilence was, by the late 1300s, a corruption that disproportionately affected the young. Leicester chronicler Henry Knighton writes of the 1361 epidemic, "*mortalitas generalis oppressit populum quæ dicebatur pestis secunda. Et moriebantur tam majores quam minores, et maxime juvenes et infantes*" [a general death, which was called the second pestilence, crushed the people. And as many great people as lesser people died, and especially youths and children].[50] So, too, does the *Anonimalle* chronicler bewail the "*secunde pestilence parmy Engleterre la quel fuist appelle la mortalite des enfauntz*" [second pestilence throughout England, which was named the mortality of children],[51] a sentiment seconded by the Grey Friars of Lynn, who note that "*infantes in magno numero delevit*" [it exterminated children in great numbers].[52] The epidemic of 1361—the "*pestilentia puerorum*" [children's plague][53]—would prove the demographic pattern for outbreaks through the second half of the fourteenth century and into the fifteenth, a decades-long span in which successive waves of plague increasingly affected groups that had no opportunity to develop a resistance to it, namely those living in isolated communities or born after the initial epidemic.[54] Samuel Cohn writes, "More than class or sex, the most persistent and consistent change with late medieval plague across Europe was the age of its victims. Like many other infectious diseases, medieval plague, after striking virgin-soil populations, tended to kill those who had not been previously exposed to it the next time around. As a consequence, after several strikes, it became domesticated as a disease largely of children."[55]

Most likely written in the 1380s, when repeated outbreaks of plague most intensely affected the young, *Pearl* might be seen as attuned both to the personal tragedy of one girl's death and to the profound cultural rupture of the

---

49. This cyclicality is powerfully reiterated in the final poem of the manuscript, *Sir Gawain and the Green Knight*, when the poet marks the passage of the year from Gawain's decapitation of the Green Knight to the Knight's promised repetition of Gawain's blow (*Gaw.* 495–535).

50. Knighton, *Chronicon Henrici Knighton*, 2:116.

51. *The Anonimalle Chronicle*, 50.

52. "A Fourteenth-Century Chronicle from the Grey Friars at Lynn," 275.

53. *Chronicon Abbatie de Parco Lude*, 38.

54. Further chronicle evidence supports the continued susceptibility of children to the disease: a third wave of pestilence in 1369 and a fourth in 1374 were both regarded as particularly deadly for children in the *Anonimalle Chronicle* (58, 124), while Walsingham, *Historia breuis Thomæ Walsingham*, notes how the "fifth pestilence" of 1390–91 killed "*iuuenum præcipuè, & puerorum*" [especially young people and boys] (277).

55. Cohn, *The Black Death Transformed*, 212.

pestilence in the earthly figure of the Pearl Maiden, a child who "lyfed not two
3er in oure þede" [lived not for two years in our land] (483) and whose corporeal form—though spotless in the paradise of the Dreamer's vision—exists
in the terrestrial *erbere* as a body covered in *clot*, marred by *moul*, and over-
spread with *spysez*. A precious gem, a beloved daughter—the pearl takes on
the additional valence of a young casualty of the pestilence, a single representative of the countless children taken by the disease, one of a hundred thousand whose "flesch be layd to rote" [flesh is laid to rot] (958).[56] But, of course,
she is more than that. The pearl is also the redeemed Christian soul, the kingdom of Heaven, the gift of God's grace, and even, as the "maskellez bryd þat
bry3t con flambe" [immaculate bride, as bright as flame] (769), the spotless
body risen from the grave at the sounding of the last trumpet.[57] Simultaneously flawed and *maskellez*, the Pearl Maiden is thus a figure whose perfection
can be realized only through her physical decay. This signature paradox—one
that the poem continually reinscribes as it conflates the spotty and the clean,
the body and the spirit, the earthly child and the queen of heaven, the wounds
of the crucified Christ and the wool of the Lamb—is what allows *Pearl* to cling
to the earthly even as it reaches toward the transcendent, to create beauty and
even perfection from the spot. It is the same paradox that opens the possibility
that the poem is subtly engaged with the pestilence, a disease of black spots
and buboes and living decay that emerges here both as an occasion for earthly
despair and a means to heavenly bliss.

In its language, its painstaking structure, and its maddeningly intricate
poetics, *Pearl* does more than simply consider the paradoxes of bodily death
and ghostly rebirth within the evolving context of the pestilence, more than
offer the solace of spiritual redemption in the face of grievous human loss.
Rather, the poem comes to embody and assimilate the very spots that evoke
the plague, taking into its poetic form the same flaws and mouls that it alternately reveals and occludes on the body of the dead girl, on the body of the
dying Christ, and on the Dreamer himself, whose body slumps upon the
earthly spot of the garden. Readers have long noticed that *Pearl*'s almost perfect form is riddled with provocative inconsistencies: the "extra" stanza in the

---

56. See also Freidl and Kirby, "The Life, Death, and Life of the Pearl-Maiden."

57. While it stops its exploration in the mid-thirteenth century, a decade before the emergence of the plague in Europe, Bynum's *The Resurrection of the Body in Western Christianity*
is suggestive here, particularly her central understanding of medieval Christian eschatology as
expressing "not body-soul dualism but rather a sense of self as psychosomatic unity. The idea
of person, bequeathed by the Middle Ages to the modern world, was not a concept of soul
escaping body or soul using body; it was a concept of self in which physicality was integrally
bound to sensation, emotion, reasoning, identity—and therefore finally to whatever one means
by salvation" (11).

fifteenth stanza group, which gives the poem a Jerusalem-appropriate 1212 lines;[58] the break in concatenation in stanza groups twelve and thirteen, which works to reinforce the link between "Jesus" (87–88n721) and "*ryȝt*" (720);[59] and so forth. Indeed, the poem's entire semantic strategy is predicated on the necessary flaw of the metaphor itself, what Stanbury calls "metaphor as a 'planned category mistake' in which linguistic limits and categories are willfully broken to engage new possibilities . . . a set of meanings over and beyond the literal."[60] As with the Dreamer's instructive misapprehension of the Pearl Maiden's teachings, the mistake of the metaphor becomes instrumental to the means by which the poem creates meaning, just as it is instrumental to *Pearl*'s theological probing and aesthetic beauty. Inasmuch as *Pearl* is a poem *about* spots, it is also a poem *of* spots, a work that, we might say, becomes pestilential as it reveals the hard-won beauty to which pestilence gives way.

THE VOCABULARY OF SALVATION AND THE SPOTTY BEAUTY OF IMPERFECTION

As the language and imagery associated with the plague seep through the poem, they mingle with *Pearl*'s prevailing narrative of mortality and resurrection in critical ways, inhabiting the poem and touching equally upon the dead girl *cum* Pearl Maiden and upon the wounded Christ of the Passion *cum* radiant Lamb. The spots that first appear in group one, for example, reappear when Christ calls the Pearl Maiden to him—"Cum hyder to Me, My lemman swete, / For mote ne spot is non in þe" [Come to me my sweet love, for no flaw or blemish is within you] (763–64)—and, still more suggestively, when the Dreamer remarks that the moon holds no power in the New Jerusalem because "to spotty ho is, of body to grym" [she is too spotty, and her body too grim] (1070), a description that reinforces the disease and corporeal degradation to which the vulnerable human *corpus* is subject. Moreover, *Pearl* exploits a rich array of synonyms for the word *spot*, many of which similarly evoke

58. There have been several studies of the numerology of *Pearl*, most recently Condren, *The Numerical Universe of the Gawain-Pearl Poet*. *Pearl*'s numerical structure is also considered in Fritz, "*The Pearl*: The Sacredness of Numbers"; Fleming, "The Centuple Structure of the *Pearl*"; and tangentially in Martin, "Allegory and Symbolism," especially 337–38.

59. Andrew and Waldron, among other editors, emend "Jesus" to "Ryȝt" in order to preserve the formal regularity of the poem's link words. Their emendation notwithstanding, I would argue that the identification of Jesus with "Ryȝt" may just as easily be another carefully planned "error" on the part of the poet. Given that *Pearl* exists in only one manuscript, this textual crux is patently unsolvable (Andrew and Waldron, *The Poems of the* Pearl *Poet*).

60. Stanbury, "Introduction," *Pearl*, 3.

the physical symptoms of the plague, as well as to the shifting relationship between earthly flaw and cosmic perfection. Thus, the followers of the Lamb become "þys *motelez* meyny" (925)—this flawless, place-less, spotless multitude. Meanwhile, the New Jerusalem emerges as

> þe borȝ þat we to pres
> Fro þat oure flesch be layd to rote,
> Þer glory and blysse schal euer encres
> To þe meyny þat is withouten mote.
> (957–60)

> [the city we fly to when our flesh is laid to rot; there glory and bliss shall forever increase to the spotless multitude.]

The New Jerusalem thus becomes sanctuary and final destination of those whose spotty bodies, like the body of the Pearl Maiden herself, are laid to rot within the ground, subject first to the physical shocks of disease and then to the postmortem ravages of the grave. Within the heavenly city, however, the whole host of maidens exist without a spot—without a physical location on the earth, without a spiritual blemish to keep them from the presence of the Lamb, without a spot to link them to the pestilence.

That such language should be used to describe the Pearl Maiden and her fellows in the New Jerusalem is not surprising: the relationship that the poem proposes between the "flesch . . . layd to rote" [flesh . . . laid to rot] (958) and the "meyny þat is withouten mote" [spotless multitude] (960) only amplifies the paradox created jointly by the Dreamer, who laments in the opening stanza group that his pearl is "clad in clot" [covered in clods] (22), and the Pearl Maiden, who declares herself to be "vnblemyst" [unblemished] (781) and "wythouten blot" [without spot] (781).[61] The Maiden's assertion that the *grym* body of the moon cannot affect the New Jerusalem additionally recalls how the earthbound Dreamer cannot "tempte [the] wit" [test the wisdom] (904) of the Maiden because he is "mokke and mul among" [among muck and earth] (905), a poignant reminder of the longing for communion—both human and divine—that propels the Dreamer's lament and animates *Pearl*'s understated sacramental conclusion. Such statements highlight the perfection of those souls allowed within the heavenly city, and they reinforce the concomitant imperfection of those kept outside; however, they also reify the paradox of the

---

61. Freidl and Kirby, in "The Life, Death, and Life of the *Pearl*-Maiden," note that *blot* may be "particularly significant since *blot* is considered to be a borrowing from OFr. *blo(s)tre*, a boil" (375).

body itself. Transient, prone to disease, ever subject to "fylþe oþer galle" [filth or gall] (1060), the body in *Pearl* reveals the gross decay that is a product of its flawed mortality *and* shows how that decay becomes necessary to immortality. Within *Pearl*'s multivalent (and plague-inflected) language, such a focus would have offered the poem's fourteenth-century readers a consolation not unlike the one offered to the Dreamer himself. Just as the evident formal and aesthetic beauty of the poem absorbs and then transcends the *spottez* and *clottez* of its imperfect poetic form, so does the resonant soteriological framework that *Pearl* invokes—the promise of eternal beauty emerging from the spotted body—provide a means to assimilate the devastating losses of the plague into a consoling cultural-religious discourse, one shaded by the imagery and the language of pestilent disease.

The contradictions of the body become still more crucial when the poem turns to consider Christ himself. Throughout the poem, the figure of Christ, like the spotty and spotless Maiden, oscillates between the radiant Lamb with its single life-giving wound and the scourged man of the flesh who "schede Hys blode" [shed His blood] (741) and suffered "with payne" [with pain] (954) in the earthly Jerusalem. But despite these oscillations, the poem also insists that the Christ of the Passion and the Lamb are the same. It is precisely the single bleeding wound on the Lamb that gives eternal life to the heavenly city's "spotleȝ perleȝ" [spotless pearls] (856), precisely the flaw in the flesh that redeems the faithful. The very perfection of the Lamb, the wellspring of life offered by his blood, is coterminous with the rent in his side, the single wound within the flawless form:

The Lombe delyt non lyst to wene;
Þaȝ He were hurt and wounde hade,
In His sembelaunt watz neuer sene,
So wern His glentez gloryous glade.
(1141–45)

[No one could help but see the Lamb's delight. Though He was hurt and had a wide wound it never showed in his face, so glorious and glad was his gaze.]

Here, the paradox of perfection's necessary imperfection is made incarnate in the life-giving Lamb, whose delight and perfection are evident despite ("þaȝ") the still-flowing wounds of his crucifixion. Unlike the Maiden's body, which the Maiden insists is transcended by her redeemed soul, the corporeal wounds of Christ are one with his celestial perfection. Within the figure of the wounded Lamb, the rent side—the spot, the flaw, the open "wounde ful wyde and weete" [wound so wide and wet] (1135)—is inseparable from the "wolle quyte so ronk and ryf . . . þat mot ne masklle moȝt on stretche." [white wool so luxuriant and thick . . . to which neither spot nor flaw might cling] (844, 843).

In exploring the coexistence of imperfection and flawlessness, *Pearl* also reveals its affinity with the remaining poems in its manuscript. *Cleanness* in particular develops a deeply ambiguous relationship with the spots of the body and the soul, one that complicates its assertion that those who "any vnclannesse hatz on, auwhere abowte" [have any uncleanness anywhere] (30) are denied the beatific vision. While it is fiercely critical of the physical and spiritual sins detailed in its exempla, *Cleanness*'s explicitly typological structure also insists upon the complex relationship between such "fylþez" [filths] (14) and Christ's "clannes" [cleanness] (1087), especially in Christ's ministrations to the sick: "For whatso He towched also tyd tourned to hele, / Wel clanner þen any crafte cowþe devyse" [For whatsoever He touched turned to health, and became much cleaner than any human craft could devise] (1099–100). *Cleanness* also shares with *Pearl* a recognition of the stark beauty engendered by—and embedded within—the biblical punishments that Christ's incarnation promises to supersede. In its depiction of the Flood, for example, the doomed antediluvians experience an emotional and even spiritual apotheosis just before their drowning. We witness with increasing sympathy the "frendez [who] fellen in fere and faþmed togeder, / To dryȝ her delful destyné and dyȝen alle samen" [friends who came together and embraced one another, to suffer their doleful fate and to die together] (399–400), the lovers who resign themselves "to ende alle at onez and for euer twynne" [to end their lives at the same moment and part forever] (402), and the mothers and children who "heterly to þe hyȝe hyllez . . . haled on faste" [fled as quickly as they could into the high hills] (380).[62] Generations later, the idolatrous and drunken Belshazzar achieves a similar moment of grace when he glorifies the prophet Daniel with a "coler of cler golde" [collar of pure gold] (1744), declaring him "heȝest of alle oþer saf onelych tweyne" [highest of all men in the court, except for two] (1749). Even Lot's wife is provided with a moment of subtle dignity when, apparently out of sympathy for those dying in Sodom, "ho bluschet to þe burȝe" [she glanced toward the city] (982), her all-too-human transgression against God's command.

---

62. The pronounced sympathy that the poem accords to the antediluvians has attracted significant critical attention, and I will address it myself in my chapter on *Cleanness* below. See Reading, "Ritual Sacrifice and Feasting," suggests that our sympathy for the victims is part of a pattern of ritual sacrifice, one that requires the Flood itself to register as "an undeserved but necessary thing, evoking an intense feeling of pity" (282). See also Calabrese and Eliason, "The Rhetorics of Sexual Pleasure and Intolerance"; Wallace, "*Cleanness* and the Terms of Terror."

Analogous moments of redemption and transcendence emerge from the physical filths and imperfections detailed in both *Patience* and *Sir Gawain and the Green Knight*. Jonah is at his most spiritually compliant when he is vomited onto the shore near Ninevah, his body and clothes "sluchched" [soiled] (*Pat.* 341) from the "ramel ande myre" [muck and mire] (279) of the whale's belly. So, too, do the Ninevites most comport with the divine when they purify themselves through acts of physical abasement, covering their bodies with dust and ash to bring themselves closer to God. And of course, Sir Gawain achieves his most ecstatic emotional and spiritual release at the moment he receives his signature physical blemish, the "nirt in þe nek" [nick in the neck] (*Gaw.* 2498) that he earns from the Green Knight's third stroke, the "schene blod" [bright blood] (2314) that "blenk on þe snawe" [shone on the snow] (2315). Such passages, which present imperfection as coterminous with an overwhelming emotional and spiritual consummation, resonate with *Pearl*'s apotheosized and bleeding lamb, whose perfection is likewise predicated upon his horrifying and beautiful wound. So, too, do they resonate with the structure of the poem's dream, which, as Stanbury notes, provides the Dreamer with "a kind of visual *jouissance* that culminates in his attempt to cross the stream and fracture the divide between his body and the object of his gaze."[63] These dramatic conjunctions of physical imperfection and spiritual completion, so central to the soteriological concerns of all four poems, are rendered in language and imagery reminiscent of the plague—the spots and bruises of the crucified Christ in *Pearl*; the physical scourges that await Jonah in the belly of the whale; the burst of red blood against white snow and the nick in Gawain's neck; the septic waters of the Flood and the Dead Sea.

With that said, I do not want to imply that the wound in the side of the *Pearl*'s Lamb *is* simply a running plague sore, any more than I want to assert that the Dead Sea *is* a one-to-one analogue for a suppurating carbuncle. Nor do I want to argue that Christ himself is merely the poet's stand-in for a plague victim. The bruises and wounds of Christ were common images well before the arrival of the pestilence, as were the waters of the Flood and the Dead Sea; their significance in the poems is multivalent and complex. Nonetheless, the metaphorical flexibility of such visual and literary images—the spotty and tortured Christ who ascends spotless from his tomb; the pearly Lamb whose bleeding wound offers life to the Christian faithful—allows them to absorb and mediate the ongoing experience of the plague, a process though which both image and experience are mutually recontextualized. Just as Grünewald uses the physical marks of contemporary disease to inform his sixteenth-

---

63. Stanbury, "Feminist Masterplots," 100.

century altarpiece, so, too, does the writer of *Pearl* saturate his meditations on salvation and rebirth with language and imagery evocative of the plague. Whether this saturation represents a conscious strategy by the poet or reflects his unconscious immersion in a world beset by pestilence, the poet situates the disease within the totalizing frame of Christian soteriology while simultaneously revivifying the ahistorical discourse of Christian soteriology by revealing its relevance to the contemporary pandemic.

For *Pearl*—both as an elegy for a young girl and as a universal allegory of Christian salvation—the net result is twofold. By insinuating its lament for the child into an existing soteriological framework that emphasizes the emergence of flawless "goste" [spirit] (63) from spotty body, the poem offers a consolation that accords with the losses of the pestilence and that reestablishes the redemptive promise of the "makelez Lambe þat al may bete" [matchless Lamb that may make all things better] (757). At the same time, by implicitly comparing the suffering of Christ to the suffering of those ravaged by plague, the poem grounds the Passion and the Resurrection in physical terms that would have been particularly evocative for English readers familiar with the symptoms of the disease. As both elegy and allegory—as both personal lament and public lesson—*Pearl* heightens its affective potential by absorbing the language and imagery of the pestilence into its mingled discourses. Much like *Cleanness* and its Old Testament exempla, *Pearl* not only evokes the plague experience through its subtle and recursive references to the *spottez* and *moulynge* of the flesh; it comes to embody that experience within its own poetics, assimilating the disease into its own textual body, resonating with and then transcending its cankers, bloody sores, and signal imperfections. The poem thus forces its readers to confront, in its delicate aesthetic beauty and in its moments of imagistic and narrative abjection, the paradoxically twinned biological and soteriological ends of the pestilence, the physical and emotional suffering linked with the ecstatic release of salvation, the failed spotty body that opens out to radiant eternal life.

Nonetheless, the cold human comfort that *Pearl* offers and the still more austere spiritual lesson it strives to teach prove difficult to reconcile with the raw fact of death itself. As David Aers writes, death stands in *Pearl* as "a massive challenge to human identity, the disclosure of an utter powerlessness framing our will to control others, our environments, and ourselves."[64] It is precisely this challenge that the Dreamer registers as he struggles to square his own searing grief with an intransigent divine will. Indeed, as late as the

---

64. Aers, "The Self Mourning," 56.

poem's concluding stanza group, the Dreamer acknowledges the ongoing tension between these two powerful drives, admitting his continued personal turmoil even as he putatively, ruefully submits to God:

> I raxled, and fel in gret affray
> And, sykyng, to myself I sayd:
> "Now al be to þat Pryncez paye."
> (1174–76)

[I awoke restlessly and fell into great consternation, and sighing, I said to myself, "Now let all be given to the satisfaction of that Prince."]

The Dreamer also struggles with the reality of death when he first sees the Pearl Maiden in the bejeweled otherworld of his vision. At once a "faunt" [child] (161) and a "mayden of menske" [lady of courtly grace] (162), the Pearl Maiden gradually emerges as the lost pearl itself, the jewel and the girl buried in the garden. Initially overjoyed that he has been reunited with his pearl—"Suche gladande glory con to me glace" [such gladdening exaltation then glided over me] (171)—the Dreamer quickly succumbs to a new wave of dread, apparently fearing that he may again lose what he seems to have found:

> More þen me lyste my drede aros:
> I stod ful stylle and dorste not calle;
> Wyth yȝen open and mouth ful clos
> I stod as hende as hawk in halle.
> I hoped þat gostly watz þat porpose;
> I dred onende quat schulde byfalle,
> Lest ho me eschaped þat I þer chos,
> Er I at steuen hir moȝt stalle.
> (181–88)

[More than I wished, my dread arose. I stood motionless and dared not call out. With eyes open and mouth fully closed, I stood as courteous as a hawk in hall. I thought that her purpose must have been spiritual; I dreaded at once what might happen if the one I saw there escaped the moment before I could stop her.]

Aers locates in this moment "a double fear—the fear that 'so strange a place' may signify unknown changes and, decisively, the fear of loss, the fear that she

on whom he now gazes will elude him again."[65] Such a reading justly highlights
the emotional and psychological responses to which the Dreamer is necessarily subject, perhaps even revealing a posttraumatic inarticulacy that borders in
this instance on paralysis. However, the fear of loss that the Dreamer evinces
here also indicates his inability to distinguish the "gostly" from the physical,
the transcendent domain of God from the earthly—and specifically aristocratic—domain of the "hawk in halle" [hawk in hall] (184), of the English
court itself.[66] Even within the spiritual otherworld of his vision, the Dreamer
is unable to reconcile the atemporality of the Pearl's eternal existence with his
own knowledge of temporal loss, with the inevitable series of ruptures and
bereavements pursuant to earthly life.[67]

This manifestly human failure is central to *Pearl*'s narrative progress; it
precipitates "the narrator's acts of passionate misreading and misinterpre-
tation," and it propels the central dialogue between the Pearl Maiden and
the Dreamer.[68] Less immediately apparent is how the loss that the Dreamer
alternately experiences and fears is consistently figured in the terms of personal abandonment, both the pearl's abandonment of the jeweler and, more
obliquely, his own abandonment of the pearl. No sooner does the Dreamer
invoke his loss than he describes how the pearl "fro me yot" [slipped away
from me] (9). In a similar fashion, the Dreamer declares that he "wyste neuer
quere [his] perle watz gon" [never knew where his pearl was gone] (376), again
emphasizing the pearl's agency in fleeing, as well as his own crisis of unknowing and loss. Most poignantly, when he recognizes the Maiden gathered with
her fellows at Christ's feet, the Dreamer laments, "Þen saȝ I þer my lyttel quen
/ Þat I wende had standen by me in sclade" [Then I saw there my little queen,
whom I thought had still been standing next to me in the valley] (1148–49),
a final abandonment that precipitates the Dreamer's ill-fated effort to rejoin
(or perhaps to reclaim) his daughter across the river. But despite his ongoing
sense of abandonment, the Dreamer also suggests his own agency in the loss
of the pearl: his foundational lament, "Allas! I leste hyr in on erber" [Alas! I
lost her in a garden] (8), echoes across the poem with a sense of personal culpability that is never fully effaced. These lingering senses of abandonment and
personal culpability are redoubled by the expressly courtly mode of the poem
itself, which constantly forces us to refigure the implicitly familial relationship
between the Pearl Maiden and the Dreamer as the hierarchical relationship
between a "mayden of menske, ful debonere" [debonair lady of courtly grace]

---

65. Aers, 60.
66. See Spearing, *The Gawain Poet*, especially 147–50.
67. Aers, "The Self Mourning," 62.
68. Stanbury, "Introduction," 4.

(162) and a "joylez jueler" [joyless jeweler] (252) whose gentility she questions. Aranye Fradenburg recognizes courtly discourse as operating within "an economy of sacrifice as well as prosthesis," in which "a great man risks a little prestige when he condescends to courtly friendship with a lesser man, and a lesser man risks what rank he has by approaching a greater man."[69] Within *Pearl*, the jeweler's insecure social and spiritual status is consistently overwhelmed by the luminescent certitude of the Maiden's heavenly queenship. The risk of courtly loss, which Fradenburg situates within "the court's special claim to *jouissance*—its pursuit, its travail, even its passionate self-extinction," is everywhere reinscribed.[70]

Such are the contradictory terms in which we must finally understand the Dreamer's *drede*, a polyvalent word that evokes the patently human anxieties surrounding bereavement and abandonment, articulates the posttraumatic paralysis and inarticulacy that follows profound loss, acknowledges the structures of sacrifice inherent within the courtly nexus, and also gestures toward the "drede of Dryȝtan" [dread of the Lord] (*Cl.* 295) appropriate to the presence of the divine. Might this *drede* also intimate the fear of contagion that the poem raises in its opening stanza group?[71] Again, we can only speculate; however, it is worth noting how closely the memorable phrase "I stod as hende as hawk in halle" [I stood as courteous as a hawk in hall] resonates with the description Machaut provides of himself in *Jugement dou Roy de Navarre*, waiting out the plague in Paris "*comme un esprevier qu'on mue*" [like a hawk in moult].[72] The confluence of these emotional, social, theological, and even pestilential possibilities is most fully realized in the Dreamer's declaration, "More þen me lyste my drede aros" [More than I wished, my dread arose] (181). Here, confronted with the daughter he believed to be beneath the ground, now transcendent, queenly, and perfected, the Dreamer registers at once a painful human desire to be with his lost pearl, a profound fear of the

---

69. Fradenburg, *Sacrifice Your Love*, 100.

70. Fradenburg, 80.

71. The Dreamer's ongoing fear of contagion may additionally be suggested by the word *galle*, which the Dreamer uses in relation to the Pearl Maiden just after he reveals his "drede." It is, as Freidl and Kirby rightly point out (395), yet another synonym for spot; however, it also means "poison or venom." *MED*, s.v. "galle" n.(1), n.(2).

72. Machaut, *The Judgment of the King of Navarre*, 22–23 (l. 460). Machaut's terror of contagion comes to the fore earlier in the poem, when he writes, "*Je ne fui mie si hardis / Que moult ne fusse acouardis*" [I was not at all so brave / That I did not become very cowardly] (20–21, ll. 433–34). To my knowledge, this sympathy between the *Pearl*-Poet's work and Machaut's more overt response to the plague in *Navarre* has not yet been explored.

I would also note here that the Dreamer's emphasis on standing "Wyth yȝen open and mouth ful clos" (*Pe.* 183) may offer an oblique allusion to theories of plague transmission through vision, discussed more fully by Fumo in "The Pestilential Gaze," especially 130–35.

Maiden's ghostly purpose, a sudden recognition of the sacrifices demanded of his position within both the earthly and heavenly courts, a suffocating combination of remorse over her loss and resentment over his own abandonment, and perhaps even a shock of fear over the possibility of contagion.

It is difficult to imagine a more paradoxical collision of responses, or a more poignant one for a parent grieving the loss of a child. As a number of chroniclers and poets attest, however, these were precisely the responses occasioned by the Black Death and its recurrences. Gabriele de' Mussis's *Historia de Morbo*, which documents the first wave of the pandemic to strike continental Europe, recalls the cries of children suffering from plague, abandoned by parents too terrified to approach them. So, too, does it capture the sense of abandonment felt by parents whose children had either died of the disease or fled from fear of it.

> *O pater cur me deseris, esto non immemor geniture. . . . O Mater ubi es, cur heri mihi pia modo crudelis efficeris. Que mihi lac vberum propinasti, et nouem mensibus, vtero portasti. . . . O, filij, quos sudore et laboribus multis educauj cur fugitis.*[73]

> [O father, why have you deserted me? Do you forget that you engendered me? . . . O mother, where are you; why are you cruel to me now when you were tender yesterday? You gave me milk from your breasts and for nine months carried me in your womb. . . . O children, whom I raised with much sweat and labor, why have you fled?]

In a similar account of the pestilence in Oxfordshire, one chronicler relates how "*vix aliquis infirmum ausus est contingere*" [hardly anybody dared to touch the sick],[74] while in Scotland, John of Fordun notes that the plague generated "*tanto horrore*" [such horror] that "*filii parentes, in extremis laborantes, et e converso, metu quodam contagionis, veluti a facie lepræ vel colubri fugientes, non auderent visitare*" [sons would not dare to visit their parents, even in the pains of death, because of the dread of contagion, fleeing as if from the presence of leprosy or from a serpent].[75] The dissolution of the bond between parent and child is further detailed by Boccaccio, who recounts with incredulity how "*era con sí fatto spavento questa tribulazione entrata ne' petti degli uomini e delle donne, che . . . quasi non credibile, li padri e le madri i figliuoli,*

---

73. Gabriele de' Mussis, *Historia de Morbo*, 53.
74. Geoffrey le Baker, *Chronicon Galfridi le baker de Swynebroke*, 99.
75. John of Fordun, *Chronica gentis Scotorum*, 369.

quasi loro non fossero, di visitare e di servire schifavano" [men and women alike were possessed by such a visceral terror of this scourge that . . . believe it or not, mothers and fathers would avoid visiting and tending their children, they would virtually disown them],[76] and by Machaut, who describes how *"li fils failloit au pere, / La fille failloit a la mere, / La mere au fil et a la fille / Pour doubtance de la morille"* [father lacked son, / Mother lacked daughter, / Son and daughter lacked mother / Because of fear for the plague].[77] These same fissures in social and familial relations are, I would suggest, negotiated by *Pearl*'s Dreamer, a father who both celebrates and mourns his lost daughter, who simultaneously desires and dreads her presence, and whose ready combination of fear and guilt leads him to remark that she is without *galle*—without flaw, without spot, without sore, without venom, and without bitterness at the paralyzing human *drede* her earthbound father exhibits.

And what of the other maidens, "a hondred and forty þowsande flot" [a hundred and forty thousand in a host] (786), radiant and spotless beneath "legyounes of aungelez" [legions of angels] (1120), surrounded by "ensens of swete smelle" [sweet smelling incense] (1121)? As the poem nears its conclusion and the Dreamer gazes upon the heavenly court of the New Jerusalem, *Pearl* widens the aperture of its poetic lens, taking in not only one young bride of the Lamb but many young brides, a multitude of spotless maidens gathered under his "lombe-ly3t" [lamb/lamp light] (1046). The figure of "an hundreþe þowsande, / And fowre and forty þowsande mo" [a hundred and forty-four thousand] (869–70) has a scriptural precedent in the Book of Revelation, but for late medieval readers, the expressly apocalyptic image of thousands upon thousands of maidens gathered in new life at the foot of the Lamb—their earthly bodies, like that of the Dreamer's daughter, moldering in the *clot* and *moul* of the grave—must have resonated as well on a human, even a communal level. Such a multitude of heavenly souls, I would suggest, could not help but bring to mind the scores of thousands killed by a disease so virulent that *"les vives ne purroint enseveler les mortz"* [the living were not able to bury the dead].[78] Finally, it is this moment of personal, spiritual, and civic revelation, when the Pearl Maiden slips from the Dreamer's side and reappears in the Holy City "among her ferez" [among her companions] (1150), that the poem at once fully embraces and radically transcends the elegiac and allegorical modes that readers have traditionally ascribed to it. As elegy, the poem mourns the loss of a beloved child even as it celebrates her ascension into an eternal para-

---

76. Boccaccio, *Decameron*, 16 (Waldman, 10).

77. Machaut, *The Judgment of the King of Navarre*, 15–16 (ll. 333–36).

78. *The Anonimalle Chronicle*, 30. The cliché reappears in many chronicle accounts of the plague.

dise where her body is at last free of the spots of her disease. As allegory, it offers a compelling vision of salvation in which the pearl, the unsullied and penitent Christian soul, is called through Christ's sacrifice to join her fellows in eternal life. But in the context of the ongoing pandemic, the elegy in these final lines also surpasses the expression of personal grief for an individual, offering a lament not for one but for countless children, whole generations— an elegy for England itself, even for the whole dying world. And considered in the same context, the poem's allegory likewise overreaches its immediate soteriological valences to comment also upon the eschatological and the apocalyptic, speaking not only to the salvation of the individual soul but evoking the decades following the first wave of the plague, when, as Laura Smoller has noted, successive outbreaks of the disease were seen as "key signs and portents [heralding] the nearness of the apocalypse."[79]

This shift from the soteriology to eschatology—from salvation to apocalypse—is a dramatic one in *Pearl,* but as with the poem's language and imagery, it comports with our understanding of the medieval response to the Black Death. A broad spectrum of English and continental writers, chroniclers and poets alike, saw the plague as a harbinger of the Apocalypse. William Dene of Rochester, author of the *Historia Roffensis,* regards the terrifying extent of the mortality as evidence that Gog and Magog—comrades of the Antichrist and dark heralds of the Second Coming—had already returned to the known world.[80] Similarly, an Anglo-Latin lyric from the late fourteenth century known as "On the Pestilence" deploys rhetoric commonly associated with the Apocalypse: "*Fortes Christi milites modo recesserunt; / Sathanæ satellites templum subverterunt; / Laceras et debiles oves perdiderunt*" [The powerful warriors of Christ have now retreated; / Satan's courtiers have overturned the temple; / they have lost the wounded and disabled sheep].[81] In Italy, Boccaccio captures a looming sense of millennium when he discusses how frightened citizens fled plague-ravaged Florence believing "*la sua ultima ora esser venuta*" [its last hour had come].[82] And in the Malvern Hills, William Langland specifically associates "pokkes and pestilences" [poxes and plagues] (B.XX.98) with the coming of the Antichrist. *Pearl,* too, can be read in the company of these works and in the context of this particular cultural trauma. A poem simultaneously invested in Christian salvation, earthly loss, and the struggle to rec-

---

79. Smoller, "Plague and the Investigation of Apocalypse," 163. For a succinct overview of the millenarianism associated with the pestilence, see Lerner, "The Black Death and Western European Eschatological Mentalities."

80. See *Historia Roffensis,* in Horrox, *The Black Death,* 73.

81. "On the Pestilence," 280.

82. Boccaccio, *Decameron,* 15 (Waldman, 10).

oncile human grief with the divine will, *Pearl* might also be recognized as a meditation on the personal, soteriological, and even eschatological shocks that the pestilence inflicted on England throughout the second half of the fourteenth century, a work engaged with an ongoing trauma at once local and universal, timely and eternal, crushingly immediate and harrowingly apocalyptic.

PART 2

Beyond the Symptomatic

Considering the Plague in Fourteenth-Century England

CHAPTER 3

Flight and Enclosure in *Patience*

It is important that we not overlook that any epidemic
proceeds from the divine will, in which case we
can only counsel to return humbly to God.

—Report of the Medical Faculty of Paris, Oct. 7, 1347[1]

WRITTEN IN THE shadow of the 1829 cholera pandemic, Edgar Allan Poe's "Masque of the Red Death" is a grotesque of Boccaccio's *Decameron*. The would-be *brigata* of Poe's short story, a group of one thousand debauched aristocrats led by the eccentric Prince Prospero, takes refuge from epidemic disease not by traveling to an airy Tuscan villa but by sealing themselves into a fortified abbey, resolving "to leave means neither of ingress or egress to the sudden impulses of despair or of frenzy from within."[2] But while Boccaccio's ten youths return to Florence with health and spirits intact, Poe's thousand courtiers meet an altogether grislier fate. At the stroke of midnight during an opulent masque, an unknown guest, costumed as a victim of the Red Death, appears inside the abbey. Most of the revelers draw away in horror, but Prospero, enraged by the costume, attacks the stranger before suddenly dropping dead himself. Desperately and irrationally courageous, the remaining guests then rush toward the figure and strip off his robes, only to discover no one underneath. "And now," Poe concludes, "was acknowledged the presence of the Red Death. He had come like a thief in the night. And one by one dropped

---

1. "*Amplius pretermittere nolumus quod epidimia aliquando a divina uoluntate procedit, in quo casu non est aliud consilium nisi quod ad ipsum humiliter recurratur.*" "The Report of the Medical Faculty of Paris," 156.

2. Poe, "The Masque of the Red Death," 670–71. A recent overview of critical responses to the story, including references to the cholera pandemic, can be found in Haspel, "Bells of Freedom and Foreboding."

the revellers in the blood-bedewed halls of their revel. . . . And Darkness and Decay and the Red Death held illimitable dominion over all."[3]

Poe's story, like its eponymous disease, is a work of fiction; however, it resonates with the medieval plague experience in revealing ways.[4] The perceived link between plague and moral degeneracy, for instance, which Chaucer exploits in his "Pardoner's Tale," is clearly evoked in Prospero's dissolute revelers, and the symptoms of the Black Death itself—its rapid and often bloody presentation—are vividly recast in the pathology of the Red Death. But perhaps the most crucial parallels between Poe's story and the fourteenth-century pandemic are the two responses to the threat of contagion staged by Prospero's guests: their initial flight from the disease and their claustration in the "safe" locus of the abbey. For evidence of the former in the Middle Ages, we need look no further than Pampinea's argument in *The Decameron*: "*io giudicherei ottimamente fatto che noi, sì come noi siamo, sì come molti innanzi a noi hanno fatto e fanno, di questa terra uscissimo, e fuggendo come la morte i disonesti essempli degli altri onestamente a' nostri luoghi in contado*" [the best thing we can do in our present situation is to leave the city, as so many have done before us and are still doing, and go stay in our country estates].[5] For the latter, we might recall Machaut hiding from the plague in his sealed chamber like a reclusive "*esprevier qu'on mue*" [hawk in molt], as well as the strategies of quarantine and enclosure enacted by some medieval cities to manage outbreaks.[6]

Such considerations are suggestive for the third poem of the *Pearl* manuscript. A work marked by alternating episodes of flight and enclosure, *Patience* centers on the story of the reluctant prophet Jonah, his flight from God's command to preach, his three-day confinement inside a whale, and the events of his mission to Nineveh. Though largely faithful to the Latin Vulgate, the poem makes several important embellishments to its source, investing Jonah with a psychology only hinted at in the Bible and fleshing out the narrative with several original details.[7] These embellishments have, to a large degree, given modern criticism on *Patience* its shape.[8] They have been used to show

---

3. Poe, "The Masque of the Red Death," 676–77.

4. For possible medical analogues to the Red Death, see Silverman, *Edgar A. Poe: Mournful and Never-Ending Remembrance*.

5. Boccaccio, *Decameron*, 23–24 (Waldman, 16–17).

6. Machaut, *The Judgment of the King of Navarre*, 22–23 (l. 460). I discussed the phrase earlier in relation to *Pearl*'s Dreamer standing "as hende as hawk in halle" (Pe. 184).

7. See Diekstra, "Jonah and *Patience*: The Psychology of a Prophet," 205–6.

8. The watershed article in this regard is Berlin, "*Patience*: A Study in Poetic Elaboration."

the poem's consonance with homiletic and exegetical tradition,[9] analyzed to make assertions about audience,[10] considered in social contexts ranging from debates over church sanctuary to late medieval conceptions of maternity,[11] and, of course, marshalled to query the poem's titular virtue itself.[12] *Patience,* in other words, reveals its central concerns by how it develops the Latin Vulgate, how it renders the Book of Jonah into a culturally resonant work for its fourteenth-century readers.

At its core, this chapter continues this line of inquiry by reconsidering a number of interpretive problems presented by *Patience*—including its development of its biblical source and its curious use of Jonah (rather than the more obvious Job) to exemplify its central virtue—in the dual contexts of flight and enclosure, two prevalent but fraught responses to the plague in the Middle Ages. Building from the pestilential contexts developed in the first part of this study, I will speculate that just as the Old Testament exempla of *Cleanness* align with traumatic and posttraumatic responses associated with the plague's aftermath, *Patience*'s adaptation of the story of Jonah recalls how individuals and communities reacted to the plague's immediate threat, to the approach of a disease broadly understood as a manifestation of God's anger. Considered in these terms, *Patience* emerges as a poem focused resolutely on the "now," one driven not by the burdens of an unspeakable past (as is *Cleanness*) or the promise of a transcendent future (as is *Pearl*) but by a shifting series of more proximate concerns: fear, gratitude, frustration, self-preservation, joy, despair. Not simply a negative exemplar of the poem's titular virtue, Jonah becomes a figure for patterns of behavior intimately connected to the experience of the Black Death, a flawed but sympathetic figure through whom the poet explores the moral, theological, ethical, and even medical dimensions of resisting God's pestilential wrath.

This chapter will also consider how *Patience* resists the apocalyptic certainty of *Pearl* and *Cleanness,* and gestures instead toward the anxious and contingent universe of *Sir Gawain and the Green Knight,* the final poem in the Cotton Nero A.x manuscript. Such a reading is consonant with Sandra Pierson Prior's understanding of *Patience* as centered on "those who must work within history, who must cease looking to a distant, timeless future and

---

9. Tomasch, "*Patience* and the Sermon Tradition"; Hazard, "*Patience* and *The Book of Jonah*."

10. Hill, "The Audience of *Patience*"; Wolfe, "Monastic Obedience in *Patience*."

11. Spearing, "The Subtext of *Patience*: God as Mother and the Whale's Belly"; Allen, "Sanctuary and Love of this World."

12. For one among many examples, see Stock, "The 'Poynt' of *Patience*."

become instead responsive to the present reality of God and his will."[13] I situate that "present reality," however, within the cultural nexus of the medieval plague pandemic to consider the possibility that the poem tests the desperate exigencies of survival against a disease every bit as omnipresent and as terrible as Jonah's demanding God.

THE SUDDEN IMPULSES OF DESPAIR:
FLIGHT, AFFILIATION, AND GOD'S WILL

The urge to flee is a fundamental biological imperative, a reflexive response to emotional or physical threat.[14] Flight is, in this respect, coterminous not only with humanity but with animality: we have an innate urge to flee what will cause us physical or emotional trauma, what we believe will harm us, what we believe will kill us. And yet, if the *impulse* to flee is grounded in biology, the act of fleeing itself is socially and psychologically contingent, existing within a web of communal and familial affiliations, cultural expectations, and psychosocial impulses that complicate any simple equation between fear and flight.

Traditionally, flight has been understood as "nonsocial behavior" emerging from panic, a reflexive condition that has the potential to cause a "disintegration of social norms and cessation of action with reference to a group or institutional pattern [and that] sometimes results in the shattering of the strongest primary group ties and the ignoring of the most expected behavior patterns."[15] Such is the panic that Boccaccio famously describes as a response to the Black Death: "*era con sí fatto spavento questa tribulazione entrata ne' petti degli uomini e delle donne, che . . . quasi non credibile, li padri e le madri i figliuoli, quasi loro non fossero, di visitare e di servire schifavano*" [men and women alike were possessed by such a visceral terror of this scourge that . . . believe it or not, mothers and fathers would avoid visiting and tending their children, they would virtually disown them].[16] That panic, too, colors more contemporary responses to epidemic disease. Anthony Doryen, a survivor of a 2014 outbreak of Ebola hemorrhagic fever in Liberia, recounts how the disease "makes you afraid because when you get around your family, apparently

---

13. Prior, *The Fayre Formez of the Pearl Poet*, 146.

14. As early as 1915, physiologist Walter Bradford Cannon observed how the physical and physiological changes associated with both emotional and physical threat are "often distressingly beyond the control of the will," patterns now commonly known as the fight-or-flight response. See Cannon, *Bodily Changes in Pain, Hunger, Fear and Rage*, 185–87.

15. Quarantelli, "The Nature and Conditions of Panic," 270.

16. Boccaccio, *Decameron*, 16 (Waldman, 10).

you get in contact with it. It makes you go far away from your family."[17] Similar social patterns have been recognized in many other global health crises, including, most notably, the global AIDS pandemic.[18]

Recent studies of panic and mass flight, however, have pushed against this dominant paradigm, and while narratives like Boccaccio's and Doryen's still speak to the profound social rupture caused by epidemic disease, they only tell part of the story. Drawing on John Bowlby's work on attachment relationships, researchers have increasingly demonstrated that "rather than fight or flight, the typical response to danger is affiliation, that is, seeking the proximity of familiar conspecifics and places, even if this involves remaining in or approaching a situation of danger."[19] The tension that emerges between flight and affiliation, then, might be expressed as a tension between two equally ingrained responses to severe threat. One the one hand, fleeing from the familiar in an effort to avoid the danger of disease—fleeing from parents and children and entire communities—runs counter to the affiliative urge. On the other hand, moving toward such communities when they are also loci of contagion is anathema to the imperative for self-preservation that manifests as flight. This is a tension that we can see implied in several chronicle accounts of the Black Death, among them Geoffrey le Baker's description of frightened individuals who "*relicta mortuorum quondam et nunc preciosa tamquam infectiva sani fugiebant*" [fled the things left behind by the dead, formerly precious but now infectious to the healthy].[20] It is also a tension, I would suggest, that we might recognize in the first two poems of MS Cotton Nero A.x—in Lot's wife, who both flees and looks back upon the destruction of Sodom; in the doomed antediluvians, who run from the rising waters of the Flood but drown embracing their loved ones; and, more subtly, in *Pearl*'s Dreamer, who approaches the body of his dead daughter even as his spirit springs from the physical world. Within these works, the state that exists at the intersection of flight and affiliation is one of psychic and even physical paralysis. Indeed, in that respect, it is a state that recalls the "drede" [dread] (*Pe.* 181) experienced by the Dreamer when confronted with the grown figure of his lost daughter,

17. Onishi, "Ebola Turns Loving Care into Deadly Risk," *New York Times*, Nov. 13, 2014.

18. Strong, in "Epidemic Psychology," writes, "The distinctive social psychology produced by large-scale epidemic disease can potentially result in a fundamental, if short term, collapse of social order. All kinds of disparate but corrosive effects may occur: friends, family and neighbours may be feared—and strangers above all; the sick may be left uncared for; those felt to be carriers may be shunned or persecuted" (255).

19. Mawson, "Understanding Mass Panic," 98. See also Sime, "Affiliative Behaviour during Escape to Building Exits."

20. Geoffrey le Baker, *Chronicon Galfridi le Baker de Swynebroke*, 99.

a state engendered by severe trauma and expressed through bodily and linguistic inarticulacy.

As a specific response to the plague, flight occupied an ambiguous moral
and ethical space in the later Middle Ages, one reflected in a range of theoretical, medical, and religious writings. *The Decameron,* of course, uses an
episode of mass flight to structure its frame narrative, but even as Boccaccio
lays the groundwork for the departure of his genteel *brigata,* he also reveals
a caustic attitude toward flight that undercuts the supposed refinement of his
Florentine youths:

> Alcuni erano di più crudel sentimento, come che per avventura più fosse
> sicuro, dicendo niuna altra medicina essere contro alle pistilenze migliore
> né così buona come il fuggir loro davanti: e da questo argomento mossi, non
> curando d'alcuna cosa se non di sé, assai e uomini e donne abbandonarono
> la propia città, le proprie case, i lor luoghi e i lor parenti e le lor cose, e cer-
> carono l'altrui o almeno il lor contado, quasi l'ira di Dio a punire le iniquità
> degli uomini con quella pistolenza non dove fossero procedesse.[21]

> [Others there were who were totally ruthless and no doubt chose the safest
> option: there was in their view no remedy to equal that of giving the plague
> a very wide berth. On this premise any number of men and women deserted
> their city and with it their homes and neighbourhoods, their families and
> possessions, heedless of anything but their own skins, and made for other
> people's houses or for their country estates at any rate, as though the wrath of
> God, in visiting the plague on men to punish their iniquity, was never going
> to reach out to where *they* were.]

Interwoven with Boccaccio's moral indignation are several contradictory
understandings about what plague was, why it emerged, and how (and if) it
could be avoided. That the plague was contagious was recognized early during
the pandemic, and many medical authorities advised flight, even from immediate family members, as the best medicine against the disease.[22] The prominent physician Gentile of Foligno writes, "*concedo quod fugere . . . optimum in
peste particulari. Est enim hec passio venenorum venenosissima nam sua irra-
diatione et macula cunctos inficit*" [I concede that to flee . . . is best in this particular pestilence. Indeed, this disease is a most venomous of venoms, for its

---

21. Boccaccio, *Decameron,* 15 (Waldman, 9–10).

22. See Winslow, *The Conquest of Epidemic Disease:* "It was the Black Death which at last
taught the communicability of disease beyond any peradventure" (96).

spread and pollution infect everybody].[23] Another physician, Alfonso de Córdoba, likewise advises, "*hoc summum remedium est, fugere pestem, quia pestis
non sequitur fugientem*" [this is the best cure, to flee the pestilence, because
the pestilence does not follow the fugitive], while a later German tract recom-
mends, "get out quickly, go a long way away and don't be in a hurry to come
back."[24] Even the renowned physician Guy de Chauliac addresses the efficacy
of flight when he writes, "*in præseruatione non erat melius quam ante infec-
tione fugere regione*," advice repeated verbatim in a Middle English rendering
of Guy's *Surgery*: "In preseruynge þer was no bettre þan afore þe infeccioun to
fle þe contraye" [With regard to preservation, there is nothing better than to
flee the region before infection].[25]

Fear of contagion also provoked flight on a civic scale. In one well-documented example from Sicily, Michele da Piazza relates how the people of Messina "*migrare de civitate quam mori potius elegerunt; et non solum in urbem
veniendi, sed etiam appropinquandi ad eam negabatur. In aeris et in vineis
extra civitatem cum eorum familiis statuerunt mansiones*" [chose rather to go
away from the city than to die; and not only refused to come into the city but
indeed to approach it. They established lodgings with their families in the
open air and amidst the vines outside the city].[26] The diary kept by a Florentine apothecary records a similar observation: "*uscissene di molti frati e anda-
vano alle ville de'loro padri e loro parenti e amici*" [many of the *Frati* left the
city and went away to the villas of their fathers and relatives and friends].[27] In
France, the chronicle of Guillaume de Nangis notes that, for fear of contagion,
"*sacerdotes timidi recedebant, religiosis aliquibus magis audacibus administra-
tionem dimittentes*" [timid priests withdrew, abandoning the administration
of spiritual offices instead to a few brave clergy];[28] while in England, Thomas
Walsingham reports that "*villæ olim hominibus refertissimæ suis destitutæ-
sunt colonis*" [villages formerly crowded with people were destitute of their
inhabitants].[29]

---

23. Gentile of Foligno, *Singulare consilium contra pestilentiam*, unpaginated manuscript.
(Quotation is from the conclusion of *tertium capitulum*.)

24. Sudhoff, "*Epistola et regimen Alphontii Cordubensis de pestilentia*," 224; German plague
tract quoted in *The Pest Anatomized*, 3. The latter is also quoted in Horrox, *The Black Death*,
108.

25. Guy de Chauliac, *Dn. Guidonis de Cauliaco, in arte medica exercitatissimi chirurgia*, 115;
Guy de Chauliac, *The Cyrurgie of Guy de Chauliac*, 157.

26. Michele da Piazza, *Cronaca*, 83.

27. Landucci, *Diario Fiorentino dal 1450 al 1516 di Luca Landucci*, 154; translation from *A
Florentine Diary from 1450 to 1516*, ed. Jervis, 124.

28. Guillaume de Nangis, *Chronique Latine de Guillaume de Nangis*, 211.

29. Walsingham, *Historia breuis Thomæ Walsingham*, 159.

But if the plague was recognized as an illness that could hypothetically be avoided by flight, it was simultaneously understood to be a scourge sent by God, a judgment from which flight was impossible, and maybe even illicit. In fact, in the Muslim world, plague flight was specifically prohibited because the disease—qualified by fourteenth-century Syrian historiographer Abū Hafs 'Umar Ibn al-Wardī as "for the Muslims a martyrdom and a reward, and for the disbelievers a punishment and a rebuke"[30]—was seen as divinely ordained. While no explicit prohibition on flight existed in the Christian world, there remained a sense that running from the disease was immoral, uncharitable, and ultimately contrary to the will of God.[31]

The implicit impropriety of plague flight was even more pronounced when it involved civic or ecclesiastical figures, whose relationships to Christian precepts of service and *caritas* were vocationally and divinely ordained. Michele da Piazza complains bitterly in his chronicle that *"judices et notarii fexi ad testamenta facienda ire recusabant"* [judges and notaries refused to go and make wills] and, worse, that *"sacerdotes vero nullatenus ad domos infirmorum accedere timore pre nimio mortis trepidabant"* [priests would by no means approach the houses of the sick because of great fear of death].[32] The chronicler of the *Annales Pistorienses,* too, laments how "neither friar nor priest attended those wishing their services, because the disease spread from the sick to the well."[33] Certainly not all priests and civic officials (nor all members of the laity) fled in the face of contagion; on the contrary, the comparatively high mortality rates for clergy attest to just how many remained to minister to the sick. What is clear, however, is that the tension between flight and affiliation recognized by contemporary psychologists was mirrored in the fourteenth century by a tension between medical and theological opinions on flight, as well as by the conflicting priorities of survival and religious duty.

The point at which the will to survive and the duty to serve God diverge is precisely where Jonah finds himself at the beginning of *Patience.* Commanded by God to "nym þe way to Nynyue wythouten oþer speche, / And in þat ceté My saȝes soghe alle about" [take the road to Nineveh without any further speech, and sow My words all about in that city] (66–67), Jonah instead flees toward Tarshish, defying God's command in order to save his own skin. In the biblical account, no reason is offered for Jonah's flight: God tells Jonah to

30. Ibn al-Wardi, "Ibn al Wardī's 'Risālah al-naba' 'an al waba,'" 454. See also Cohn, The *Black Death Transformed,* 115–16.

31. See Horrox, *The Black Death,* 109.

32. Michele da Piazza, *Cronaca,* 87.

33. *Annales Pistorienses,* quoted in Cohn, The *Black Death Transformed,* 124.

preach, and Jonah simply turns tail.[34] In *Patience,* however, the poet adds an interior monologue in which Jonah fantasizes in gruesome detail about the agonies awaiting him in Nineveh:

> "I com wyth þose typþynges, þay ta me bylyue,
> Pynez me in a prysoun, put me in stokkes,
> Wryþe me in a warlok, wrast out myn yȝen.
> Þis is a meruayl message a man for to preche
> Amonge enmyes so mony and mansed fendes,
> Bot if my gaynlych God such gref to me wolde,
> For desert of sum sake þat I slayn were.
> At alle peryles," quoþ þe prophete, "I aproche hit no nerre."
> (78–85)

["If I show up with those tidings they'll seize me for sure, pin me in a prison, put me in the stocks, twist me into fetters and pluck out my eyes. This is a quite a message for a man to preach among so many enemies and cursed fiends, unless my gracious God would have me suffer such grief, the result of some offense for which I should be slain. Whatever the cost," said the prophet, "I will not get near to that city."]

This self-justifying speech comports with two important traditions surrounding the figure of Jonah. First it alludes to his typological status as an imperfect precursor to Christ, a link reinforced several lines later when Jonah frets that he might be "naked dispoyled, / On rode rwly torent with rybaudes mony" [stripped naked, piteously torn on a cross by a bunch of villains] (95–96).[35] Second, and more subtly, the passage gestures toward an exegetical tradition that saw in Jonah's act of disobedience a preemptive action against the Ninevites, who would eventually threaten Jonah's own people.[36] The prophet's defiance of God, then, might be understood not only as a crude attempt

---

34. Jonah 1:2–3.

35. See Friedman, "Figural Typology in the Middle English *Patience*"; Johnson, *The Voice of the Gawain-Poet,* 22.

36. This exegesis finds influential voice in Saint Jerome, who writes in *In Ionam,* "*Scit propheta, Sancto sibi Spiritu suggerente, quod paenitentia gentium ruina sit Iudaerum. Idcirco, amator patriae suae, non tam saluti inuidet Nineue quam non uult perire populum suum*" [Through the inspiration of the Holy Spirit, the prophet knows that the repentance of the Gentiles will be the ruin of the Jews. Also, as one who loves his homeland, he does not envy Nineveh's salvation as much as he does not want his people to perish]. Latin and translation both from Vasta, "Denial in the Middle English *Patience,*" 11. See also Vantuono, "The Structure and Sources of *Patience,*" 416–18.

at self-preservation but also as a principled bid to save Judea from future subjugation.

While both of these readings rightly embed Jonah's disobedience within relevant typological and exegetical contexts, I would suggest that the most striking feature of Jonah's rationale is not its consonance with patristic commentary but rather its impulsiveness, the decidedly ad hoc way that Jonah scrambles to justify his flight. If he is concerned with the future of the Jewish people, in other words, Jonah nonetheless expresses considerably *more* concern—or at least a more immediate concern—with keeping his eyes in his head, his limbs out of the stocks, and his body off the cross. What the poet emphasizes in his embellishment of the Vulgate, then, is raw panic, the terror that arises in Jonah precisely where his will to live conflicts with his responsibility to God.[37] We recognize that same panic in Jonah when he asserts, against all sense, that God cannot harm him in Tarshish (88), as well as in his equally delusional conviction that he will be safe from God's anger on the open sea (111–12), two more details original to the poet. What Jonah demonstrates then—more than Lot's wife and the antediluvians of *Cleanness* and certainly more than the vexed Dreamer of *Pearl*—is the impulse to flight unfettered by affiliation, a response to threat in which he "revert[s] automatically to primitive, highly-emotional, irrational behaviour," a purely nonsocial panic response.[38]

While Jonah's interior monologue is peppered with imagined torments, it is not suffused with the loaded puns and linguistic markers that I have suggested may align *Pearl* and *Cleanness* with the traumas of the plague. With the notable exception of the "malys" [malice] (70), "vilanye" [villainy] (71), and "venym" [venom] (71) that God ascribes to the Ninevites—a phrase that recalls "þe venym and þe vylanye and þe vycious fylþe" [the venom and the villainy and the vicious filth] (*Cl.* 574) of *Cleanness*'s Sodomites and that could also suggest what Thomas Moulton calls "the venym [venom] and the malice of the pestilence"[39]—such pestilential language is mostly absent from Jonah's flight to Tarshish. Nonetheless, the prophet's response conspicuously echoes responses to the plague recorded by both chroniclers and continental poets. Indeed, the poet's incredulity over Jonah's "wytles" [witless] (*Pat.* 113) belief that God has no power to cause harm over the ocean comes very close to Boc-

---

37. Malcolm Andrew also sees Jonah's panic imitated in the harried rhythms of the passage itself. See Andrew, "Biblical Paraphrase in the Middle English *Patience*," 51.

38. Sime, "Affiliative Behaviour during Escape to Building Exits," 22.

39. Quoted in Rawcliffe, *Urban Bodies*, 61. Moulton's fifteenth-century tract is a translation of John of Burgundy's influential treatise of 1365, and while it follows *Patience* by several decades, the linguistic parallels between the two remain striking.

caccio's dismissal of the Florentines who believe that *"l'ira di Dio"* [the wrath of God] cannot reach them outside the city walls.[40] More broadly, the central ironic thrust of *Patience*—that in attempting to flee from Nineveh Jonah ends up going there in the most foul way imaginable—finds a morbid analogue in contemporary accounts of plague-flight: the Messinese who abandoned their city only to find death waiting for them in the nearby town of Catania; the Vienese who *"ad tuciora loca se transtulerunt; sed quia prius erant infecti, propterea non poterant evadere quin ex eis quam plures morerentur"* [conveyed themselves to safe places, but because they were infected earlier as a result could not escape and many died]; the citizens of Reading, who experienced only *"fuga sine refugio . . . plurimi a facie pestilentiae fugerant infecti nec necem evaserant"* [flight without refuge . . . (as) many who fled from the face of the pestilence were infected and did not evade the death].[41] Such doomed attempts to avoid God's pestilential vengeance are mirrored in Jonah's own fruitless attempt to avoid God's "arende" [mission] (72), a patently human if spiritually deficient act that would have resonated with fourteenth-century readers familiar with both the temptation and the futility of running from the plague.

If Jonah's panicked attempt at escape implies the poet's dubious attitude toward flight, the Ninevites' contrasting reaction to Jonah's preaching further confirms it. After being unceremoniously vomited out by the whale, Jonah hustles to Nineveh and, in terms that pointedly recall the biblical calamities of *Cleanness*, foretells the destruction of the city to its inhabitants:

3et schal forty dayez fully fare to an ende,
And þenne schal Niniue be nomen and to no3t worþe:
Truly þis ilk toun schal tylte to grounde;
Vp-so-down schal 3e dumpe depe to þe abyme,
To be swol3ed swyftly wyth þe swart erþe,
And alle þat lyuyes hereinne lose þe swete.
(359–64)

[By the time forty days have fully come to an end, then shall Nineveh by its name be utterly destroyed. Truly, this town shall be knocked to the ground, dumped upside-down deep into the abyss to be quickly swallowed by the dark earth, and all that live in it to lose their lifeblood.]

---

40. Boccaccio, *Decameron*, 15 (Waldman, 10).

41. *Monumenta Germaniae Historica, Scriptorum Tomus IX*, 676; John of Reading, *Chronica Johannis de Reading*, 109.

Far more overtly than his rationale for fleeing to Tarshish, Jonah's prophesy
hums with a pestilential lexicon not unlike the one that I've suggested exists
in *Pearl* and in *Cleanness,* echoing not only the Jordan plain rising to consume Sodom and Gomorrah, where "þe grete barrez of þe abyme he barst vp
at onez" [(God) burst the great barriers of the abyss at once] (*Cl.* 963), but
also the dark waters of the Flood overwhelming the antediluvian world: "Þen
bolned þe abyme, and bonkez con ryse" [Then the abyss swelled forth, and
the banks begin to rise] (363). We might push this idea further and speculate
that the prophesy also hints at the medical language so prominent in *Cleanness,* particularly in Jonah's concluding promise, "alle þat lyuyes hereinne lose
þe swete" [all that live in it lose their lifeblood] (*Pat.* 364). The word *swete*
here primarily refers to the loss of life itself, but could it also imply the loss
of sweat? As a purgative, sweating was often advised to manage a variety of
humoral symptoms, including (but not limited to) the carbuncles and buboes
associated with bubonic plague.[42] As the Middle English version of Guy de
Chauliac's *Surgery* makes clear, a wide range of "apostemes, . . . pustules, . . .
[and] exitures" [apostemes, . . . pustules, . . . and swellings], including plague
buboes, were treated by prescribing patients "to make *swete* and to smeke out"
[to make sweat and to release out humoral vapors].[43]

Such conjecture aside, however, what remains undeniable is that unlike
Jonah, the Ninevites do not flee. Rather, and *in extremis,* they repent, prostrat-
ing themselves before God in a display of abjection and remorse.

> Þenne þe peple pitosly pleyned ful stylle,
> And for þe drede of Dryʒtan doured in hert;
> Heter hayrez þay hent þat asperly bited,
> And þose þay bounden to her bak and to her bare sydez,
> Dropped dust on her hede, and dymly bisoʒten
> Þat þat penaunce plesed Him þat playnez on her wronge.
> (371–76)

[Then the people prayed piteously in silence because the dread of God
grieved their hearts; they quickly gathered up hair shirts that bit bitterly
into the skin and bound those to their backs and their naked sides, dropped
dust on their heads, and prayed gravely that their penance would please Him
who complained against their sins.]

---

42. *MED* s.v. "swēt(e)" (n.1) a, b, d.
43. Guy de Chauliac, *The Cyrurgie of Guy de Chauliac,* 73, 85.

Nor are the ordinary citizens alone in their penitence. The king, too, exchanges his royal robes for a hair shirt and ashes, and he decrees that all Ninevites—"Vch prynce, vche prest, and prelates alle" [Each prince, each priest, and all the clerics] (389)—atone for their offenses:

> Sesez childer of her sok, soghe hem so neuer,
> Ne best bite on no brom, ne no bent nauþer,
> Passe to no pasture, ne pike non erbes,
> Ne non oxe to no hay, ne no horse to water.
> Al schal crye, forclemmed, with alle oure clere strenþe;
> Þe rurd schal ryse to Hym þat rawþe schal haue.
> (391–96)

[Children shall cease of their nursing, no matter how it grieves them, and the beast shall bite neither broomstraw nor grass, nor pass forth to pasture nor pick any herbs. Nor is any ox to eat hay, nor any horse to drink water. We shall all cry out, pained with hunger, with all of our strength; the noise shall rise up to Him so that he might have pity.]

Particularly in light of *Patience*'s narrative embellishments—the poet specifically adds babies to the call to fast and amplifies the restrictions placed on Nineveh's animals[44]—the contrast between Jonah and the Ninevites could not be sharper: Jonah attempts to avoid judgment by running from God while the people of Nineveh remain in their city and pacify him; Jonah's flight leads to a hellish journey in the belly of a whale while the Ninevites' violent penitence—one that anticipates the extreme practices of such postplague groups as the Flagellants[45]—causes God to withhold his vengeance. If *Patience* offers a comparative account of the relative merits of flight and affiliation, it clearly deems affiliation to be the more effective and more appropriate course of action.

Speculative as this pestilential reading might be, I want to insist that it is not mere *idle* speculation. Indeed, just as the central exempla of *Cleanness* were common medieval touchstones for describing the overwhelming destruction of the plague, so too was Nineveh's deliverance frequently used in sermons and *concilia* to encourage prayer and repentance against its approach.

---

44. Jonas 3:7 specifies the terms of the Ninevites' repentence: "*Homines, et jumenta, et boves, et pecora non gustent quidquam: nec pascantur, et aquam non bibant*" [Let neither men nor beasts, oxen nor sheep, taste any thing: let them not feed, nor drink water].

45. For a brief if somewhat sensationalized overview of the Flagellant movement in Europe, including the appearance of Flagellant groups in England in 1349 and 1350, see Zeigler, *The Black Death*, 84–97.

In a 1348 letter, Bishop Ralph of Shrewsbury admonished his archdeacons to *"mementote siquidem quibus fuit prophetico oraculo digne prenunciata subversio, penitenciam agentes, fuerunt ab exterminio comminato Dei judicio misericorditer liberati, dixerunt enim 'Quis scit si convertatur et ignoscat Deus, et revertatur a furore ire sue et non peribimus'"* [be mindful, therefore, of the destruction that was fittingly and prophetically foretold; (the Ninevites) performed penance, and they were mercifully freed from the threatened destruction by the judgment of God; indeed, they said, 'Who can tell if God will turn, and forgive: and will turn away from his fierce anger, and we shall not perish?']. Cognizant that plague was approaching England from France, the bishop further urged his readers to *"de peccatis suis contereantur et peniteant . . . ut misericordie Dei nos cito anticipen et avertat a populo suo hujusmode pestilenciam"* [be terrified and penitent for their sins . . . so that God's mercy may swiftly prevent and avert from his people this manner of pestilence].[46] In an similar letter from the plague outbreak of 1375, Archbishop Sudbury invoked the figure of *"Ninive civitatem a subversione precibus liberatam"* [the city of Nineveh freed from destruction by prayers], while on the Continent, a later sermon by German preacher Gabriel Biel entitled *"De fuga pestis"* similarly recalled how *"nam tali conuersione & oratione, conuersi Niniuitœ liberati sunt a subuersione suœ ciuitatis"* [by such great conversion and prayer, the converted Ninevites were freed from the destruction of their city].[47] Finally, a 1382 English prayer against the plague, composed at roughly the same time as *Patience*, was addressed directly to *"Deus, qui imminentem Ninivitis interitum sola misericordia removisti"* [God, who in your mercy alone removed the imminent destruction of the Ninevites].[48] The story of Nineveh's escape from God's judgment, in other words, was not a neutral text in the second half of the fourteenth century. On the contrary, as a common figure for deliverance from God's wrath, it was intimately connected to the experience of the Black Death, just as were the stories of the Flood, the Fall, and the Destruction of Sodom and Gomorrah.

Such connections could hardly have been unknown to the author of *Patience*. Likely a cleric attached to an aristocratic household, he would almost

---

46. Ralph of Shrewsbury, *The Register of Ralph of Shrewsbury*, 555–56. The biblical passage quoted by Shrewsbury is Jonah 3:9.

47. Sudbury, "*Commissio ad orandum pro cessatione pestilentiae*," 3:100; Biel, "*Contra pestilentiam sermo medicinalis III*," 363. Biel preached in the sixteenth century, but his reference to Nineveh confirms the persistence of this trope in sermons and other writings against the plague.

48. "*Salus populi*," col. 810. The context of this prayer is discussed in Horrox, *The Black Death*, 120–21.

certainly have been acquainted with writings like those quoted above.[49] Authorial biography notwithstanding, however, Nineveh's currency in late medieval discourses on the plague offers a possible solution to another critical dilemma that has long occupied readers of the poem, namely the poet's use of Jonah, rather than Job, to exemplify its titular virtue. James Rhodes offers one provocative rationale for this choice, positing that it "alerts us to the independence and subjectivity of the narrator. . . , and it upsets whatever preconceived notions we might have about the nature of patience."[50] I would raise the possibility, however, that for fourteenth-century readers and auditors, the image of Jonah's panicked flight twinned with the repentance and deliverance of the Ninevites would not so much have upset preconceived notions about patience as situated them within contemporary concerns about the propriety of flight and the efficacy of prayer as prophylactic measures against the plague. Once again, I do not want to imply here that we should simply consider Jonah a literal fugitive from pestilence or that we should regard the Ninevites as standins for communities choosing affiliation over flight. Nonetheless, the affinities among the biblical narrative, the lived experience of the plague, and the range of cultural references to the disease—affinities brought into relief by the poet's knowing embellishment of the Vulgate—suggest *Patience*'s subtle purchase in the Black Death, and they show how the poem might have explored its titular virtue both in broad theological terms and in the more culturally resonant terms of the ongoing pandemic.

It is finally important to note that while it articulates a generally negative attitude toward flight, *Patience* also highlights in its flawed protagonist the physiological imperative for self-preservation that makes flight comprehensible and, perhaps, forgivable. Particularly in comparison to *Cleanness*, the poem that immediately precedes it in the manuscript, *Patience* is emphatically a poem of forgiveness, both divine and human.[51] Its investigation of flight and affiliation also positions the poem differently in regard to the pandemic than either *Pearl* or *Cleanness*, both of which suggest, albeit tacitly, responses to the *aftermath* of the disease, the personal and cultural losses sustained by survivors, and the difficulty of giving voice to trauma. *Patience*, by contrast, positions itself not in the wake of the traumatic event but on its cusp. And while *Pearl*'s circular structure and *Cleanness*'s traumatic repetitions both hint at the plague's cyclical nature, *Patience*'s anxiety over the proximate future

---

49. Andrew and Waldron summarize the case for this poet's clerical identity in their introduction to *The Poems of the Pearl Manuscript*, 10–11. I will return to the clericalism of the poet and his possible audiences later in this chapter.

50. Rhodes, "Vision and History in *Patience*," 4.

51. See Benson, "The Impatient Reader of *Patience*," 147–61.

amplifies the truth that *Pearl* and *Cleanness* imply, that the trauma of the pestilence is never really in the past. This is not to say that *Patience* never looks back over its shoulder. It is, however, to suggest that even for survivors, the plague is always an event that will almost certainly happen again, a cataclysm that lurks always on the horizon. Such a shift in perspective moves us away from the inhuman certainty of *Pearl*'s Maiden and the unswerving judgments of *Cleanness*'s God and toward a poetic universe defined not by the absolute terms of past judgments or eschatological futures but by the immediate contingencies of what is happening *now*, the moment-to-moment world of human experience.

FRENZY FROM WITHIN: ENCLOSURE *AS* AND *AGAINST* FLIGHT

Jonah's flight and the Ninevites' repentance bracket the central episode of *Patience*, Jonah's three-day sojourn in the belly of a whale. As a literary set piece, the scene is a tour de force, with the poet fleshing out the Vulgate with psychologically and theologically resonant additions. Considered alongside his passage in the ship and his stint in the woodbine, however, Jonah's cetacean entombment is but one of three episodes in the poem that dramatize a site of physical enclosure, another repeated motif that, like the compulsive repetitions of *Cleanness*, implies the verbal and physical symptoms associated with the posttraumatic response. Lawrence Eldridge has argued that these three spaces—boat, whale, and woodbine—are examples of "sheltering space," loci of moribund confinement and pseudo-security that contrast with the "cosmic space" of God's creation, "the potentially liberating space of the beatitudes and of the church."[52] While it is tempting to translate Eldridge's dichotomy of "cosmic space" and "sheltering space" into a respective consideration of flight and enclosure, the two practices are less opposed than they might seem, particularly if we consider them with respect to the Black Death. To be sure, plague flight involves, at its most basic level, a movement outward, away from a perceived source of contagion and toward a space whose very openness promises antisepsis and healing. Enclosure, by contrast, involves a physical movement inward—into the closed city, the house, the room, the curtained bed. But as Cary Howie's recent meditation on the erotics of claustration reveals, the enclosed space is always in some way a permeable one, a

---

52. Eldridge, "Sheltering Space and Cosmic Space," 133. For further development of Eldridge's analysis, see Spearing, "The Subtext of *Patience*"; Bollermann, "In the Belly, in the Bower"; Pohli, "Containment of Anger."

space that, like Poe's castellated abbey, allows for egress and ingress in both mundane and unexpected ways. "Concealment is tempting," Howie writes. "I hide from you; you seek me out. What happens when concealment becomes a matter of space, the kinds of space where I hide, and where, perhaps, I seek to be sought?"[53] The body enclosed within a "sheltering space"—in the context of the plague, the body seeking shelter from contagion—is always open to corruption from a radically uncontrolled "cosmic space." Secure enclosure is as much a fantasy as effective flight, and it is born of the same impulses.

Gilles Deleuze and Félix Guattari likewise posit that flight and enclosure are not contradictory. Enclosure can be said to articulate a line of escape that exists "between points, in their midst, and no longer goes from one point to another," a line without physical motion but that constitutes flight in a metaphysical sense.[54] Within the context of a contagious pestilence whose "any point . . . can be connected to anything other," all attempts at enclosure from the Black Death become lines of flight from the disease's rhizomatic multiplicity of vectors.[55] Writing in northern Spain in 1348, Jacme d'Agramont exemplifies this idea when he encourages readers to seek refuge in *"los lochs baixs e les cambres soterranies"* [low places and underground rooms], keeping *"les finestres de les cambres e les espiylleres diligentment tanquades"* [windows and embrasures tightly shut]; it is advice that matches in intended effect, if not in kind, his alternative strategy of fleeing contagion by residing in *"los lochs alts e les montaynnes"* [high places and mountains].[56] And yet, during times of plague, as was regularly observed, neither the reality of flight nor the reality of enclosure matched its respective ideal. There was, quite simply, no such thing as a high-enough mountain or a tight-enough window.

In *Patience*, enclosure is frequently coterminous with flight. Jonah's desperate journey to Tarshish in particular is closely linked with enclosure and its associated desire for physical security. Frightened by the storm buffeting his ship, Jonah squirrels himself away below deck, seeking comfort and safety in the enclosed space of the hold. But the protective enclosure is easily penetrated by the ship's navigator, an intrusion that shatters Jonah's facile attempt at safety.

> A lodesmon ly3tly lep vnder hachches,
> For to layte mo ledes and hem to lote bryng.

---

53. Howie, *Claustrophilia*, 11.

54. Deleuze and Guattari, *A Thousand Plateaus*, 298. See also Raunig, "The Heterogenesis of Fleeing," especially 46–48.

55. Deleuze and Guattari, *A Thousand Plateaus*, 7.

56. Jaume d'Agramunt, *Regiment de preservació*, 26, trans. Duran-Reynals and Winslow, 79.

But hym fayled no freke þat he fynde my3t,
Saf Jonas þe Jwe, þat jowked in derne.
He watz flowen for ferde of þe flode lotes
Into þe boþem of þe bot, and on a brede lyggede,
Onhelde by þe hurrok, for þe heuen wrache,
Slypped vpon a sloumbe-selepe, and sloberande he routes.
Þe freke hym frunt with his fot and bede hym ferk vp:
Þer Ragnel in his rakentes hym rere of his dremes!
(179–88)

[A navigator rushed quickly under the hatch to fetch more men to cast lots, but he failed to find anyone except for Jonah the Jew, who lay hidden and sleeping. He had fled in fear from the noise of the flood into the bottom of the boat, and he lay on a board, huddled by the rudder for fear of heaven's retribution. He had fallen slobbering and snoring into a deep sleep. The man kicked him with his foot and told him to hurry up to the deck: may Ragnel (a devil) in his rattling chains wake him from his dreams!]

There is an obvious double irony in this attempt at shipboard claustration: first Jonah is in far more danger on the sea that he will ever be in Nineveh; second, and more pointedly, he causes the storm that threatens him by cloistering himself from the only thing keeping him safe, "þe face of frelych Dry3tyn" [the face of gracious God] (214). What drives both of these ironies is the simple fact that any security Jonah seeks in his manmade enclosure—from God, from natural danger, from death itself—is illusory. The false serenity of Jonah's "sloumbe-selepe" [deep sleep] (186), a phrase that both recalls the *Pearl*-Dreamer's "slepyng-sla3t" [deathly sleep] (*Pe.* 59) and anticipates Jonah's later "sloumbe-slep" (*Pat.* 466) in the woodbine, is heightened by the storm-tossed ship, "a joyles gyn" [a joyless ship] (146) that "reled on roun vpon þe ro3e yþes" [reeled erratically on the rough waves] (147) and "sweyed on þe see" [swayed on the sea] (151). Jonah senses danger where there is none and feels secure when he is in peril. The safety he imagines in his shipboard enclosure is a sham.

As a species of flight, Jonah's act of claustration is a self-deception that resonates with the similarly false promise of enclosure from epidemic disease. Like Prince Prospero's impenetrable abbey or Jacme d'Agramont's sealed chamber, the protective space of the hold is inevitably penetrated, and Jonah finds himself dragged onto the open deck, humiliated and "jugged to drowne" [adjudged to be drowned] (245), torments akin to those he was attempting to avoid in the first place. If safety exists within the world of the poem—and, as

Jonah will discover inside the whale, it *does* exist—it lies not in human efforts at claustration but in the grace and protection of the divine.[57] The physical space of the enclosure is always permeable. It is, as Howie articulates, "ambivalent in the most literal sense: enclosure wants it both ways."[58] With this in mind, we might thus venture that *Patience* manifests the same attitude toward prophylactic enclosure as it does toward flight. Neither, it implies, offers protection from a disease widely understood as a species of God's judgment.

The idea that *Patience*'s images of enclosure echo the poem's pestilential environment is, I want to propose, even more strongly suggested by Jonah's final enclosure, the woodbine. As he does at other key points in his narrative, the poet carefully transforms the simple "*hedera*" [ivy] of the Latin Vulgate into something far more elaborate:[59]

Such a lefsel of lof neuer lede hade,
For hit watz brod at þe boþem, boȝted on lofte,
Happed vpon ayþer half, a hous as hit were,
A nos on þe norþ syde and nowhere non ellez,
Bot al schet in a schaȝe þat schaded ful cole.
Þe gome glyȝt on þe grene graciouse leues,
Þat euer wayued a wynde so wyþe and so cole;
Þe schyre sunne hit vmbeschon, þaȝ no schafte myȝt
Þe mountaunce of a lyttel mote vpon þat man schyne.

(448–56)

[Never had the man had such a praiseworthy bower of leaves, for it was broad at the bottom, vaulted aloft, enclosed on either side as though it were a house, with a window on the north side and nowhere else, all enclosed in a thicket that provided cool shade. The man looked on the luxuriant green leaves that waved in a breeze so mild and cool; the bright sun shone all around it, but no shaft of light, even the size of a little speck, could shine in on him.]

---

57. We might compare the ship's hold in *Patience* to the Ark in *Cleanness,* another prominent enclosure and one that creates a very real locus of security for its cloistered inhabitants. Unlike the Tarshish-bound ship, however, the Ark was constructed by God's willing prophet, an enclosure whose efficacy reflects its divine sanction.

58. Howie, *Claustrophilia,* 15.

59. Jonah 4:6 reads, "*Et praeparavit Dominus Deus hederam, et ascendit super caput Jonae, ut esset umbra super caput ejus, et protegeret eum (laboraverat enim): et laetatus est Jonas super hedera laetitia magna*" [And the Lord God prepared an ivy, and it came up over the head of Jonas, to be a shadow over his head, and to cover him (for he was fatigued), and Jonas was exceeding glad of the ivy].

Unlike the manufactured ship's hold, the woodbine is a product of God's will; its sudden growth, miraculous shape, and evident beauty set it apart from the earlier enclosures and recall, as Elizabeth Allen writes, "God's role as artificer of both Jonah's punishment and his protection."[60] Its supernatural aspects notwithstanding, however, the woodbine is perhaps most notable for those qualities that connect it to domestic architecture—a broad floorplan and a lofted ceiling; a north-facing window to allow in cool, light drafts; walls so tightly woven that even a dust mote will not pass through. We can, as one critic has suggested, "discern here a sense of sheer fun" in these architectural details; we might, more seriously, recognize the woodbine as "a refuge from the violence and corruption that seem so inextricably part of other 'safe' spaces."[61] Neither of these readings, however, accounts for the specificity of detail that the poet brings to the biblical *hedera,* the high ceilings, the wide floor, the impenetrable walls, the single north-facing window.

If we consider them in the context of the Black Death, these architectural details gain an increased gravity, recalling the precise aspects of domestic enclosure thought to offer protection against the plague. Indeed, while the ideal of total sequestration was postulated as the best precaution against the disease (as in Jacme d'Agramont's airtight room), most plague treatises, recognizing the impossibility of such perfect isolation, encourage opening north-facing windows, as the southern wind was thought to carry corruption and disease. The report of the Paris medical faculty specifically cites the "*frequenti flatu ventorum meridionalium grossorum et turbidorum propter extraneos vapores quos secum deferunt*" [frequent blowing southern winds, great and turbulent] and their "*extraneos vapores*" [foreign vapors] as proximate causes of the pestilence, a view repeated in countless derivative tracts.[62] In the same vein, an English translation of Bengt Knuttson's treatise relates how "the south wynde . . . hurtith the harte" [the south wind . . . hurts the heart] and it advises readers "to haue the wyndowes open againste the northe and easte, and to shitte the windowes againste the southe" [to have the windows open toward the north and east and to shut the windows against the south].[63] The Veronese scholar Hieronymus Fracastorius suggests opening north-facing windows and fumigating rooms with strong-smelling flowers, while a manual from the Islamicate Iberian peninsula advises, "One should always take care to have fresh air by living in houses facing north, by filling them with cold

60. Allen, "Sanctuary and Love of This World," 124.

61. Andrew, "Biblical Paraphrase in the Middle English *Patience,*" 66; Allen, "Sanctuary and Love of This World," 125.

62. "The Report of the Medical Faculty of Paris," 154.

63. *A Litil Boke the Whiche Traytied Many Gode Thinges for the Pestilence,* 4 recto.

fragrances and aroma of flowers."[64] Read against such pervasive advice, the enclosure described in *Patience* implies less a simple bedroom than it does a structure designed to mitigate the pestilence, its open north-facing window allowing in nourishing breezes, the sweet smell of the woodbine diminishing septic vapors.[65]

We might push this speculation still further and note that the bower's "happed" [enclosed] (450) walls prevent even "a lyttel mote" [a little speck] (456) of unwanted sunlight to fall upon Jonah. In *Pearl*, mote comes not only to signify "speck" but also to imply "spot" and "sore": the Lamb's heavenly faithful are a "motelez meyny" [spotless multitude] (*Pe.* 925); the New Jerusalem is a "mote without moote" [a spot without a spot] (948). If it draws on *Pearl's* punning register while also evoking contemporary medical discourse, *Patience* might be seen as developing the biblical *hedera* into an ideal counterplague space, an enclosure that mimics, in both form and function, the strategies of prophylaxis familiar to *Patience's* fourteenth-century readers and slyly evoked in Pearl's *hortus amoenus*.

These preventative strategies might have provided some comfort in communities confronted with pestilence; however, it was still widely recognized in the fourteenth century that even the best human efforts at protection paled in comparison with the power of the divine. "*Terribilis super filios hominum Deus, cujus nutibus subdunrur omnia suae voluntatis imperio*" [Terrible to the sons of man is God, by whose command all things are subdued to his imperial will], writes one Canterbury cleric, attempting to account for the ferocity of the Black Death.[66] His words find a close analogue in the report of the Paris medical faculty: "*Amplius pretermittere nolumus quod epidimia aliquando a divina uoluntate procedit, in quo casu non est aliud consilium nisi quod ad ipsum humiliter recurratur*" [It is important that we not overlook that any epidemic proceeds from the divine will, in which case we can only counsel to return humbly to God].[67] Such humility in the face of God's will is, of course, precisely the lesson that Jonah cannot seem to learn in *Patience* itself. Miserable after his woodbine is blasted into a weed-patch and sweltering in a suspect "wynde of þe weste" [wind of the west] (*Pat.* 470), Jonah rages at God, asking to die rather than suffer further indignity:

---

64. Winslow, *Conquest of Epidemic Disease,* 141; Abū Ja'far Ahmad ibn Khātima, in John Aberth, *The Black Death,* 55.

65. While it is sometimes another name for common ivy, "wodbynde" most often refers to the honeysuckle [*Lonicera periclymenum*], well known for its sweet-smelling blossoms. See *MED* s.v. "wǫde-bǐnd(e (n.) (a, c).

66. "*Literae prioris et capituli cantuar,*" 2:738.

67. "The Report of the Medical Faculty of Paris," 156.

With alle meschef þat Þou may, neuer Þou me sparez;
I keuered me a cumfort þat now is caȝt from me,
My wodbynde so wlonk þat wered my heued.
Bot now I se Þou art sette my solace to reue;
Why ne dyȝttez Þou me to diȝe? I dure to longe.
(484–88)

[You never spare me with all of the hardship that you make. I found myself
a comfort that is now snatched away from me, my beautiful woodbine that
protected my head. But now I see that You are intent on stripping away all of
my solace. Why don't you put me to death? I have already endured too long.]

The short speech is based on the Vulgate, although Jonah's grasping self-refer-
entiality—"*I* keuered *me* a cumfort," "*my* wodbynde," "*my* solace"—is original
to the poet. In its manuscript context, Jonah's tone evokes the *Pearl*-Dreamer's
reference to "*my* lyttel quene" [*my* little queen] (*Pe.* 1147), but in *Patience* itself
that tone speaks to Jonah's stubborn belief in his own control over his physical environment, his ability to flee or sequester himself from God's anger, to
shut out heat and miasmic vapors within a leafy bower, to avoid suffering and
dis-ease.

Coming near the end of a poem in which he is supposed to have learned
obedience to God, Jonah's petulant assertion of self-sufficiency can easily be
interpreted as "a temper tantrum," a response akin to the pleading of a scolded
child.[68] I would suggest, however, that to infantilize Jonah or to belittle his
loss is misguided, particularly if we apprehend the woodbine in the context
of the plague. No mere child's playhouse, the vegetal structure described in
Patience—like the garden in *Pearl* and the purified space of Christ's nativity in
Cleanness—outlines an enclosure that promises separation from disease and
corruption of the outside world, a refuge that not only offers protection in a
generic sense but that strikingly evokes contemporary measures against the
Black Death. God's destruction of the bower may rightly remind Jonah (and
the fourteenth-century reader) that true refuge can only be granted by the
divine, but within the extratextual framework of a pandemic that killed indis-
criminately, that heavily affected those performing Christian pastoral duties,
and that increasingly struck children in its later outbreaks, the poem's concluding assertion that "patience is a nobel poynt" [patience is a noble virtue]
(531) must have read as a bitter comfort, even for the most devout readers.[69]

---

68. For such a reading, see Bollermann, "In the Belly, In the Bower," 217.
69. Allen, "Sanctuary and Love of This World," 127.

Jonah, we might surmise, grasps to his woodbine just as Gawain grasps to his flimsy green silk: both men love their lives, and both men flinch. Like *Sir Gawain and the Green Knight* then, *Patience* registers not only the failures of its central character but also the social, cultural, and human contexts that make those failures reasonable and even forgivable—that make those failures human.

GOD'S PROTECTION AND THE WHALE'S BELLY

Jonah's enclosure inside the whale is itself enclosed on a formal level by the poem's other scenes of claustration, a circular structure that suggests the narrative shape of *Pearl* as it eddies around the unspeakable trauma at its center. These elements are further enclosed by *Patience*'s narrative frame, a concrete structural *imitatio* from a poet whose work is elsewhere marked by a keen attention to formal, architectural, and numerical detail. Like the woodbine, the whale's belly is figured in the poem as a shelter, but where the latter's north-facing window and lofted ceiling evoke domestic space, the whale's cathedral-door mouth (268) and belly "brod as a halle" [broad as a hall] (272) suggest the monumental edifice of a gothic cathedral. Again, as with the instantaneous growth of the woodbine, Jonah's survival within that cetacean basilica is possible only through the intervention of God, a central feature of exegetical readings that figure Jonah's confinement in the whale as typologically preceding Christ's entombment.

But there are also important differences that set the whale's belly apart from the woodbine, not least of which is the abject filth of this divine shelter *nonpareil*. The poet's description of the interior of the whale is yet another departure from the Vulgate. At fifty-six lines, it is *Patience*'s longest poetic invention, and it is a masterpiece of nausea and disgust, rivaling in its repugnant detail the most descriptive passages in *Cleanness*. Jonah enters the beast's mouth like a "mote in at a munster dor" [dust mote into a cathedral door] (268), eventually settling in the "glaym ande glette" [slime and filth] (269) of the massive stomach.

> And þer he festnes þe fete and fathmez aboute,
> And stod vp in his stomak þat stank as þe deuel.
> Þer in saym and in sorʒe þat sauoured as helle,
> Þer watz bylded his bour þat wyl no bale suffer.
> And þenne he lurkkes and laytes where watz le best,
> In vche a nok of his nauel, bot nowhere he fyndez

No rest ne recouerer, bot ramel ande myre,
In wych gut so euer he gotz.
(273–80)

[And there he sets his feet and gropes about, and stood up in the stomach
that stank like the devil. There in grease and filth that reeked like hell, there
his bower was appointed so that he would suffer no sorrow; and then he
lurks around and seeks in every corner of his belly for a good shelter, but
nowhere does he find rest or recovery—only muck and mire wherever he
goes in those guts.]

If *Cleanness*'s description of the Cities of the Plain and the Dead Sea—with its
"smod" [filth] (*Cl.* 711), "spitous fylþe" [disgraceful filth] (845), and "ȝestande
sorȝe" [yeasty filth] (846)—marshals a "rhetoric of revulsion"[70] that intimates
both the symptoms and miasmic causes of the plague, might the "glaym ande
glette" [slime and filth] (*Cl.* 269) and "ramel ande myre" [muck and mire]
(279) of the whale's stinking belly do the same? Such a conjecture would be
difficult to prove of course, but at the very least, the belly is a space marked
by "the disgusting," which Sianne Ngai shows to be "perceived as dangerous
and contaminating."[71] So too does the description of the whale's belly align
with a "poetics of disgust," one aligned with contagion and sepsis.[72] Particularly within a cultural and textual environment whose best science understood
disease to be spread by "*vapores malos putridos et venenoso*" [bad, putrid, and
poisonous vapors], Jonah's fishy enclosure may not be just infernal, as so many
critics have argued, but also pestilential.[73] Perhaps the poem's particular "poetics of disgust," then, also scans as a poetics of plague.

    If the whale's belly, as I've considered above, does articulate such a pes-
tilential space, Jonah's immediate response to his confinement in it, a short
appeal to God without precedent in the Bible, may carry a similar pestilential
charge:

Now, Prynce, of Þy prophete pité Þou haue.
Þaȝ I be fol and fykel and falce of my hert,
Dewoyde now Þy vengaunce, þurȝ vertu of rauthe;
Thaȝ I be gulty of gyle, as gaule of prophetes,
Þou art God, and alle gowdez ar grayþely Þyn owen.

----

70. Calabrese and Eliason, "The Rhetorics of Sexual Pleasure and Intolerance," 264.
71. Ngai, *Ugly Feelings*, 336.
72. Ngai, 345.
73. "The Report of the Medical Faculty of Paris," 154.

Haf now mercy of Þy man and his mysdedes,
And preue Þe ly3tly a Lorde in londe and in water.
(282–88)

[Now, Prince, have pity on Your prophet. Though I am foolish and fickle and
false of my heart, withdraw now Your vengeance through the virtue of your
pity. Though I am guilty of guile, as the most wretched of prophets, You are
God, and all graces are truly Your own. Have mercy now on Your man and
his sins, and show Yourself readily a Lord on land and in water.]

Critics have struggled to account for this addition, a redundant and essentially
selfish preamble to the prayer from the belly that, as Lynn Staley Johnson
remarks, strikes the reader as "not a prayer of repentance but a bargain."[74]
Self-serving as it is, however, the entreaty has more than a little in common
with the hasty and sometimes ad hoc prayers offered against the pestilence.
Consider, for instance, a prayer from a 1382 mass against the plague (a mass,
it should be noted, that also invokes Nineveh as an example of God's potential for mercy): "*Ecclesiæ tuæ, quæsumus, omnipotens Deus, munus placatus
intende; et misericordia tua nos potius quam ira præveniat; quia si iniquitates nostras observare volueris, nulla poterit creatura subsistere, sed admirabili
pietate qua nos fecisti, opera mannum tuarum non sinas interire*" [O almighty
God, we ask, kindly give us the gift of your church; and come before us in your
mercy rather than anger; because if you choose to observe our iniquities, no
creature could survive; but because of the remarkable tenderness with which
you created us, do not permit the work of your hand to die].[75] Of similar tim-
bre are a 1375 call to prayer by Archibishop Sudbury, who claims that in times
of plague "*Oratio enim est instans praesidium*" [prayer is in fact an immediate
protection],[76] and a 1348 call to prayer by the Archbishop of York, who ensures
that such "*orationibus*" [orations] will lead God to "*iram Suam avertat, pesti-
lentiamque et infectionem hujusmodi amoveat et repellat*" [avert his anger, and
withdraw and drive away the pestilence and infection].[77] In both content and
style, Jonah's own hurried plea for deliverance from the pestilent enclosure of
the whale—"dewoyde now Þy vengaunce" [withdraw now Your vengeance]
(284); "haf now mercy of Þy man and his mysdedes" [have mercy now on Your
man and his sins] (287)—mimics these desperate entreaties. Such a prayer

---

74. Johnson, *The Voice of the Gawain-Poet*, 11. For a similar assessment of the entreaty, see
Allen, "Sanctuary and Love of This World," 123.

75. "*Salus populi*," 811.

76. Sudbury, "*Commissio ad orandum pro cessatione pestilentiae*," 2:100.

77. Zouche, "A Letter from Archbishop Zouche," 396.

may not attain the ideal of "a humble petition arising from spiritual poverty,"
but in its immediacy and spiritual lack, as well as in its situated-ness within a
moment of pronounced need, it rings out with the same desperate energy as
intercessionary prayers against the plague.[78]

Particularly given the nature of the prayer, what the enclosure of the
whale's belly performs within the text is a fundamental inversion of expectations, both Jonah's and the reader's. Protected by God even in the direst of circumstances, Jonah is never safer than when he is "wanlez of wele in wombe of
þat fissche" [hopeless and joyless in the belly of that fish] (262), certainly not
beneath the creaking boards of the ship nor even nestled into the woodbine.
There is, of course, something slightly comical in the fact that Jonah's safest
enclosure is also the vilest, but the contrast between Jonah's discomfort and
security also amplifies the central didactic point that prophylaxis is ultimately,
and solely, God's to provide.[79] If we speculatively place the poem into the context of the pestilence, *Patience* might thus be seen as offering both rebuke and
consolation to its readers. It implies the inefficacy of flight and enclosure by
articulating the dubious moral and theological stakes of circumventing God's
vengeance; however, it also reaffirms the possibility of God's protection in the
foulest, and even the most pestilent, spaces: the city of Nineveh; the "rokkez
ful roȝe" (254) of the ocean floor; the belly of a nauseated whale.[80] Moreover,
by emphasizing not the apocalyptic wrath of God but his capacity for forgiveness, *Patience* draws back from the moral and theological rigidity of *Cleanness*
and *Pearl* and opens a space for human imperfection—for fear, desire, anger,
mistrust, and even faithlessness—amidst the most strenuous demands of the
divine will.

CLERICAL FLIGHT AND THE ECONOMICS OF DEATH

Thus far I have avoided any sustained discussion of *Patience*'s frame, a first-
person address that explicitly joins the first and last of Christ's beatitudes:
"Thay arn happen þat han in hert pouerté, / For hores is þe heuen-ryche to
holde for euer" [They are blessed that have poverty in their heart, for theirs
is the kingdom of heaven to have forever] (13–14), and "Þay ar happen also

---

78. Davis, "What the Poet of *Patience* Really Did to the Book of Jonah," 276.

79. Allen, "Sanctuary and Love of This World," refers to the whale as "a suggestively hellish,
yet in the end relatively harmless, beast" (123).

80. The poet surmises that the presence of Jonah in the whale's gut makes the creature feel
"wamel at his hert" [sick in his heart] (300), a detail that is confirmed when the whale "brakez
vp þe buyrne" [vomits the man up] (340) on the shore near Nineveh.

þat con her hert stere, / For hores is þe heuen-ryche, as I er sayde" [They are also blessed that can steer their heart, for theirs is the kingdom of heaven, as I said before] (27–28). By isolating and linking these two "sunderlupes" [beatitudes] (12) in his own poetic voice, the poet reinforces established exegetical connections between poverty and patience, and he also establishes a narrative persona insistently marked by poverty, noting, "syn I am put to a poynt þat pouerté hatte, / I schal me poruay pacyence and play me with boþe" [Since I am put in a situation where I must have poverty, I shall equip myself with patience and amuse myself with both] (35–36).[81] In this way, the narrative frame of *Patience* has been recognized as offering a broadly pastoral address, one that exhorts the ideal of a mixed life comprised equally of solitary devotion and outwardly directed works, "two modes of living . . . whose dual motive was charity—showing love of God through contemplation and love of one's neighbor through actions."[82] Such an understanding of the poem's frame accords with the demands placed on a poet who was likely a cleric in the service of a noble household and who had to balance the contemplative aspects of the religious life with outwardly directed pastoral duties. It also accords with the poem's central exemplum, the story of a would-be prophet who refuses to preach in the face of dangers both real and imagined.[83] In concluding this chapter, I want to consider how such a narrative stance might align not only with a broad clerical context but also with narrower contexts specific to clerical work during the Black Death.

Pastoral duties were dangerous during outbreaks of the plague, not because of angry Ninevites or superstitious sailors but because the work itself placed priests in close proximity with the sick at their most contagious. The sacrament of Extreme Unction in particular, which involved anointing the dying with oil, would have offered a point of contagion unique to clergy, bringing them into intimate contact with infected individuals. This increased risk of contagion does not necessarily mean, as conventional wisdom has held, that mortality rates among the clergy were *always* higher than those of the general population; indeed, the factors that increased the possibility of infection in the clergy seem sometimes to have been offset by other factors, such as the clergy's comparatively favorable living standards.[84] Nonetheless, in light of the plague's recognized contagion and of the very real potential of person-to-person transmission, the performance of clerical duties took on a deeply

---

81. See Schmidt, "Imagery and Unity of Frame and Tale."

82. Bowers, "Ideal of the Mixed Life," 16. For a dissenting view, see Irwin and Kelly, "The Way and the End Are One," 49.

83. See also Bowers, "Ideal of the Mixed Life," 15.

84. Benedictow, *The Black Death,* 342–50.

threatening cast during plague outbreaks. As Benedictow notes, "To the extent that the parish priests personally discharged their spiritual obligations of administering last rites to their parishioners when the Black Death broke loose in their local communities, they would have a particularly high degree of exposure to infection."[85] The psychological and physical pressures that such exposure placed on clerics across the ecclesiastical spectrum would have been significant. Indeed, the performance of pastoral work during times of plague might even be regarded as a site of trauma in its own right, a space in which clerics were repeatedly asked to face, in excruciatingly intimate and physical terms, the full calamity of the pandemic.

The plight of the clergy during outbreaks is well documented in medieval sources, as are clerical reactions (both principled and ignoble) to the advance of the disease. Gabriele de' Mussis relates in his *Historia de Morbo* how "*sacerdos attonitus, ecclesiastica sacramenta timidus ministrabat*" [the dazed priest fearfully administered the sacraments of the church], and he further notes in an anecdote how quickly the disease spread among those who had contact with the dying: "*Qui dam ibi suum volens condere Testamentum notario, et presbitero confessore, ac testibus omnibus auocatis mortuus est. et die sequenti omnes pariter tumulati fuerunt*" [One man (in Bobbio), wishing to compose his will, died with the notary, confessor priest, and everyone called to witness (the will). And it followed that all of them were buried together].[86] More cynically, an anonymous Flemish chronicle records that for fear of contagion, "*nec presbyteri confessiones infirmorum audiunt, nec sacramenta eis dantur*" [priests do not listen to the confessions of the sick, nor do they offer them the sacraments], while, in a more sympathetic mode, Benedictine abbot Giles le Muisis writes, "*pro certo curati ac capellani confessiones audientes et sacramenta ministrantes, clerici etiam parrochiarum, et cum infirmos visitantes, de talibus multi decesserunt*" [to be sure, of the priests and chaplains who heard confession and administered the sacraments, and also the parish priests, and those who visited the sick with them, many such died].[87] Michele da Piazza claims that many unscrupulous religious refused to minister to the infected, but he also relates the high mortality rates of those who did, writing that "*Fratres . . . Ordinis minorum at Predicatorum et aliorum ordinum accedere volentes ad domos infirmorum predicatorum, et confitentes eisdem de eorum peccatis,*

---

85. Benedictow, 346–47.

86. Gabriele de' Mussis, *Historia de Morbo*, 53, 52. Samuel Cohn, Jr., offers a concise summary of clerical responses to the Black Death, including several of those that I mention here. See Cohn, *The Black Death Transformed*, 121.

87. *Breve Chronicon Clerici Anonymi*, 17; Gilles li Muisis, *Chronicon majus Aegidii Li Muisis*, 2:381.

et dantes eis penitentiam juxta velle sermus divinam justitia, adeo letalis mors ipsos infecit, quod fere in eorum cellulis de eis aliqui remanserunt" [Franciscans and Dominicans and other orders who were willing to come near the houses of the sick, and confess them of their sins, and give penance, and be willing to preach divine justice, were themselves infected with the death, so that hardly any were left in their cells].[88] Finally, in England, the Bishop of Bath and Wells records that in his own bishopric *"non inveniantur presbyteri, qui velint devotionis zelo, aut pro stipendio aliquo curas praedictorum locorum subire, et infirmos visitare, eisque sacramenta ecclesiastica ministrare; forsitan propter infectionem, et contagionis horrorem"* [priests cannot be found, for devotional zeal or for wages, to go to those places and visit the sick, take on the responsibility for those (infected) places and visit the sick and also to administer the sacraments of the church; on account of infection and the horror of contagion].[89]

If we bear such contemporary accounts in mind, the virtue invoked in *Patience*'s memorable first line—"Pacience is a poynt, þaȝ hit displese ofte" [Patience is a virtue, even though it often displeases] (1)—assumes an additional significance that informs (but does not replace) our understandings of patience as the "patient endurance" and "obedience to God" demanded of willing preachers.[90] Indeed, for the clerical audience implied by the poem's prologue, even the most common pastoral duties—hearing confession, preaching, administering Extreme Unction—required not only "patient endurance" but also the emotional and psychological self-control to enter a situation that was quite literally life threatening. The tasks demanded of clerics during plague time—tasks evoked in the noisome "ernde" [mission] (52) of *Patience*'s prologue and amplified into Jonah's prophetic calling in the central exemplum— might thus be considered as more than mere run-of-the-mill duties. Indeed, even a minor foray into a pestilent space could lead to infection and to death.

Can we read Jonah's terror at completing his own *ernde*, then, as well as his unsuccessful attempts at flight and self-enclosure, as embedded both within the clerical contexts of the poem's prologue *and* within the pestilential contexts that haunted the vocational spaces occupied by both the poet and his audience? Such a reading is a conjectural one, but considering it nonetheless allows us to recognize Jonah's dread—so frequently derided as excessive by

---

88. Michele da Piazza, *Cronaca*, 83.

89. *"Mandatum Radulphi, episcopi Bath et Wellen de confessionibus tempore pestilentiae,"* 2:745. It is also worth noting that the Bishop of Rochester threatened suspension for clerics who refused to serve during plague time, for which see Gasquet, *The Black Death of 1348 and 1349*, 121.

90. Wolfe, Monastic Obedience in *Patience*, 504; Hill, "The Audience of *Patience*," 106.

contemporary critics—as more comprehensible. It is, in these terms, a dread
that gives voice to the trauma confronted by plague victims, as well as to the
profound fears of those required to work on, what were in the later Middle
Ages, the vanguard of contagion. Moreover, considering Jonah's terror in the
context of the pestilence shapes his flight itself—which the poem presents
by turns as ineffective, humorous, morally dubious, contrary to God's will,
and psychologically understandable—into a negative exemplum not only for
patience in general but for the far more stringent self-control demanded of
clerics during times of pestilence. Such self-control, as Jonah's behavior suggests, must have been difficult to muster.

Furthermore, while such clerical and pestilential contexts may inform the
poem, the strong link that the prologue makes between patience and poverty
also implies a more inclusive social concern that reaches beyond them, one
that transcends the poem's immediate clerical milieu much as *Pearl* transcends
its courtly identity to reflect a wider range of social and cultural losses. The
narrator's identification with *pouerté* has proven divisive in *Patience* criticism,
sparking a long-running debate over the precise nature of the term. Indeed,
while the poverty discussed in the poem has most often been taken to refer
to "poverty of spirit" or "poverty of heart," it can also be recognized as refer-
ring to the pressures of physical and economic poverty.[91] As J. J. Anderson
observes, the poverty ascribed to the poet is not simply disagreeable but also
imposed: "Physical poverty was often thought of in such terms, but never spiritual poverty."[92] I would thus maintain that, at the very least, *Patience* allows
the reader to apprehend *both* spiritual and economic poverty in its use of the
term.

In this respect, and as much as pastoral work posed palpable dangers during plague time, poverty itself—the kind endured by the majority of England's
population—was more dangerous still. Benedictow's précis of the living conditions of England's poor is revealing in this respect and is worth quoting at
length:

> The hovels of the peasants [in the countryside] were built in wattle and daub,
> i.e., with interlaced rods and twigs or branches in walls and roofs that were
> plastered with clay or mud, materials that offered no real resistance to the
> movement and settling of rats. Inside, there were grossly unsanitary condi-
> tions: pigs and chickens and even cows and sheep would live in the same

---

91. Charles Moorman inaugurates this reading of spiritual poverty in "The Role of the
Narrator in *Patience*," 92. For poverty as physical and economic deprivation, see Anderson,
"The Prologue of *Patience*."

92. Anderson, "The Prologue of *Patience*," 283–84.

rooms as the peasant household who would sleep on hay directly on the earthen floor. Higher temperatures and much filth and dirt were living conditions very much to the liking of house rats. . . . Much the same can be said about the urban housing of the poor and destitute classes.[93]

Demographers and historians have regularly noted the "supermortality among the poor and destitute classes" during outbreaks of plague.[94] Literary critics like Kathy Lavezzo have similarly shown that while late medieval rhetoric describing death as a "great leveler" suggested that the plague might strike any class at any point; the reality was that death attended to England's indigent populations with a ferocity often spared members of the upper classes, a "reciprocal intensification of death and poverty" that made the disease particularly harrowing and particularly traumatic for the poor.[95] Even contemporary chronicles, whose concerns more often lay with princes than with peasants, recognize the connection between poverty and plague mortality. Ranulph Higden's *Polychronicon*, for instance, describes the seemingly universal horrors of England's 1348 outbreak—"*vix decima pars hominum superstes erat relicta*" [hardly a tenth part of the people were left living]—but also notes that "*pauci vel quasi nulli domini vel magnates in ista pestilentia decesserunt*" [only a few, actually almost none, of the lords and magnates passed away in that same pestilence].[96] The chronicle of Geoffrey le Baker likewise observes that "*pauci proceres moriebantur*" [only a few nobles died] but that "[vulgus] *innumerum, et religiosorum atque aliorum clericorum multitudo soli Deo nota, migravere*" [innumerable common people and a multitude of religious as well as other clerics only known to god departed].[97] Such pronouncements are by no means universal. Many chronicles across Europe held—and not without good cause—that the pestilence killed "*e grandi e piccioli*" [both grandees and commoners].[98] Taken as a group however, chronicle accounts offer compelling evidence that a relationship between poverty and mortality was not only present but also widely acknowledged during the time of the pandemic.

Poignantly, by positing a concrete link between the economic condition of poverty and the clerical virtue of patience, the poet might be seen as recognizing the increased threat of contagion bourn mutually by his own ecclesiastical class and by the indigent poor. On the one hand, this rhetorical move may

93. Benedictow, *The Black Death*, 348.
94. Benedictow, 262.
95. Lavezzo, "Chaucer and Everyday Death," 263.
96. Higden, *Polychronicon Ranulphi Higden Monachi Cestrensis*, 8:355.
97. Geoffrey le Baker, *Chronicon Galfridi le Baker de Swynebroke*, 99.
98. Morelli, *Ricordi*, 109.

seem out of keeping with the other poems in the *Pearl* manuscript, particularly *Pearl* and *Sir Gawain and the Green Knight,* which lavish attention on the physical and social appurtenances of the upper class in order to articulate their courtly milieu. Indeed, it may even seem out of keeping with aspects of *Patience* itself, which implies its own stake in court culture by imagining the eight beatitudes as a parade of well-appointed "dames" (31–33). But on the other hand, the affiliation that the poet proposes between his own clerical class and those suffering in poverty offers an intriguing mirror to the social position of *Pearl*'s jeweler, a figure of the middle-class whose futile attempts to enter the kingdom of Heaven are paralleled by his anxious and sometimes oppositional relationship with the aristocratic Pearl Maiden. Taken together, *Pearl*'s hesitant address to the aristocracy and *Patience*'s similarly halting embrace of the peasantry further inscribe the poet within a social and cultural middle space, investing him with a Janus-like hierarchical location, at once grasping and sympathetic, simultaneously upwardly mobile and downwardly oriented.[99] As he considers the affinities between clerics who perform pastoral work and the poor who often receive it, the two groups most dramatically affected by the plague and least empowered to flee from it, the poet of *Patience* emerges as a figure whose explicitly courtly poetry is tempered by surprisingly populist concerns.

This argument should not be taken to suggest that the poet of *Patience* offers some kind of overt cry for the plight of England's poor. On the contrary, the poem remains securely positioned at the intersection of the courtly and the clerical, where Christian virtues masquerade as courtly ladies and where righteous submission to poverty, in both of its senses, is an important part of the poet's didactic thrust. Nonetheless, if *Patience* is, as I conjecture here, a poem that draws energy and depth from its pestilential historical context, it can also be seen as a poem that acknowledges the struggles of England's poor and the additional dangers that poverty brought during a time of plague. Moreover, the poem recognizes that such struggles and fears exist within not only a religious context but a human one as well, and while it ultimately intones against flight and enclosure on theological terms, it also concedes, and even forgives, the impulse toward them, be it flight from God's command or enclosure from the judgment he sends in the form of pestilence. Though not yet incarnate in the person of Christ, the God of *Patience* nonetheless emerges as a deity who seems to exist not above the world but within it, who recognizes human frailty and endures the immediate and sometimes selfish actions

---

99. Lavezzo remarks in "Chaucer and Everyday Death" how Chaucer occupies a similar social location, though a less clerically oriented one, and emerges "as what we might anachronistically call a traditional intellectual possessed of certain protoliberal impulses" (284).

of humans in crisis. In this way, *Patience,* unlike the repeatedly apocalyptic *Cleanness* and the theologically inflexible *Pearl,* becomes a poem not defined by God's wrath but by God's mercy. Its focus on the questionable decisions that human actors make under stress and its insistence on God's capacity to forgive provides an important counterweight to *Pearl* and *Cleanness,* one that shifts readers toward the more indeterminate and contingent world imagined by the manuscript's final poem, *Sir Gawain and the Green Knight.*

CHAPTER 4

Sex, Death, and Social Change in
Sir Gawain and the Green Knight

> What are we to do now, brother?
>
> — FRANCESCO PETRARCH, *EPISTOLÆ DE REBUS FAMILIARIBUS*[1]

NEAR THE END of Fitt One of *Sir Gawain and the Green Knight*, in the bewildering caesura that follows the Green Knight's exit from Arthur's court, the narrator poses a deceptively straightforward query: "What þenne" [What then] (462)? The question is ludic in its simplicity but devilish in its impossibility, and as Arthur and Gawain stand in the vacuum left by the Green Knight, their only answer is an ambiguous and uneasy laughter, an incongruous response that strains to assimilate the spectacle of the beheading into the comfortable schema of Arthur's Yuletide feast.[2] Indeed, no sooner does the Green Knight ride headless from the king's hall than Arthur soothes his court and queen "wyth cortays speche" [with courteous speech] (469), reasserting the festivities with an extra helping of food and claiming the intruder's axe as an exotic wall trophy.[3] In Arthur's Camelot, the visceral shock of a botched beheading is transformed into yet another "vncouþe tale" [strange tale] (93) told before dinner, and the traumatic violence of the contest itself dissolves into the "enterludez" [interludes] (472) and "kynde caroles" [courtly carols] (473) enjoyed by the guests. The promise of Gawain's death, too, is sublimated

---

1. "*Quid vero nunc agimus, frater?*" Petrarch, *Epistolæ de rebus familiaribus et variæ*, 13. This quote is from Petrarch's preface to the collected letters and addressed to "Socrates," or Lodewijk Heyligen, a Flemish Benedictine monk to whom Petrarch wrote many of his letters and eventually dedicated his collected *Epistolæ de rebus familiaribus*. See Tournoy, "The Enigmatic Socrates."

2. On the ambiguity of laughter in the poem, see Longsworth, "Interpretive Laughter in *Sir Gawain and the Green Knight*."

3. For the axe as a substitute for the missing head, see Cohen, *Of Giants*, 145–46.

into the "mete and mynstralcie" [food and merriment] (484) of the Christmas banquet, a portent of doom accepted as a jovial holiday game.

If, as I have discussed throughout this study, one customary response to traumatic events is to suppress them from consciousness, then *Sir Gawain and the Green Knight* stages in its first fitt the alarmingly casual mechanism by which institutional power moves to effect and maintain that suppression.[4] But like the mute gaze of Lot's wife toward the destruction of Sodom, the question "what þenne?" opens a space in which to consider not the erasure of trauma but rather its determined persistence. Locally, the question acts as a hinge between the poem's most vivid moment of bodily violence and its assured repetition; more broadly, it impels readers, both medieval and modern, to query the convenient amnesia that Arthur's laughter promotes. In the succeeding fitts, the poem repeatedly, if implicitly, reiterates that same unanswerable question: when Gawain crosses himself in the bitter Wirral, and Hautdesert materializes before him; when he resists (three times) sexual congress with the Lady, refuses (almost three times) the gifts she offers, and fully satisfies (only twice) his exchange with her husband; when he ignores the porter's advice to flee and instead rides toward the Green Chapel—what then? Such dramatic contingencies provide *Sir Gawain and the Green Knight* with its anxious narrative energy, and they reveal within the poem the social and religious mores of a decaying seigneurial culture, the fluid borders between court and hinterland, and, most materially for this chapter, the divergent gender and economic hierarchies of Camelot and Hautdesert. "What þenne?" becomes a question that suggests the profound social, spiritual, sexual, and psychological stakes of the work.

The question also marks *Sir Gawain and the Green Knight* as a poem whose ultimate point of focus is not Arthur's stifling laughter but the fissures and uncertainties that it seeks to occlude, the looming threats to an ambitious Camelot still in its first age and the sometimes violent fractures—registered variously as physical, linguistic, and psychic—within its highly stratified social milieu. Scholarly attempts to trace those fractures have informed much of the criticism surrounding the work, and they have revealed the poem as drawing from, in Christine Chism's words, "a historical moment that resonates with contemporary tensions . . . between a royal court becoming increasingly alienated from traditional seigneurial modes of chivalry and a conservative and insecure provincial gentry, whose status, livelihoods, and careers were

---

4. See Herman, *Trauma and Recovery*, 1.

increasingly coming to depend upon careers at the royal court."[5] Underlying these contemporary tensions, however—indeed, a key driver of the new realities confronting England's aristocratic courts—is the ongoing demographic shift precipitated by the Black Death. This chapter thus considers the cultural changes that the Black Death catalyzed within England, particularly those changes to the social and economic roles assumed by aristocratic women in the late fourteenth century. In doing so, it makes a conjectural case that many of the disjunctures dramatized by *Sir Gawain and the Green Knight,* particularly its pressing reversals of gender hierarchies and its ambivalence over female desire and sexual agency, resonate with what were understood in the fourteenth century to be lingering symptoms and proximate causes of the pandemic.

Finally, the question "what þenne?" comports with the generic shift that *Sir Gawain and the Green Knight* inaugurates in its particular manuscript sequence, away from the allegorical and exemplary modes of *Pearl, Cleanness,* and *Patience* and toward the more secular mode of Arthurian romance. This generic shift, I want to argue, is important to the recuperative logic of *Sir Gawain and the Green Knight* individually and of the four poems as a group. Indeed, as Geraldine Heng shows, "The impetus of romance . . . is toward recovery—not repression or denial—but surfacing and acknowledgement through stages of transmogrification, and the graduated mutating of exigency into opportunity." Such an effort at recovery, at developing "a *safe* language of cultural discussion" within the romance, aligns the poem in important ways with *Cleanness* and *Patience,* both of which, I have suggested, deploy biblical episodes to evoke the trauma of the Black Death and to speak the plague's unspeakable losses.[6] Is it possible that *Sir Gawain and the Green Knight* uses the resources of Arthurian romance to similar ends? In this chapter, I propose to take that possibility seriously by considering how the poem, like those preceding it in the manuscript, might reveal itself to be concerned with the cultural and psychic ruptures caused by the ongoing trauma of the plague. I will further speculate on how the poem registers several key social and economic upheavals confronting England in the immediate wake of the pandemic, how it implies the riven processes of cultural change and recovery that followed, and finally how it insinuates the crisis of the Black Death into the mythic sweep of British history itself.

---

5. Chism, *Alliterative Revivals,* 66. It is important to note that in recent years, critics have pushed against the Eurocentric definitions of center and margin and have rightly advised that we embrace a more global view not only of the poem but of the Middle Ages as a construct. See, especially, Ng and Hodges, "Saint George, Islam, and Regional Audiences."

6. Heng, *Empire of Magic,* 3.

ENGENDERING THE BLACK DEATH:
MORGAN LE FAY AND THE PLAGUE ECONOMY

Once dismissed as a peripheral character,[7] Morgan le Fay is now recognized as crucial to the major concerns of *Sir Gawain and the Green Knight*. Several significant articles in the 1980s and 1990s, most notably by Sheila Fisher and Geraldine Heng, succeeded in shifting Morgan from critical margin to poetic center, situating her within a knot of female relationships and desires that inscribe a feminine shadow narrative to Gawain's own progress, a knot that, as Fisher suggests, reveals how "women constitute a threat to the chivalric code that is simultaneously sexual, political and economic."[8] Later critics have built on this groundbreaking work to read Morgan variously as a queer presence within Bertilak's court, a figure of sovereignty and latent Celtic spirituality, and a marker of Gawain's conflicting genealogical and feudal obligations.[9] Chism likewise identifies Morgan as reflecting geographical and cultural tensions between court and hinterland, while Randy Schiff, similarly attentive to the nuances of geography, regards her as a product of the Northwest Midlands' careerist economy."[10] These latter two analyses, which situate Morgan historically as well as theoretically, serve as my point of departure here; however, rather than focusing on the spatial rift between Arthur's Camelot and Morgan's Hautdesert, I want to begin by considering the temporal interval between the poem's central two loci, the year-long gap between axe strokes.

A poem famously "steeped in time,"[11] *Sir Gawain and the Green Knight* insists not only on the geographical fissures that crisscross its landscape—the rocks and crags of the Wirral, the forbidding scar of the Green Chapel—but also on the temporal fissures that divide its characters and key events, fissures where, as Richard Godden remarks, "the future and the past collide in the present."[12] Time functions in the poem not simply as continuum but as rift, a mode of division that the poet emphasizes in one of his most justifiably celebrated passages: "A ȝere ȝernes ful ȝerne, and ȝeldez neuer lyke; / Þe forme to þe fynisment foldez ful selden" [A year ȝernes very quickly, and it yields never

---

7. Derek Brewer, for example, states in "The Interpretation of Dream, Folktale, and Romance" that the poem is "self-evidently the story of Gawain: Morgan and Guinevere are marginal, whatever their significance to Gawain" (570).

8. Fisher, "Taken Men and Token Women," 72. See also Heng, "Feminine Knots"; Fisher, "Leaving Morgan Aside."

9. Respectively, Ashton, "The Perverse Dynamics of *Sir Gawain and the Green Knight*"; Donnelly, "Blame, Silence, and Power"; Twomey, "Morgan le Fay at Hautdesert."

10. Chism, *Alliterative Revivals*, chapter 3; Schiff, *Revivalist Fantasy*, chapter 3.

11. Bloomfield, "*Sir Gawain and the Green Knight*: An Appraisal," 18–19.

12. Godden, "Gawain and the Nick of Time," 154.

the like; the beginning seldom matches to the end] (498–99). Such a temporal geometry does not promise a reassuring cycle in which season and history comfortably reassert themselves year after year. Rather, it inscribes time as an erratically fractured circuit where past and future misalign in unexpected ways and where, in the single word ȝernes, the year both rushes forward to the promise of the future and yearns backward for the losses of the past.[13] Such a broken chronotope establishes a temporal present defined by contingency and mired in ambiguity. Unlike Gawain's geometrically endless pentangle, which "vmbelappez and loukez" [interlaces and rejoins] (628) its own beginnings at every perfect vertex, the shape of time is always broken in *Sir Gawain and the Green Knight,* its uncertain movement toward tomorrow charted not by some prescient and connective vision of the present but by the frayed, retrospective vision of so many used up ȝisterdayez:

> Þenne al rypez and rotez þat ros vpon fyrst,
> And þus ȝirnez þe ȝere in ȝisterdayez mony
> And wynter wyndez aȝayn, as þe worlde askez,
>> No faȝe,
>> Til Meȝelmas mone
>> Watz cumen wyth wynter wage.
>> Þen þenkkez Gawan ful sone
>> Of his anious uyage.
>
> (528–35)

[Then all ripens and rots that grew in the beginning, and thus ȝernes the year in many yesterdays, and winter winds around again as the world surely demands, until the month of Michaelmas came in with winter's promise. Then Gawain once again thinks about his troublesome journey.]

Traced in these lines are not only the regular seasonal and civic rhythms that count the clock in Arthur's court—the measured arc from "crabbed Lentoun" [crabbed Lent] (502) to "soft somer" [soft summer] (510) to "heruest" [harvest] (521) to "Meȝelmas" [Michaelmas] (532)—but also events that play an uneasy counterpoint to them, the Lenten fast "þat fraystez flesch" [that tests the body] (503), the "greuez" [groves/graves] (507) that grow green in the spring, the "droȝt [and] dust" [drought and dust] (523) that hamper manorial production. Falling, moreover, between the decapitation of the Green Knight and Gawain's follow-up journey, the passage asks us to recognize Arthur's

---

13. *MED,* s.v. "irennen" v. 1, 3 (to run, to elapse); s.v. "yernen" v. 1 (to long for).

Camelot and Morgan's Hautdesert as separated by the passage of time and its attendant pleasures and traumas, by a full year of "werre and wrake and wonder" [war and destruction and amazement/disaster] (16).[14] When he journeys from Camelot to Hautdesert, Gawain can be said to journey not just from center to margin but from today to tomorrow, from a conservative court steeped in the unquestioning display of masculine power to a more fluid cultural arena whose uncanny *now* may adumbrate one future for Arthur's realm.[15]

A seat of bald ostentation and egregious excess, Arthur's court has rightly been recognized as an idealized feudal site reflecting the intricate courtly forms and social mores of fourteenth-century aristocratic society, a "version of the ideal aimed at by any of the great courts of Western Europe in the later Middle Ages."[16] And yet, even as a projection, the Camelot of the poem proposes a vision of the English aristocratic court as it ideally existed—and as it could *only* exist—*before* the demographic and social upheavals precipitated by the Black Death. Hautdesert, by contrast, a site divided from Arthur's by both distance and time (as well as by the traumatic visitation of the Green Knight himself), is a court whose differences from Camelot comport with important cultural shifts occasioned by the plague. This is not to suggest that Camelot is in any literal sense early Edwardian while Hautdesert is late Edwardian or Ricardian; rather, it is to recognize that many of the hallmarks of these two courts align with specific economic and social indicators of preplague and postplague England. Within the context of this de facto temporal disjuncture, I want to propose that we might recognize Hautdesert, in several key respects, as a postplague *fynisment* of Camelot's preplague *forme*.

Prominent among the cultural shifts that followed the plague were changes in both the status and roles of women. To be certain, Caroline Barron's claim that postplague England offered a political and economic "golden age" for women is an overstatement;[17] however, historical studies do show that the decades-long labor shortage caused by the Black Death increased economic

---

14. Chism notes the contrast between Arthur's youth and Morgan's advanced age as reinforcing the relative maturity of Hautdesert's court in *Alliterative Revivals*, 68–70.

15. Lynn Arner, also attentive to the temporal interplay within the poem, proposes in "The Ends of Enchantment" that Hautdesert and the Wirral are in fact the revenants of an England *before* Camelot, arguing that "the frontier is a primitive [*sic*] terrain that has yet to develop into a cultivated region resembling Arthur's kingdom" (86). I disagree with the argument that Hautdesert simply represents Camelot's past. Indeed, the circularity of time within the poem forces past and future to touch: the up-to-the-moment castle of Hautdesert exists within a wilderness that borders on the primordial. These qualms notwithstanding, Arner's broader point that the poem insists on a temporal rift between the two realms is an important one.

16. Spearing, *The Gawain Poet*, 181. See also Mann, "Courtly Aesthetics and Courtly Ethics," 241; Bowers, *The Politics of Pearl*, 17.

17. Barron, "The 'Golden Age' of Women in Medieval London."

and social opportunities for some women, granting them broader participa-
tion in a depleted work force and allowing access to jobs once held only by
men.[18] Repeated spikes in mortality in the late fourteenth century also affected
customs related to landholding, as women inherited lands and rents more
frequently than in earlier decades. One case study of Essex in the plague year
of 1349, for instance, finds land moving more often from husband to widow
than from father to son, while a similar study focused on the 1370s and 1380s
shows women succeeding 60 percent of childless male landowners, statistics
that suggest how postplague demography put new pressures on increasingly
outmoded models of inheritance and land transfer.[19] Marriage patterns, too,
were affected by the plague, as single women increasingly deferred marriage,
and widows more commonly chose not to remarry. It is, of course, difficult
to know whether this change reflected a lack of potential husbands, a surfeit
of economic opportunities, or a combination thereof; however, civic records
from the late fourteenth and early fifteenth centuries confirm that women
tended to remain unmarried longer, perhaps opting to exercise a hard-won
economic power rather than to surrender it to a husband.[20] Chaucer's Wife
of Bath, who oscillates between the economic power of widowhood and the
impulse toward remarriage, speaks to this specific cultural crux, as does the
anxiety she evokes in many of her fellow pilgrims.

With these social changes in mind, it is important also to note that while
the lower classes may have gained some economic traction from the postplague labor shortage, the lives of peasant women immediately following
the Black Death remained bound to patterns of subsistence living similar to
those before the crisis.[21] Indeed, for England's working poor, the trauma of
the plague brought only more trauma: the loss of family, the dissolution of
community, and, more intangibly, the potential loss of faith, an issue explored
by both *Pearl* and *Patience*. The most dramatic beneficiaries of postplague
economic and social changes were the women of the aristocracy and, perhaps more significant, women in the emergent middle class. Thus, when we
consider how the demographic crisis of the Black Death promoted social and

---

18. See especially Mate, *Daughters, Wives and Widows after the Black Death*; Goldberg,
Women, Work, and Life Cycle in a Medieval Economy.

19. Respectively, Schofield, "The Late Medieval View of Frankpledge and the Tithing System: An Essex Case Study," 413; Platt, *King Death*, 50. See also Mate, *Daughters, Wives and
Widows after the Black Death*, 1.

20. Goldberg, *Women, Work, and Life Cycle in a Medieval Economy*, 210, 272–78. See also
Razi, *Life, Marriage, and Death in a Medieval Parish*.

21. My analysis is informed by Bennett, "Medieval Women, Modern Women." See also
Payling, "Social Mobility, Demographic Change, and Landed Society"; Archer, "Women as
Landholders and Administrators."

economic mobility, we are necessarily considering a relatively small, nonrep-
resentative subset of England's population. Judith Bennett stresses, moreover,
that any such demographic changes should additionally be understood as "a
short-term phenomenon, confined to the peculiar circumstances of a population ravaged by disease."[22] And yet, that particular subset of the population
and those particular circumstances—the English aristocracy and a disease-
ravaged economic landscape—are directly relevant to the audience of the
courtly *Sir Gawain and the Green Knight*. If there was ever a group poised to
recognize and participate in "the unusual opportunities and agency enjoyed
by some women during the 100–150 years after the first major outbreak of
plague," it was the readers of this intricate Arthurian romance.[23]

It is against this backdrop that I want to situate the character of Morgan
le Fay. Dowager, sorceress, crone, companion to the lady of the manor—Morgan emerges belatedly as the central locus of Hautdesert's courtly power and
the guiding intelligence behind the Green Knight himself. She is, moreover,
a woman whose shadowy presence is invested with both a numinous magical
force and a frank economic one.[24] Bertilak, in his guise as the Green Knight,
first reveals the extent of Morgan's influence, disclosing his own identity in
the process:

"Bertilak de Hautdesert I hat in þis londe.
Þurȝ myȝt of Morgne la Faye, þat in my hous lenges,
And koyntyse of clergye, bi craftes wel lerned—
Þe maystrés of Merlyn mony ho hatz taken,
For ho hatz dalt drwry ful dere sumtyme
With þat conable klerk; þat knowes alle your knyȝtez
       At hame.
   Morgne þe goddes
   Þerfore hit is hir name;
   Weldez non so hyȝe hawtesse
   Þat ho ne con make ful tame.
(2445–55)

[Bertilak of Hautdesert I am (called) in this land, through the power of
Morgan le Fay, that lives in my house; and by cleverness of study and by

---

22. Bennett, "Medieval Women, Modern Women," 162.

23. McIntosh, *Working Women in English Society*, 252.

24. David Lawton notes in "The Unity of Middle English Alliterative Poetry" that Morgan's
presence at the head of the banquet table shows an "unwonted respect for a dowager [which]
presages an unusual power structure at Hautdesert" (90).

well-learned crafts, she has taken many of the powers of Merlin, for she has
sometimes had intimate relations with that excellent clerk, as is known to all
your knights at home. Morgan the goddess, therefore, is her name; there is
no one of such high prowess that she cannot fully tame.]

Schiff reads this description's "uneasy awareness of magnified female economic power" in the regional context of the militarized Northwest Midlands,
and he convincingly argues that Morgan's identity as a powerful magnate
reflects a careerist society in which the absence or death of soldier-lords created socioeconomic gaps that were filled by women.[25] While I fully agree with
Schiff that Morgan gives voice to a moment in which women filled sudden
lacunae in authority, military careerism was not the only cause of that power
vacuum in late fourteenth-century England. As I've recounted above, the
economic dynamics that Schiff describes were similarly (and arguably more
fundamentally) precipitated by the plague. With that in mind, we might consider whether those same aspects that link Morgan to a regional culture of
careerism also link her more broadly to a national postplague environment,
one in which aristocratic women expanded their authority by exploiting a
changed demographic landscape.

It should be noted here that military careerism and the Black Death were
not mutually exclusive; each exacerbated the demographic pressures caused by
the other, and both created the same sorts of economic and social opportunities for late fourteenth-century women, particularly widows.[26] In that respect,
those details that link Morgan's cultural power to a regional careerist economy—her de facto inheritance of "Þe maystrés of Merlyn" [the powers of Mer-
lin] (2448), her "heȝly honowred" [highly honored] (949) status within the
court, and her aristocratic bona fides as "Arþurez half-suster" [Arthur's half-
sister] (2464)—also align her with the postplague conditions of aristocratic
women. In other words, if Morgan's character suggests the outlines of a war
widow from Cheshire, it likewise suggests the outlines of a dowered plague
widow. And yet, *Sir Gawain and the Green Knight* further hints that Morgan may be not only a beneficiary of her specific demographic situation but
also, at least in part, a cause of it—that she has generated her own sphere of
power through what the poem figures as her "predatory feminine sexuality."[27]
Morgan emerges, then, as both creator and exploiter of her particular cul-

---

25. Schiff, *Revivalist Fantasy*, 73.

26. By its very nature, the militarism of Cheshire would also have created *proportionately*
more widows to widowers than the Black Death, even if fewer widows overall, as the mortality
caused by military activity was sex specific.

27. Chism, *Alliterative Revivals*, 91.

tural environment. This key distinction exists beyond Morgan's affinities with careerist widows, and it begins to hint at a matrix of moral and medical discourses that are bound inextricably to the Black Death.

Throughout this study, I have alluded to several reputed causes of the medieval pandemic, and I have traced some of them through the Cotton Nero A.x poems: the biblical apocalypse in *Pearl*; the broadly defined (but sexually tinged) filth of *Cleanness*; the callow faithlessness that Jonah demonstrates in *Patience*. Of these putative causes, none was more commonly cited by medieval thinkers and moralists than illicit sexuality, the cardinal sin of lechery. Writing in 1362, one English chronicler blames the "*dira Domini flagellatio*" [dire scourge of God] on those who wasted God's gifts "*in sævitiam, superbiam, luxuriam, et gulam*" [in cruelty, arrogance, lechery, and gluttony].[28] John of Reading amplifies this point when he blames the disease on men who "*virgines deflorare, sponsarum ac matronarum castitatem violare*" [ravish virgins and violate the chastity of brides and matrons], while other moralists fault priests who trade benefices "*pro pecunia, pro mulieribus et quandoque pro concubinia*" [for money, for women, and sometimes even for concubines].[29] More comprehensive still, Thomas Brinton, Bishop of Rochester, writes in a 1375 sermon that that plague most grievously affected the English because they had indulged in "*furtum, rapina, gula, luxuria, incestus, et adulterium*" [theft, rape, gluttony, lechery, incest, and adultery], and he laments that "*ex omni parte est tanta luxuria et adulterium quod pauci de suis vxoribus contentantur, sed vnusquisque post vxorem proximi sui hinnit . . . fetentem detinet concubinam quod est horribile et pessima dignum morte*" [from all parts there is such great lechery and adultery that only a few men are content with their own wives, but each one brays after his neighbor's wife . . . or reserves a fetid concubine, which is horrible and deserving of a most low death].[30] To be sure, the moral failings blamed for the Black Death extended beyond lechery—plague treatises cite a broad host of sins as causes—but sexual licentiousness was clearly seen as paramount among them.

If lechery was believed to be the moral cause of God's vengeance, female sexuality in particular was cited by many (male) authorities as the apogee of such sinful behavior. Indeed, in the earliest account of the plague's arrival in

---

28. *Eulogium (Historiarum sive Temporis)*, 3:231.

29. John of Reading, *Chronica Johannis de Reading*, 168; Von Herford, *Liber de rebus memorabilioribus sive Chronicon Henrici de Hervordia*, 128.

30. Brinton, *The Sermons of Thomas Brinton, Bishop of Rochester*, 1:216. For narrative evidence of an increase in incest caused by sexual imbalances that followed the Black Death, a situation that Brinton might be alluding to in his sermon, see Cohn, *The Black Death Transformed*, 130. In that regard, it is worth noting that *Sir Gawain and the Green Knight* alludes to the damning incest between Morgan and Arthur at lines 2464–66.

Europe, Gabriele de' Mussis blames the disaster squarely on women, chastising them for their sexual openness and demanding repentance: *"dominarum pomposa vanitas, que sic uoluptatibus Imiscetur, freno moderata procedat"* [let the pompous vanity of ladies, which thus grows into voluptuousness, be slowed and checked].[31] Writing in response to an outbreak several decades later, Yorkshire chronicler Thomas Burton similarly recounts several suspect tournaments to which *"vocatis ad hæc dominabus, matronis, et aliis mulieribus generosis. Nec fuit tamen ibidem vix ulla domina seu matrona viro suo proprio sed alteri deputata, qua pro suæ libidinis impetu ad tempus abutebatur"* [ladies, wives, and other noble women were invited, and yet in those places scarcely any lady or wife was with her own husband but instead was with another, who used her at that time for his violent lusts].[32] Burton's observation is seconded by Henry Knighton, who connects the disease to *"dominarum cohors"* [a cohort of wives] who *"corpora sua ludibriis et scurrilosis lasciviis vexitabant"* [vexed their own bodies with trivialities and scurrilous lasciviousness], women who *"nec deum verebantur nec verecundam populi vocem erubescebant, laxato matrimonialis pudicitiæ fræno"* [neither dreaded God nor blushed with shame at the people's reproof, but relaxed the bond of marital chastity].[33]

At times during the plague crisis, female licentiousness was posited as both cause *and* effect of the Black Death. In its account of the epidemic of 1361, Ranulph Higden's *Polychronicon* relates how plague widows *"quasi degeneres sumpserunt maritos tam extraneos quam alios imbecilles et vecordes"* [as if degenerate, took as their husbands foreigners and other imbeciles and madmen].[34] John of Reading also decries women's moral laxity in the wake of the catastrophe: *"maxime tamen dolendum fuit de vita muliebri; nam relictae, priorum maritorum amore oblito, in homines extranos, plures in consanguineos, irruentes, impudicitiae falsos procreabant heredes, (sed et in multis locis ut dicebatur, fratres sorores acceperunt in uxores) qui fuerunt in adulterio generati"* [the greatest sadness was from women's behavior; those left behind, forgetting their earlier love in marriage, ran to foreign men, or, many times, to relatives (in many places brothers took sisters in marriage) and wrongfully produced heirs who were begotten in adultery].[35] In these assertions of female sexuality as both cause and result of illness, we can recognize how a corrosive late medi-

---

31. Gabriele de' Mussis, *Historia de Morbo*, 55.

32. Burton, *Chronica Monasterii de Melsa a Fundatione usque ad Annum 1396*, 3:72. The connection that Burton proposes between the ravages of plague and the inviting sexuality of women is implicit but unmistakable.

33. Knighton, *Chronicon Henrici Knighton*, 2:57–58.

34. Higden, *Polychronicon Ranulphi Higden Monachi Cestrensis*, 8:411.

35. John of Reading, *Chronica Johannis de Reading*, 150.

eval antifeminism was wrapped around the contours of a cyclically recurring disease, generating a rationale for the pandemic that was misogynistic and gynophobic in equal measure.

Her "blake chyn" [pale chin] (958) wrapped in a chalk-white wimple and her "lyppez . . . soure to se" [lips . . . disgusting to see] (962–63), Morgan le Fay does not project the seductive female sexuality described in so many chronicle accounts of the Black Death. That role, as I will discuss later in this chapter, falls to the Lady, whose "bry3t þrote, bare diplayed" [bright throat, openly displayed] (955) heightens the decrepitude of Morgan's "rugh ronkled chekez" [rough wrinkled cheeks] (953) and "blake bro3es" [black brows] (961).[36] The mingled description in which the two women are first described, however, ends in a quatrain that lingers less on the inviting figure of the Lady than on Morgan's own body, a moment that suggests how Morgan, though not physically alluring to Gawain, might manifest a sexual potency that transcends the knight's limiting heteronormative desire:

> Her body watz schort and þik,
> Hir buttokez bal3 and brode;
> More lykkerwys on to lyk
> Watz þat scho hade on lode.
> (966–69)

[Her body was short and thick, her buttocks *bal3* and broad; more delicious to look upon was the one she led with her.]

In its attention on Morgan's hips and posterior, these lines articulate a powerful female presence that exists apart from the bounded carnal desires of the poem's hero, a sexualized body whose relationship to the male gaze is decidedly other than that of courtly object of desire. Indeed, the very presence of Morgan's body serves in this passage to shift Gawain's gaze toward the lady herself. In that respect, Morgan's body not only resists being appropriated and constrained by Gawain, it also works to refocus his own desire, to bend and redirect it to Morgan's will. It is a small moment of control that subtly anticipates Morgan's immense authority over Hautdesert itself.

Also notable within this description is the adjective *bal3*, meaning bulging, stout, or round, a word that appears in only two other passages in the poem,

---

36. The description of the two ladies of Hautdesert has been discussed often in criticism, a tradition initiated by Derek Pearsall, who influentially describes their contrasting appearance in terms of a rhetoric of *descriptio feminae*. See Pearsall, "Rhetorical 'Descriptio,'" 129–34, and Narin, "Rhetorical Descriptio and Morgan la Fay in *Sir Gawain and the Green Knight*."

both of which are strongly suggestive of female sexuality. First, as Gawain arms himself to face the Green Knight, the narrator recounts how "he hade belted þe bronde vpon his *balȝe* haunchez, / Þenn dressed he his drurye [the Lady's girdle] double hym aboute" [he had belted the sword upon his bulging haunches, then wrapped the love token around himself twice] (2032–33).[37] In this context, *balȝe* conveys the muscular bulge of Gawain's haunches just as they are being wrapped in the Lady's feminine (and arguably apotropaic) "luf-lace" [love lace] (1874). This imposition of the womanly girdle atop Gawain's manly thighs and phallic *bronde* implies, at the very least, the limits of Gawain's masculine chivalric virtues. More pointedly, by enfolding his *balȝe* haunches in the lady's silk—a garment that the Lady produces for Gawain from "vmbe hir sydez . . . vnder þe clere mantyle" [around her hips . . . beneath her sheer mantle] (1830–31)—Gawain implies the primacy of a feminine sexuality within the social milieu of Hautdesert, the efficacy and *potentia* of the female body within Morgan's cultural ambit.

The poet uses the word again at an equally crucial moment in the poem, Gawain's first puzzled glimpse of the Green Chapel:

a lawe as hit were,
A *balȝ* berȝ bi a bonke þe brymme bysyde,
Bi a forȝ of a flode þat ferked þare;
Þe borne blubred þerinne as hit boyled hade.
(2171–74, emphasis added)

[A little mound, as it were, a *balȝ* barrow by a slope beside a streambank,
by a channel of a river that passed there: the stream burbled in it as though
it has boiled.]

Gawain himself expresses bewilderment about "quat hit be myȝt" [what it might be] (2180), but to many readers the chapel appears to be a barrow, a type of funerary mound favored in Celtic and Anglo-Saxon Britain.[38] Such

---

37. As a signifier for bulging, masculine muscles, the use of the word here bears comparison to its appearance in *Parlement of the Thre Ages*, in which the allegorized figure of youth is describes as a "bolde beryn" who was "balghe in the breste and brode in the scholdirs" (ll. 110–12).

38. Dominique Battles provocatively links the Anglo-Saxon figures of the barrow and the mere to the site of the Green Chapel, articulating how "the entire terrain of the Green Chapel, including its remote, wild location, the cold starkness of the setting, the unnatural 'boiling' water, and the expectation of death at the hands of a monster who owns giant weapons, all suggest powerful associations with Anglo-Saxon literary tradition" (Battles, *Cultural Difference and Material Culture*, 24).

a structure certainly comports with the deathly connotations of the site, a place where "my3t aboute mydny3t / Þe Dele his matynnes telle" [the devil might perform his mass around midnight] (2187–88). At the same moment, like Morgan's "buttokez bal3 and brode" [buttocks bal3 and broad], the Green Chapel also cuts a sexual, even genital image, as though the corporeal terrain of Morgan's body has been mapped onto the forbidding landscape itself. The "anatomical geography" of the bal3 has been outlined by Robert J. Edgeworth, and while his point-to-point labeling of the site may seem overly schematic, his observation that the site is evocative of the female genitalia remains a useful one.[39] Envisioned in these terms, the poem figures the reappearance of the Green Knight through the entrance of the barrow as a birth: when the Green Knight "comez of a hole" [comes out of a hole] (2221) to challenge Gawain, he literally emerges from the mouth of an earthly womb to strike his long-deferred blow.

I would like to suggest that such a site might also, albeit obliquely, be suggestive of the Black Death for a fourteenth-century audience. At the very least, we might surmise that the mound itself follows *Cleanness*'s Dead Sea and *Pearl*'s *spot* to evoke the symptoms of the disease, bulging from the ground with gurgling fluids like some autochthonous suppurating bubo. Less speculatively, however, we might also consider how the Green Chapel's terrestrial female body merges with other aspects of the landscape: the "creuisse of an olde cragge" [crevasse of an old crag] (2183) where "þe borne blubred þerinne as hit boyled hade" [the stream burbled in it as though it has boiled] (2174); a place of "ru3e knokled knarrez with knorned stonez" [rough gnarled crags with jagged stones] (2166) where the "mist muged on þe mor, malt on þe mountez" [mist lay upon the moors and melted over the mountains] (2080).[40] While the sin of lechery and the sexual female body, both evoked by the site, were regularly regarded as an overarching *moral* cause of God's pestilential retribution, the earth itself, fractured and vaporous, was understood as the *physical* mechanism through which the plague emerged. While acknowledging that "*epidimia aliquando a divina uoluntate procedit*" [any epidemic proceeds from the divine will], the report of the Paris Medical Faculty detects the disease in "*vapores malos putridos et venenosos . . . a paludibus lacubus profundis vallibus*" [bad, putrid and poisonous vapors . . . from swamps, lakes, and

---

39. Edgeworth, "Anatomical Geography," 106–7. See also Chism, *Alliterative Revivals*, 106.

40. Some readers have taken the poet's descriptive precision as evidence that the Green Chapel is based on a real place, such the rocky ravine of Ludchurch or the cave at Wetton Mill, both located in the Peak District near the border of Chester and Staffordshire. See respectively Elliott, "Landscape and Geography," 105–17; Kaske, "Gawain's Green Chapel and the Cave at Wetton Mill."

deep valleys]; similarly, a German treatise, which opens by pondering "*utrum mortalitas, que fuit hijs annis, fit ab ultione divina propter iniquitates hominum vel a cursu quodam naturali*" [whether the mortality, which exists in these years, happens by divine vengeance because of men's iniquities or advances because of nature], sees the pestilence surfacing when subterranean pressures force "*spiritus seu vapor per rimas terre*" [airs or vapors through fissures in the earth] and specifies that the disease is most pronounced "*in cauernis et ventribus terre*" [in caverns or in the womb of the earth].[41] On the Iberian peninsula, Jacme d'Agramont writes, "*Encara pot venir aquesta mesexa pestilencia de part de la terra. Car dintre en la terra se fan moltes euaporacions dumiditats per la qual cosa naxen e ixen grans fonts e rius dalts putxs e daltes montaynnes*" [Pestilence can come from the earth, because many humid vapors are formed in the interior of the earth which is the cause of the source and issue of great fountains and rivers from high places and mountains].[42] Likewise, an early English treatise finds danger in miasmas from "standing water in diches or sloughs."[43] With its cracked landscape, ominous vapors, and surging waters, the Green Chapel is strikingly similar to the *loci pestilentes* imagined in late medieval plague treatises and medical tracts. Perhaps by twinning such literal topographic features with the form of the female body, the poet inaugurates a site that appears overwhelmingly pestilent, a "chapel of meschaunce" where the reputed moral and physical causes of the Black Death not only coexist but are fused into a single terrifying spot. When Gawain goes looking for his death, this is what he finds.

Connections between sexuality and mortality have long been acknowledged in *Sir Gawain and the Green Knight*, as have the various deathly associations of the Green Chapel itself. What I am suggesting here is that those connections may be more specific to the recurring trauma of the plague than previous readers have recognized, that the poet has developed the moral and physical universe of his romance in terms that resonate with fourteenth-century fears surrounding the Black Death. Morgan's seigneurial efficacy, figured in the poem as both economic and magical, is shaped by a series of distinctive demographic circumstances associated with England's immediate postplague environment. Her superior role within the hierarchy of Hautdesert, her rich widow's inheritance (both pecuniary and supernatural), and her practiced ability to make any man fully tame likewise point toward her identification with the figure of the plague widow. At the same time, the poem also reveals

---

41. "The Report of the Medical Faculty of Paris," 154, 156; Sudhoff, "*Pestschriften aus den ersten 150 Jahren nach der Epidemie des 'Schwarzen Todes' 1348*," 44, 50, 48.

42. Jaume d'Agramunt, *Regimen de preservació*, 11, (Duran-Reynals and Winslow, 67).

43. *A Litil Boke the Whiche Traytied Many Gode Things for the Pestilence*, 2 verso.

Morgan to be the architect of her own ascendency, and the threatening sexual contours of her body, reiterated in the yonic geography of the Green Chapel, emerge as the very thing that both threatens Gawain's life and confirms her own mystical efficacy. By insinuating the historical, moral, and medical discourses that surround the plague into Hautdesert's environment—by allowing the economic and demographic to filter into the mythical and the psychological—the poem can be seen to create a pestilent world that simmers with threat and potential, a mutable social environment that challenges the rigid masculine norms of Arthur's court. We might push this possibility even further and regard this locus as a space in which the traumatic passage of the Black Death and the changes it catalyzed could be acknowledged and interrogated, a space that drives the poem itself toward "recovery" rather than "repression or denial."[44] But even without taking that relatively conjectural stance, the possibilities evoked by such pestilential spaces invest *Sir Gawain and the Green Knight*'s complex investigations of gender, hierarchy, sexuality, and chivalric identity with an urgent currency for late medieval readers, themselves caught up in an environment riven by sudden, fundamental, and often traumatic cultural shifts.

Might we even see these pestilential implications extending to the Green Knight himself? A figure created "þurȝ myȝt of Morgne la Faye" [though the power of Morgan le Fay] (2446) with the explicit purpose of causing death—he was made "for to haf greued Gaynour and gart hir to dyȝe" [to have grieved Guinevere and to terrify her to her death] (2460)—the Green Knight appears to us as a creature born twice, first from the magic of Morgan herself and second from the genital aperture of the Green Chapel. Whatever he may signify—and critical analyses have read him as confessor, embodiment of nature, gender-distorting defiler of chivalry, and Islamo-Christian saint[45]—he is primarily described in Fitt Four as an unrelenting engine of death:

> He cheuez þat chaunce at þe Chapel Grene,
> Þer passes non bi þat place so proude in his armes
> Þat he ne dyngez hym to deþe with dynt of his honde;
> For he is a mon methles and mercy non vses.
> For be hit chorle oþer chaplayn þat bi þe chapel rydes,
> Monk oþer masseprest, oþer any mon elles,

---

44. Heng, *Empire of Magic*, 3.

45. See, respectively, Pugh, "Gawain and the Godgames," 541; Rudd, "The Wildernes of Wirral," 52; Ashton, "Perverse Dynamics," 57; Ng and Hodges, "Saint George, Islam, and Regional Audiences," 292–94.

Hym þynk as queme hym to quelle as quyk go hymseluen.
(2103–9)

[He brings about that contest at the Green Chapel, and no one, no matter how powerful in arms, passes by that place that he won't strike to the
death with a blow of his hand; for he is an immoderate man, and he uses
no mercy. Be it a laborer or a chaplain that rides by the chapel, a monk or a
priest or anyone else, it would seem to him as pleasant to kill him as to be
alive himself.]

Unlike the lengthy description of the Green Knight from Fitt One, which
invites readers to marvel over his dazzling clothing and wild appearance, this
later warning by Gawain's porter is striking for its *lack* of visual detail, its sin-
gular focus on the knight as killer. Evacuated from the description are the filigreed axe and the holly bob, which promise conflict and peace in perplexingly
equal measure; gone too are the "kyngez capados" [kingly cape] (186) and the
embroidered "bryddes and flyȝes" [birds and butterflies] (166), the fashion-
able "tryfles" [trifles] (165) that lend the knight a patina of courtly splendor
within Arthur's court.[46] And whereas the Green Knight is noted in the opening fitt for his flawless physique (145), Gawain's porter pays heed here only
to his daunting size and strength, failing even to mention his signature hue.
Stripped of the nuances that alternately signal his otherness from Camelot's
knights and perform his essential courtliness, the Green Knight emerges in
the porter's description in stark, unvarnished terms: "Aȝayn his dyntez sore
/ Ȝe may not yow defende" [Against his powerful blows you cannot defend
yourself] (2116–17).

Suggestively, the porter's description bears more than a passing resem-
blance to one of the few passages in Middle English verse to directly address
the pestilence, the description of *Deeth* in Chaucer's "Pardoner's Tale":

Ther cam a privee theef men clepeth Deeth,
That in this contree al the peple sleeth,
And with his spere he smoot his herte atwo,
And wente his wey withouten wordes mo.
He hath a thousand slayn this pestilence.
And, maister, er ye come in his presence,
Me thynketh that it were necessarie

---

46. For one analysis of the significance of the Green Knight's courtly clothing, see Craymer,
"Signifyng Chivalric Identities," 51.

For to be war of swich an adversarie.
(*CT* 6.675–82)

[There came a secret thief that men call Death, that in this country slays all
the people, and with his spear he split his heart in two and went his way
without another word. He has slain a thousand people, this pestilence. And,
master, before you come into his presence, I think that it is necessary to be
wary of such an adversary.]

Lingering in his "habitacioun" [habitation] (6.689) outside of town and eager
to kill "man and womman, child, and hyne, and page" [man, woman, child,
servant, and page] (6.688), the Pardoner's *privee theef* serves, as Peter Beidler
notes, to "[call] up a host of responses from [Chaucer's] contemporary audiences, most of whom would have known about the plague at firsthand."[47] I
don't want to suggest with this comparison that the Green Knight, like Chaucer's *Deeth*, is a straightforward figure for the plague; he is far too complex
for such an oversimplified reading. Nonetheless, it is possible to see how—
with his miasmic lair, his reputation for invincibility, and his indiscriminate
choice of victims—he could conjure similar responses from fourteenth-century readers. Indeed, I would push this idea somewhat further to suggest that
the porter's description might also give voice to pestilential fears that remain
otherwise unspoken within *Sir Gawain and the Green Knight*: the monstrous
killer that cannot be named, the trauma of the past and its assured repetition,
the unstoppable advance of the death.

The poem's concluding twist, that the Green Knight is actually Lord Bertilak himself, comports with this speculative reading. Despite the abject fear
generated by the plague, the disease also existed, particularly in its later outbreaks, as what Jeffrey J. Cohen might call a terror "that lurks like a familiar
stranger at the threshold of the hall,"[48] an epidemic engendered mysteriously
by sin and generated in the deepest fissures of the earth but spread by routine,
everyday contact, the breath of a parent or the embrace of a child, the casual
touch of a friend, the courtly kiss of a lover. Boccaccio registers this duality
in *The Decameron*, locating the plague's origin in the distant *"parti orientali"*
before recounting the ease and intimacy with which it spread through the city
of Florence:

---

47. Beidler, "The Plague and Chaucer's Pardoner," 257.
48. Cohen, *Of Giants*, 28.

E fu questa pestilenza di maggior forza per ciò che essa dagli infermi di quella
per lo comunicare insieme s'avventava a' sani, non altramenti che faccia il
fuoco alle cose secche o unte quando molto gli sono avvicinate. E più avanti
ancora ebbe di male: ché non solamente il parlare e l'usare cogli infermi dava
a' sani infermità o cagione di comune morte, ma ancora il toccare i panni o
qualunque altra cosa da quegli infermi stata tocca o adoperata pareva seco
quella cotale infermità nel toccator transportare.[49]

[And the plague gathered strength as it was transmitted from the sick to the
healthy through normal intercourse, just as fire catches on any dry or greasy
object placed too close to it. Nor did the trouble stop there: not only did the
healthy incur the disease and with it the prevailing mortality by talking to
or keeping company with the sick—they had only to touch the clothing or
anything else that had come into contact with or been used by the sick and
the plague evidently was passed to the one who handled those things.]

That the threat of death in *Sir Gawain and the Green Knight* might assume the
shape of both monstrous "half-etayn" [half-giant] (140) and courtly gallant is,
in this respect, very much in keeping with the paradoxically opposed forms
of the plague itself, a disease as common as it was mysterious, as intimate as
it was global.

SAFE SEX IN THE FOURTEENTH CENTURY: THE LADY OF HAUTDESERT AND THE MEDICAL RESPONSE

From her first appearance in the poem, the Lady of Hautdesert features as
an active subject, not merely as the passive object of Gawain's desire: "Þenne
lyst þe lady to loke on þe kny3t; / Þenne com ho of hir closet with mony cler
burdez" [Then the lady desired to gaze upon the knight; then she came out of
her chancel with many ladies in waiting] (941–42). The Lady looks because she
desires ["lyst"] to look, observes Gawain from a distance before she even steps
out from the chancel that hides her from view. In a calculated reversal of so
many medieval romances, the Lady of Hautdesert fixes the knight in *her* line
of vision, refusing reduction to what Slavoj Žižek has memorably called that
"'black hole' around which the [male] subject's desire is structured."[50] From
this first appearance, she projects an agency that neither Gawain nor the poet

49. Boccaccio, *Decameron*, 13 (Waldman, 7–8).
50. Žižek, "Courtly Love, or, Woman as Thing," 94.

can fully sublimate into the homosocial structures of the masculine court, returning the gaze Gawain levels at her, meeting his desire with her own, and using the profoundly limited expectations implicit in his overdetermined chivalric code to manipulate the Pentangle Knight to her own ends.[51] As Heng puts it, "The Lady's calculated projection of an erotic female body fuels excitation by playing off Gawain's desire to see, his impulse to look, against her provision of something that desires to *be* seen, a desirable self-display for her own private purposes."[52] She wears her traditionally appointed role of courtly object not as an ornament but as a disguise, one behind which she can act powerfully upon (and in concert with) her husband's unsuspecting guest.

The Lady, we eventually learn, acts on the orders of her husband, Bertilak; he in turn acts at the behest of Morgan, dowager and goddess. These revelations complicate the dynamic among these characters beyond any simple object/subject binary. Nonetheless, the high degree of agency that the Lady projects within the realm—her active role in the management of the estate, her considered autonomy (both social and erotic), and her surprising level of independence from her husband—reflects the shifting social realities of late fourteenth-century England just as the roles assumed by Morgan herself do. Indeed, in the periods of economic and social uncertainty that followed the Black Death, married women often held more cultural influence than has commonly been recognized, and even if they lacked the degree of economic autonomy available to widows, they exercised significant control both inside and outside the domestic sphere. Studies comparing the roles of married women before and after the plague consistently demonstrate that married women played more active economic and seigneurial roles in the years following the disease than in the period preceding it.[53] Particularly in a regional economy like the Northwest Midlands, where the frequent absence of careerist lords had already strained traditional gender hierarchies, the postplague demographic crisis further encouraged aristocratic marriage patterns that, if not economically and socially equal in the modern sense, were at least

---

51. See also Stanbury, *Seeing the* Gawain-*Poet*, 97–98: "Where [*Sir Gawain and the Green Knight*] differs markedly [from the other three poems in its manuscript], however, is in its repeated emphasis on the *returned* gaze. As they look . . . characters adopt a wide variety of visual postures that range from non-reciprocated stares, ceremonial or iconic and worshipful gazes, to evaluative mutual gazes, as in the Green Knight's first challenge, and to reciprocal and erotic glances."

52. Heng, "A Woman Wants," 109–10.

53. Goldberg, *Women, Work, and Life Cycle in a Medieval Economy*, 358–59. See also Mate, *Women in Medieval English Society*, 62.

conducted with an ethos of social parity.[54] Margery McIntosh encapsulates the situation succinctly: "The atypical demographic conditions that pertained between 1348–49 and around 1500 allowed (or forced) some women to take a more active and independent part in the public economy than was to be true by 1620 and than had probably been true in 1300."[55]

For the Lady of Hautdesert, such social and economic roles come together in her bedchamber exchanges with Gawain, which, tellingly, she conducts in the absence of her husband and feudal lord. Much of the narrative force of these verbal exchanges lies in their simmering eroticism, but the bedroom scenes also, if less obviously, implicate the Lady as a commercial and economic agent, whose words are heavily inflected with the language of the marketplace. In her three encounters with Gawain, the Lady deploys a "commercial vocabulary" that mingles potently with the oaths and flatteries of her courtly "luf-talkyng" [love talk] (927).[56] Not only does she praise Gawain for his knightly "prowes" [prowess] (1249), she also assesses his "prys" [price] (1249); not only does she present her girdle as a love token, she also advertises its worthiness, describing it as a bargain item whose "littel" [small] (1848) appearance belies its hidden "costes" [value] (1849). Indeed, the arguments that the Lady uses to convince Gawain to accept the girdle come straight from an introductory marketing textbook. If only you knew what this little piece of cloth could do, she tells the knight, you would "prayse [it] at more prys, parauenture" [praise it as of higher value, perhaps] (1850). Sexualized and fetishized as it is, at the end of the day the girdle is an alluring sale item offered by an assured mercantile agent. And while the Lady's commercial acumen alone may not link the poem to the plague, her engagement in the ad hoc marketplace of Gawain's chamber reflects the particular economic environment of postplague England, one in which opportunities opened for women to develop a more pronounced economic and social presence in a changing cultural milieu.

If the Lady of Hautdesert can thus be seen to echo the cultural and economic roles assumed by some aristocratic wives after the Black Death, the sexual presence that she strikes in her bedroom exchanges likewise gives voice to the moralistic concerns over female sexuality we have already seen embodied in Morgan, concerns exacerbated in the later fourteenth century by per-

---

54. Mate, in *Daughters, Wives and Widows after the Black Death*, shows that after the Black Death, men "were likely to spend more time away from home than they had done in earlier periods, leaving their wives freer to make their own decisions concerning the management of the family land and its income" (197–98).

55. McIntosh, *Working Women in English Society*, 251. See also Archer, "Women as Landholders and Administrators," 150.

56. Shoaf, *The Poem as Green Girdle*, 2.

ceived links between sex and plague. Bertilak's wife would, we might imagine, easily take her place among Henry Knighton's matrons, who *"laxato matrimonialis pudicitiæ frœno"* [relaxed the bond of marital chastity] and invited God's pestilential judgement.[57] While the sexual threat presented by Morgan is occluded by her mask of age, the Lady herself, "more lykkerwys on to lyk" [more delicious to look upon] (968), renders her desire in surprisingly frank terms, telling Gawain, "3e ar welcum to my cors, / Yowre awen won to wale, / Me behouez of fyne force / Your seruaunt be, and schale" [You are welcome to my body, to take for your own pleasure. I am happily forced to be your servant, and I shall be] (1237–40). As many critics have asserted, the erotic charge of the bedroom scenes hinges on the verbal interplay that the Lady instigates with Gawain.[58] I want to stress, however, that the poet equally emphasizes the Lady's presence in physical terms, implicating not only the linguistic terrain that she navigates with the knight but also the physical terrain: the gauzy bed curtains that she slips through to "bynde [Gawain] in [his] bedde" [bind Gawain in his bed] (1211); her "cheke ful swete" [sweet cheek] (1204) and her "þrote þrowen al naked" [throat laid all bare] (1740); the kisses she claims and the lacy girdle she slides from against her skin. The verbal encounters between the Lady and Gawain are always informed in the poem by the presence of the physical body itself, as well as her promise of (and his resistance to) the physical act of sex.[59]

As we have already seen, sexual desire and illicit sex were commonly associated, on moral and religious grounds, with the onset of the plague. I speculated earlier in this chapter that such associations inform the poet's depiction of Morgan and the Green Chapel itself, and they are no less present in the figure of the Lady. But even setting aside its metaphysical and moral dimensions, intercourse was considered dangerous during times of plague because of the bodily exertions it required. Put simply, coitus was unsafe because, as Thomas Moulton's plague treatise states, it "bothe openeth the pores and destroyethe the kynde naturall" [both opens the pores (to pestilential vapors) and destroys the natural humoral balances].[60] The report of the Paris Medical Faculty, considered the most definitive contemporary work on the disease, warns that *"corpora . . . magis preparate ad huiusmodi pestifere impressionis receptionem*

57. Knighton, *Chronicon Henrici Knighton*, 58.

58. Heng, "A Woman Wants," 108–9.

59. The potential for Gawain and the Lady to engage in physical sex is further heightened in the poem by Gawain's somewhat spotty sexual reputation within the larger corpus of Arthurian works. See Brewer, "Sources I," 243–55; Whiting, "Gawain: His Reputation, His Courtesy and His Appearance," 189–234.

60. Moulton, *The Myrrour or Glasse of Helth*, B.vi.verso.

sunt corpora calida et humida" [bodies most prepared to receive this pestilential impression are hot and moist bodies], and it specifically advises avoiding "*exercito coituque superfluis ac balneo*" [superfluous exercise, coitus, and
bathing].[61] Bengt Knutsson, too, cautions that plague readily affects bodies that
are "hote disposed" [disposed to heat], including those of "men that abusen
theym self with wemen" [men that abuse themselves with women], and Jacme
d'Agramont insists that it is "*esquiuar ab gran diligencia jaure carnalment ab
fembra*" [important that man abstain from carnal intercourse with a woman],
further noting that "*car ja sie ço que fer exces en la cosa damont dita en tot
temps sie cosa de gran dampnatge al nostre cors. Empero en aytal temps asseyn-
naladament e notable fa gran dan e gran dampnatge*" [to go to excess in these
matters is at all times of great danger. But, especially in (plague) times, it does
signally and notably great harm and damage].[62]

Clearly, such scientific admonitions against intercourse comport with the
concerns of moralists who saw plague linked to sexual sin, but the medical
language in which they are expressed signals a crucial difference in the two
discourses, even as that language broadens the putative dangers of sex during
plague time.[63] For *Sir Gawain and the Green Knight* specifically, such medical
advice implicates the sexuality of the Lady in pestilential terms that critics
have not previously recognized. Within the narrative, she obviously poses a
moral and spiritual quandary for Gawain, and her expressions of desire, made
doubly illicit by her marital status and her husband's role as host, put pressure
on the precepts of sexual purity implied by his pentangle and his image of the
Virgin.[64] But in light of medical warnings against sexual intercourse during
outbreaks, the strictly corporeal dangers of the Lady's "cors" are also suggestive. Gawain's resistance to sexual congress, presented in the poem as a game
of brinksmanship with its own distinct set of delights, might thus be recognized as more than an ethical or religious stance, more even than an assertion
of chivalric value. It is also a *physical* decision that, during a time of pestilence,
would have been seen as having important prophylactic value.

The fact that Gawain and the Lady do not have sexual intercourse further underscores the ethos of contingency on which the poem depends, the
central question of "what þenne?" What if, readers find themselves wonder-

---

61. "The Report of the Medical Faculty of Paris," 156.

62. *A Litil Boke the Whiche Traytied Many Gode Thinges for the Pestilence*, 3 recto and 4
recto; Jaume d'Agramunt, *Regiment de preservació*, 30 (Duran-Reynals and Winslow, 83).

63. See also Cohn, *The Black Death Transformed*, 242: "The only activity scorned by the
preachers that the doctors also warned against was sex."

64. For the pentangle virtues, see especially Gallagher, "'Trawþe' and 'Luf-Talkyng' in *Sir
Gawain and the Green Knight*"; for Gawain's status as Bertilak's guest, see Shedd, "Knight in
Tarnished Armour," 6–7; for sexual chastity, see Spearing, *The Gawain Poet*, 194–96.

ing, Gawain and the Lady *had* engaged in sex? What then of the fulfillment of the exchange game? What then of Morgan's plan? What then of Gawain's head? Such questions beg to be asked, and as narrative possibilities they are vital to the responses that *Sir Gawain and the Green Knight* has elicited from modern (and presumably medieval) readers.[65] Sir Gawain, of course, never does have sex with the Lady, nor is he ever constrained to "swap we so" [make an exchange] (1108) with Bertilak. And yet the possibilities attendant on the poem's paths not taken linger, as do their uncertain social, sexual, and perhaps medical consequences.

Such unfulfilled *potentiae* reveal themselves most sharply at the very moment that they are foreclosed, in the Green Knight's long-deferred axe blow. Indeed, all potential outcomes lead inexorably to that one result, the single cut on Gawain's pale neck, the spray of bright blood on the icy ground. Just before he reveals himself as "Bertilak de Hautdesert" (2445), the Green Knight ascribes Gawain's wound to a lack of "lewté" [faith] (2366); however, he also asserts that any failure the wound might signify is mitigated by Gawain's innate love of life:

As perle bi þe quite pese is of prys more,
So is Gawayn, in god fayth, bi oþer gay kny3tez.
Bot here yow lakked a lyttel, sir, and lewté yow wonted;
Bot þat watz for no wylyde werke, ne wowyng nauþer,
Bot for 3e lufed your lyf—þe lasse I yow blame.
(2364–68)

[As the pearl is of more value than the white pea, so is Gawain, in good faith,
compared to other fine knights. But here you lacked a little, sir, and wanted
faith; but that was not for skillful deeds or for wooing either, but because you
loved your life. For that I blame you the less.]

Gawain himself identifies similar failings, citing his "vnleuté" [unfaithfulness] (2499), "couardise and couetyse" [cowardice and covetousness] (2508), and "vntrawþe" [unfaithfulness] (2509) as reasons for the wound; such damning self-appraisals have also been echoed by modern critics seeking the root of Gawain's failure.[66] But I would suggest that we should also consider—and

---

65. See for one, Boyd, "Sodomy, Misogyny, and Displacement."

66. For a good précis of these responses up to 1995, see Blanch and Wasserman, *Forme to Fynisment*, 156–57n5. More recent assessments have continued to offer a broad range of reasons for Gawain's nick, and Chism is certainly justified in highlighting the "multivalent interpretations" (*Alliterative Revivals*, 108) that the poem encourages in its concluding moments, as well

this is particularly salient if the poem draws from discourses surrounding the Black Death—the root of Gawain's success, not just the fact of the cut but also the fact that the head is still attached at all.

These two issues are closely related, but the second provocatively inverts the first, asking us to focus on the decisions that allowed for Gawain's survival rather than on the failures that contribute to his "schame" [shame] (2504). Nicholas Watson writes, "While it may be that [Gawain] has not entirely lived up to the ideals figuratively inscribed on his shield, he has only 'lakked a lyttel'; if he has lied by omission, he has also heroically resisted sex with Bertilak's wife."[67] That resistance to sex, considered in both its moral and physical dimensions is pivotal in relation to the plague. Gawain has behaved in ways that comport with the advice of innumerable plague manuals by avoiding lechery as both a metaphysical sin and a carnal act, securing his soul through repentance and confession, and shielding his body from physical exertions thought to leave the body susceptible to corruption.[68] Moreover, while he may reveal a momentary lack of *lewté* in keeping the Lady's girdle, he nonetheless marches toward his near-certain death at the Green Chapel, confronting a space redolent of the plague and its terrifying denizen with a faith never mustered by the skittish protagonist of *Patience*. For all of the poem's thematic and discursive complexity, it is ultimately difficult to disagree with the Green Knight in his assessment: Gawain succeeds overwhelmingly, erring only because he wants so desperately not to die, because he is human and alive.[69]

Gawain's flaw is thus the same flaw demonstrated by *Pearl*'s Dreamer, a figure whose own attachment to the piebald joys and traumas of life makes it impossible for him to absorb the teachings of an apotheosized Maiden who finds value only in the certainty of the New Jerusalem. Rendered more physically, the nick that Gawain bears in his neck—a "wemme" [blemish] (*Pe.* 221) coterminous with his humanity itself—comports with the *spots*, *mouls*, and *motes* that animate the opening poem of the manuscript. Moreover, like *Pearl*'s spot, the "nirt in [Gawain's] nek" [nick in Gawain's neck] (*Gaw.* 2498) is rich

---

as in her assessment of Gawain as a "knight nicked by human failure in a fellowship of chivalric ideologues."

67. Watson, "The *Gawain*-Poet as a Vernacular Theologian," 293.

68. Gawain, in fact, goes to mass after each bedchamber encounter (1311, 1558, 1876–84), and the extent of his shrift is specifically indicated after the third: "Þere he schrof hym schyrly and schewed his mysdedez, / Of þe more and þe mynne, and merci besechez, / And of absolucioun he on þe segge calles; / And he asoyled hym surely and sette hym so clene / As domezday schulde haf ben diȝt on þe morn" [There he brightly shrove himself and showed his misdeeds, the large and the small ones, and he beseeches mercy and calls on the man for absolution. And he assoiled him as thoroughly and made him as clean as if Judgement Day had been set to fall the next morning] (1880–84).

69. See also Johnson, *The Voice of the* Gawain-*Poet*, 85.

with possible pestilential overtones, not least because of its specific location on the body. Along with the groin and the armpit, the cervical lymph nodes, located on either side of the neck, were the most common sites for bubonic infection, and the appearance of buboes on the neck was regularly noted by physicians and chroniclers alike, as when Giovanni Morelli relates how victims were stricken "*di certo enfiato che venia con gran doglia e con repente febbre o nell'anguinaia o sotto le* ditella o nella gola, da piè dell'orecchie" [with great pain and a rapid fever which derived from a certain swelling either in the groin, under the arms, *or in the throat at the bottom of the ears*].[70]

Wounds on the neck also feature vividly in medieval and Renaissance art that engages with the plague. In one particularly harrowing painting from the fifteenth century, Hainaut artist Josse Lieferinxe depicts a plague victim in visible distress, his hand cupped gingerly over a swelling in his right cervical lymph node (see figure 4.1). A comparable late medieval image from the votive Chapelle Saint-Sébastien in Lanslevillard, France, likewise focuses on a cervical bubo as it is lanced by a physician (see figure 4.2). Metaphorical representations of the plague, which often use arrows or darts to depict infection, also highlight the lymphatic clusters of the groin, armpit, and neck. Most of the dead in the monumental "Triumph of Death," now housed in Palermo's Palazzo Abetellis, have thin arrows extending from their necks, each a subtle reminder of the presentation of the disease (see figure 4.3). So, too, does the young plague victim in Giovanni di Paolo's more intimate rendering of the same motif (see figure 4.4). Finally, images of Saint Sebastian, the most prominent of plague saints, regularly depict the arrows of his martyrdom piercing his neck, clear visual references to the clinical presentation of the bubonic plague. A late medieval engraving attributed to the Master of the Playing Cards depicts the saint with one dart emerging from his cervical lymph node and a second lodged in his rib cage (see figure 4.5). A later image of Saint Sebastian by Il Sodoma also focuses on common sites of bubonic infection, specifically the neck and the upper thigh (see figure 4.6).

For readers familiar with the physical tokens and artistic representations of the disease, would Gawain's wounded neck have evoked a telltale symptom of the Black Death? Again, we can only speculate; however, it is certain that the imagery of Gawain's final encounter with the Green Knight aligns with visual rhetoric associated with the disease. "Snyrt . . . on þat on syde" [Cut . . . on the one side] so that "þe schene blod ouer his schulderes schot to þe erþe" [the bright blood shot to the earth over his shoulders] (2312–14), Gawain might even be said to evoke the physical characteristics of plague survivors,

---

70. Morelli, *Ricordi*, 288, translated in Cohn, *The Black Death Transformed*, 94. Emphasis mine.

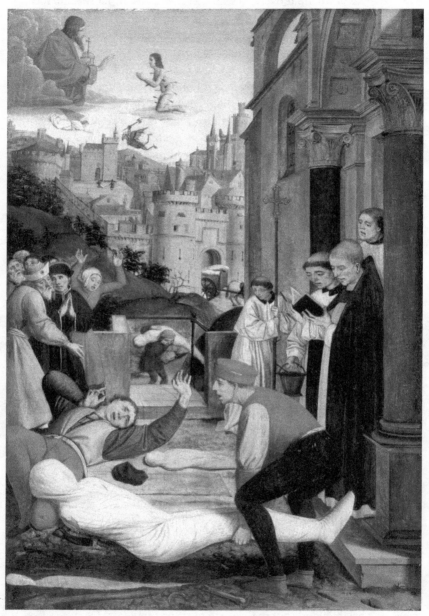

FIGURE 4.1. Josse Lieferinxe. Saint Sebastian Interceding for the Plague Stricken. Used with permission from the Walters Art Museum, Baltimore.

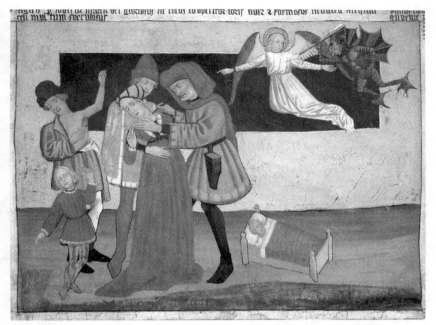

FIGURE 4.2. Scenes from the Life of St. Sebastian: The Saint Healing a Woman from the Plague. Used with permission from Scala / Art Resource, New York.

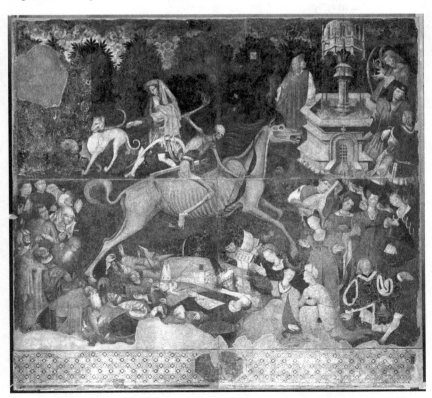

FIGURE 4.3. The Triumph of Death. Used with permission from Scala / Art Resource, New York.

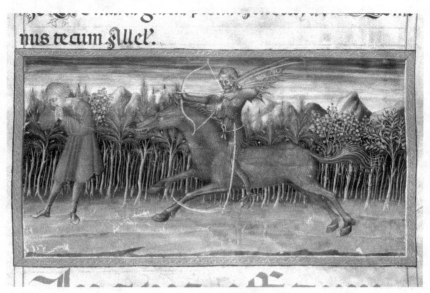

FIGURE 4.4. Giovanni di Paolo. The Triumph of Death (Death Assailing a Young Man). Used with permission from Scala / Art Resource, New York.

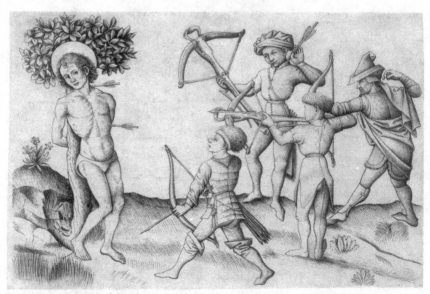

FIGURE 4.5. Master of the Playing Cards (attributed). Saint Sebastian. Used with permission from the Metropolitan Museum of Art, New York.

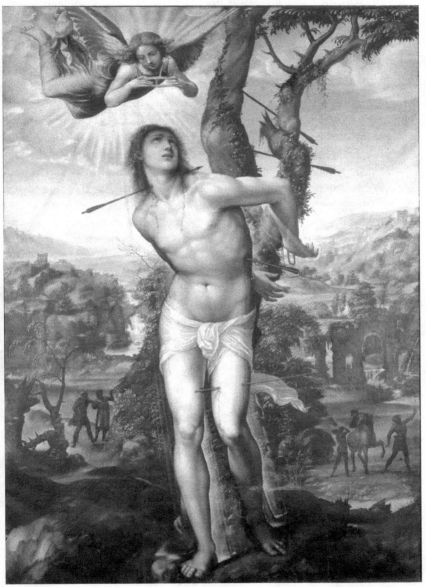

FIGURE 4.6. Il Sodoma. The Martyrdom of Saint Sebastian. Used with permission from Scala / Art Resource, New York.

their necks cut by physicians to expel toxic humors (see especially fig. 4.2) or simply torn by the internal pressure of the buboes. Given these imagistic contexts, Gawain's journey can, in its way, be considered as miraculous as Jonah's three-day progress in the whale's belly or the Ninevites' salvation—a miracle of survival against overwhelming odds.

Gawain is no biblical figure however. Neither patriarch nor prophet, his identity is constructed around the values championed by the fourteenth-century English aristocracy, the codes of sacrifice and chivalry and courtly refinement to which the poem's own medieval audience so publicly aspired. His "failure" at the Green Chapel may rightly articulate the limitations of his geometrically inflexible chivalric ethos, and it may further suggest the pre-eminence of female authority in the cultural milieu limned by Hautdesert; however, his "success" highlights the efficacy (if not the perfection) of his pentangle virtues, his resistance to sex with Bertilak's wife in accordance with the tenets of his code (and the advice of countless plague treatises), and his stalwart confrontation with his own mortality.[71] The imperfect success that Gawain achieves, then, clearly implicates the poem's courtly audience. So too, perhaps, does the sliver on his neck, the blood over the shoulders of the still-living body, the lingering threat of death, and the uncertain promise of survival. On the one hand, the bleeding wound reveals the limits of Gawain's chivalric virtues; on the other hand, the still-attached head affirms them on ethical, religious, and physical grounds, perhaps even celebrating them as prophylaxis against the pestilence.

THE QUEEN, THE LORD, AND
THE PRESSURES OF CONSERVATISM

The pronounced ambivalences of *Sir Gawain and the Green Knight* are rendered within the double crucible of the poem's two main settings, the separate but mutually penetrable spaces of Camelot and Hautdesert. A site geographically removed from Camelot, Hautdesert is defined by its de facto temporal disjuncture from Arthur's court, a gap that I have proposed may insinuate a future for Camelot that aligns with postplague cultural shifts. Such alignment is most dramatically suggested by the roles taken on by Hautdesert's

---

71. In this respect, I agree with Watson in "The *Gawain*-Poet as a Vernacular Theologian": "As 'active' rather than 'contemplative' Christians . . . Gawain and his colleagues can never in practice achieve the perfection to which they must aspire, but must expect to live their lives in a cycle of venial sin, repentance and penance, and perhaps spend time in purgatory before finally attaining heaven" (293).

aristocratic women, and those roles could not contrast more sharply with the position of Camelot's own queen. All but indistinguishable from the gems and tapestries that surround her on the dais, Guinevere demonstrates neither the commanding authority of Morgan nor the sexually inflected economic agency of the Lady. She is instead a witheringly passive presence, functioning mainly to enhance Gawain's knightly status at the holiday feast and to reflect the sumptuous excess of the court.[72] Dominated by Arthur's avuncular laughter and surrounded by knights whose patrilineal identities are written into their very names (109–15), Guinevere, like the world that she inhabits, reflects neither the loosening social restrictions nor the expanding economic opportunities available to aristocratic women in the second half of the fourteenth century. On the contrary, she reifies the stringent gender hierarchies and cultural conservatism that prevailed in England before the Black Death.

It is within this specific cultural environment, of course, that Gawain's pentangular identity first takes shape. As Carolyn Dinshaw has shown, that identity is dependent on the implementation of an "intensely rule-governed" code of aristocratic behavior and constituted by a series of performative acts that are "conventional and iterable, not freely chosen but constrained by birth, class status, and other structures of the normative."[73] At every point, the blueprint for Gawain's chivalric performance—a patriarch's "endeles knot" [endless knot] (630), which yokes the male-gendered attributes of "fraunchyse" [generosity] (652), "felaȝschyp" [fellowship] (652), and "cortaysye" [courtesy] (653) to the explicitly spiritual virtues of "clannes" [cleanness] (653) and "pité" [piety] (654)[74]—is coterminous with Camelot's entrenched gender hierarchies and homosocial chivalric ideology, the same social patterns reasserted by the constrained figure of the queen and the structured games of the Christmas feast. Ideologically as well as physically, the king's errant nephew begins his progress in Camelot.

Equally important, Gawain also *ends* his progress in Camelot, surrounded by the "lordes and ledes þat longed to þe Table" [lords and knights that belonged to the (Round) Table] (2515). It is significant, then, that while Hautdesert may be removed from Camelot geographically and temporally, it is also enclosed by Camelot poetically, a site physically marginal and formally central, existing on the hazy edge of Arthur's court and also at its core.

---

72. Schiff writes in *Revivalist Fantasy* that "Guinevere plays little role beyond that of beautifying Camelot's hall and being an unwitting object of Morgan's hostility" (92).

73. Dinshaw, "A Kiss Is Just a Kiss," 213.

74. For this fifth pentad, see Morgan, "The Significance of the Pentangle Symbolism," especially 775–79.

Structurally, Hautdesert thus has much in common with the numinous lost object of *Pearl*: it is the traumatic site that Camelot cannot speak (even the name "Hautdesert" is deferred until line 2445) but around which it exists. Despite his belated adoption of the green girdle as a heraldic device, despite being physically and psychologically marked by his experiences in Bertilak's realm, Gawain could no more be a knight of Hautdesert than the Dreamer of *Pearl* could remain with the Maiden in the celestial otherworld. Chastened, deflated, and changed by his journey—a journey, I have suggested, that takes Gawain through a world charged with both pestilential threat and postplague aftermath—Gawain remains a son of Arthur's hall.

And so again, "what þenne?" How does the pentangle knight move forward from the crisis presented by the Green Knight and his uncanny seigneurial demesne? Or, to put the question in terms proposed by Francesco Petrarch, "*Quid vero nunc agimus, frater? Ecce iam fere omnia tentavimus, et nusquam requies*" [What are we to do now, brother? Alas, now nearly everything is lost, and nowhere is there rest].[75] How does an aristocratic court, a feudal society, an entire culture move forward from the trauma of the plague? What might the future look like for Arthur and his Round Table after the Black Death?

A realm that incorporates many of the social and economic changes of the postplague world, a realm that both subtly empowers its two central female characters even as it suggests the pestilential implications of such sexual and economic autonomy, Hautdesert offers one possible answer. Gawain himself, however, seems to cling to a different future, one that looks a lot like the past he left behind when he first set out on his "anious uyage" [troublesome journey]. (535). Indeed, while he seems to experience something of a rebirth after his near-beheading—"Neuer syn þat he watz barne borne of his moder / Watz he neuer in þis worlde wy3e half so blyþe" [Not since he was a baby born of his mother was he ever in this world half so joyful] (2321–22)—Gawain ultimately gives voice to a vision of female agency filigreed with duplicity and threat, one culled from antifeminist rhetoric and energized by perceived links between women and plague. Indicative of that darker vision is Gawain's infamous misogynistic invective, a point at which the poem's submerged antifeminist discourse rises startlingly to the surface.

> Bot hit is no ferly þa3 a fole madde
> And þur3 wyles of wymmen be wonen to sor3e;
> For so watz Adam in erde with one bygyled,
> And Salomon with fele sere, and Samson, eftsonez—

---

75. Petrarch, *Epistolæ de rebus familiaribus et variæ*, 13.

Dalyda dalt hym hys wyrde—And Dauyth, þerafter,
Watz blended with Barsabe, þat much bale þoled.
Now þese were wrathed wyth her wyles, hit were a wynne huge
To luf hom wel and leue hem not, a leude þat couþe.

(2414–21)

[But it is no wonder if, through the wiles of women, I be made a fool and
be brought to sorrow; for so was Adam of old beguiled by one, and Solomon with several, and Samson again—Delilah dealt him his fate—and David
afterward was deluded by Bathsheba, which brought much sorrow. Since
these men were troubled with their wiles, it would be a huge advantage if a
man could love them well and believe them not.]

Critics have often noted how these lines conflict with Gawain's supposed dedication to the Virgin Mary and with the virtues of the pentangle itself.[76] Within
the traumatic contexts developed in this study, the sudden invective might
additionally be recognized as a belated response to the profound violence that
Gawain has experienced, an unbidden reaction to a traumatic experience that
he cannot fully suppress. This conjecture is not meant to excuse the rank anti-
feminism of these lines; Gawain is, I would submit, every bit the unrepentant
misogynist that he appears. Nonetheless, the explosive nature of the tirade
suggests the reappearance of submerged fears and anxieties, even the reasser-
tion of traumatic violence itself.

I want to propose here, however, that Gawain's outburst might also be recognized as implying fears over the pestilence, perhaps even offering a poetic
space in which the Black Death can be subtly disclosed. Certainly, we can
speculate that in its reference to Gawain's own birth, the lines reflect links
between female sexuality and plague death implied in the figure of the Lady,
as well as in the Green Chapel's pestilent landscape and Morgan's social and
economic milieu. We might also recognize pestilential connotations in the
judgements befalling the four biblical men that Gawain cites: Adam, whose
transgression with Eve first ushered death into the world; Sampson, whose
seduction by Delilah led to his torture and death; Solomon, whose submission to his wives' seductive idolatry caused God to rend his kingdom; and
David, whose illicit desire for Bathsheba culminated in murder and tragedy,
including the death of David and Bathsheba's son by a divinely ordained ill-

---

76. Morgan offers a brief summary of responses in "Medieval Misogyny and Gawain's Outburst Against Women," 265–66. See also, Clark and Wasserman, "Gawain's 'Anti-Feminism'
Reconsidered," 57, 63.

ness. Gawain's "wyles of wymmen" [wiles of women] (2415) are freighted with
more than just betrayal and deception. They are acts whose very carnality
engenders—by sin, by violence, and (in the case of David and Bathsheba) by
disease—death itself. In these respects, we might recognize Gawain's outburst
as a logical continuation of fears over female sexual agency that were exacerbated by the Black Death.

Following this line of thinking, Gawain's whiplash invective is also necessarily rooted in a profound and disturbing social conservatism, an appeal,
as David Aers notes, "for male solidarity in the face of the common enemy,
the one who is . . . an essential element in the making of masculine identity
and the one secretly feared by even the best honourmen."[77] Within the additional contexts suggested by the pandemic, however, we might also regard it
as a reactionary assault on the social and economic power that many women
gained in the wake of the plague, as well as an attack on women's agency as
a putative trigger for the disease itself. Indeed, it is precisely the active desire
of women that Gawain most strenuously rails against, even ascribing it to
Bathsheba, who is neither a seducer nor a betrayer but rather a passive victim
of David's unconstrained lust. Informed first by a well-established tradition
of medieval antifeminism (whose expression in both Latin and vernacular
discourse shaped medieval views on gender) and second by an acute environment of fear (in which women's bodies, sexuality, and agency were aligned
with the realities of pandemic disease), Gawain's diatribe is a strenuously
conservative repudiation of social change.[78] Rather than revealing any shift
in character or outlook, the outburst powerfully affirms Gawain's continuing
stake in the preplague gender hierarchies of Camelot, as well as a concomitant disavowal of the comparatively powerful postplague roles assumed by the
women of Hautdesert.[79]

Similar male anxieties over female power—political, sexual, seigneurial,
and economic—are evident throughout the poem, even if they are expressed
in less vitriolic terms. Bertilak registers his unease with Morgan's supremacy
even as he acknowledges her power over him,[80] and he reveals an abiding
discomfort with her sexual agency by noting that she gained her knowledge

77. Aers, *Community, Gender, and Individual Identity*, 171.

78. For the ubiquitous and all-permeating nature of medieval antifeminist texts, see Bloch,
"Medieval Misogyny"; Batt, "Gawain's Antifeminist Rant, the Pentangle, and Narrative Space,"
especially 137.

79. For an opposing view, see Cherewatuk, "Becoming Male, Medieval Mothering, and
Incarnational Theology," 19.

80. Schiff, *Revivalist Fantasy*, 73. See also Fisher, "Taken Men and Token Women," 95.

when she "dalt drwry ful dere" [had intimate relations] (2449) with Merlin.[81]
He also implies his discomfort with female power in Hautdesert when he
insists that he alone was responsible for his wife's overtures to Gawain:

> For hit is *my* wede þat þou werez, þat ilke wouen girdel.
> *Myn* owen wyf hit þe weued, *I* wot wel forsoþe.
> Now know *I* wel þy cosses and þy costes als,
> And the wowyng of *my* wyf. *I* wroȝt hit *myseluen*;
> *I* sende hir to asay þe.
> (2358–62, emphases mine)

> [For it is *my* garment that you wear, that same woven girdle. *My* own wife
> gave it to you, *I* know it well in truth. And *I* know well your kisses and also
> your actions, and the wooing of *my* wife. *I* wrought it *myself*. *I* sent her to
> test you.]

The Green Knight protests too much. While his words seem meant to reassert
his feudal lordship and economic mastery (note the emphasis on "costes"),
Bertilak's declaration comports neither with his revelation of Morgan as the
guiding intelligence behind the plot nor with the Lady's own assertions, in
action and speech, of her social and sexual independence.[82] Instead, his claims
of control seem merely to compensate for the diminished role he plays in
the social and economic milieu of Hautdesert. Morgan and the Lady are not
Guinevere, and their active presence within Hautdesert cannot, despite Bertilak's best efforts, be reduced to her passive one within Camelot.

Bertilak's failed bid to elide Hautdesert's ingrained female authority is further extended by Arthur himself when Gawain reappears at court. Like the
Green Knight's headless exit from the banquet hall, Gawain's return is dominated by the sound of avuncular laughter—"alle þe court als / Laȝen loude"
[all the court laughs loudly] (2513–14)—a stifling response that recalls Arthur's
reaction to the Green Knight's beheading, as well as the jocular games of the
poem's opening scenes. Moreover, the king "comfortez" [comforts] (2514) his
nephew with soothing speech, much as he earlier comforted his Queen, a figure who, it should be observed, is conspicuously absent from Gawain's home-
coming. Such small but notable details underscore the hegemonic masculinity
of Arthur's court. Ultimately, however, it is the Round Table's adoption of the

---

81. In their edition, Andrew and Waldron gloss the line as "she has formerly had very
intimate love-dealings with that excellent scholar" (297n2447–51).

82. Warner considers this interpretive crux in "The Lady, the Goddess, and the Text," 334–
35. See also Battles, "Amended Texts, Emended Ladies."

girdle that attests most powerfully to Camelot's suppression of the sexuality
and feminine agency defining Hautdesert. First appearing in the poem as "a
lace . . . þat leke vmbe hir sydez, / Knit vpon hir kyrtel, vnder þe clere mantyle" [a lace . . . that was cinched around her sides, secured upon her garment,
beneath the bright mantle] (1830–31)—a garment evoking a female sexuality associated both with "life and regeneration" and with moral and physical
peril[83]—the green silk is worn by Gawain "in syngne of [his] surfet" [as a sign
of his surfeit] (2433) before it is adopted by the knights of Arthur's court as
a "bauderyk" [baldric] (2516), a garment traditionally aligned with the masculine pursuits of hunting and military display.[84] The Round Table's assumption of the girdle performs, or at least seems meant to perform, the triumph
of Camelot's "broþerhede" (2516) over the more fluid gender aggregations of
Hautdesert, a celebration of the strict preplague social and sexual hierarchies
that prevail in Camelot and a dismissal of the postplague shifts visible in Morgan's domain.[85]

    Seen through the long lens of history, this masculine reappropriation of
female power is chillingly prescient, as the social and economic opportunities that emerged for women in the wake of the pestilence proved not to be
lasting ones.[86] In one telling assessment, P. J. P. Goldberg details how in the
mid-fifteenth century, men increasingly "sought to preserve their own position in a period of recession by excluding competition from female labour,"
a process that forced women back into the more rigid marital and economic
norms of the preplague period and that further solidified their roles in succeeding generations.[87] Thus, if we can read Hautdesert as responding to the
question "what þenne?" by articulating and even embodying the opportunities for women that emerged in the immediate aftermath of the plague, we
might similarly recognize Camelot as rolling them back, asserting England's
ingrained patriarchal structures and their agglomerated conservative pressures. In this respect, Gawain's return from Hautdesert to Camelot, his return
from a potential future to an uncertain present, thus adumbrates the clamp-

---

83. Fisher, "Taken Men and Token Women," 85.

84. See *MED*, s.v. "bauderīk" n. 1.

85. Aers, in *Community, Gender, and Individual Identity*, defines this "exuberant and fra-
ternal honouring of Gawain" as "an affirmation of the solidarity in the upper-class community,
its ceremonies, its virtue, and its goals, an affirmation confidently projected into a future . . .
which includes the poet's present" (175).

86. Bennett, "Medieval Women, Modern Women," 162–64.

87. Goldberg, *Women, Work, and Life Cycle in a Medieval Economy*, 7. Similar assessments
can be found in McIntosh, *Working Women in English Society*, 252; Mate, *Daughters, Wives and
Widows after the Black Death*, 193.

down on women's postplague agency that occurred as England moved into the early modern period.

But while the knights' collective attempt to transform a feminine lace into a martial embellishment suggests an act of masculine appropriation, the image of all that hard, manly armor wrapped up in lacy green cloth also bespeaks a different dynamic, one in which the feminine refuses to be constrained by masculine court mores but rather overwrites them.[88] Partially concealing armor that bears the knights' individual heraldic designs, the many identical girdles that Arthur's company wears not only inscribe the "presence" of women within the court but also reveal women's power to define, to circumscribe, and even to homogenize male knighthood. In this respect, the girdle is a material continuation of the objectifying "loke" [look] (941) that the Lady first fixed upon Gawain from her chancel, one that constrains and even remakes Camelot's chivalric masculinity. Read through the more pestilential lens I have suggested here, however, this intimate garment also suggests the possibility of a potent female sexuality, one commonly understood in the fourteenth century as the moral and physical cause of the disease. Indeed, in this respect, the object that arrives in Camelot and that swiftly finds a new host in "vche burne of þe broþerhede" [each man of the brotherhood] (2516)— an object that scans as a marker of female agency, an erotic memento, one knight's surfeit, and all Camelot's glory—functions precisely as a contagion. Spreading from Gawain to the other members of the round table, the girdle subtly evokes the swift advance of the plague through the household, the estate, the urban center, the community. Read in the most stringent and moralistic terms, the poem implies that by introducing into Camelot the material germ of illicit sexuality, Gawain effectively dooms Arthur's court to the very future that he has just experienced.

Richard Godden has shown how that the green girdle comes from a space out of time with Camelot, a possible future just beyond its vision.[89] I want to stretch Godden's point further still and suggest that this future—one aligned with cultural shifts associated with the Black Death—is not simply signified by the green lace but emerges symptomatically from it, developing around the infected object and metastasizing throughout the court. Indeed, the contagious presence of the luf-lace" [love lace] (1874) raises the possibility of what we might call a sexual-pestilential loop, a situation in which a token of female sexuality begets plague, which in turn leads to greater social and economic independence for women, which in turn encourages an increasingly

---

88. See Fisher, "Taken Men and Token Women," 99; Aers, *Community, Gender, and Individual Identity*, 173–75.

89. Godden, "Gawain and the Nick of Time," 168.

active expression of female sexuality, which in turn promises to promote more
plague. The circular structure of *Sir Gawain and the Green Knight* then, which
both mimics the cyclical nature of plague outbreaks and suggests the posttraumatic repetitions of those affected by the cataclysm, ultimately serves to
reiterate the deeply misogynistic terms in which the disease was understood
in the fourteenth century.

The reading I have proposed here sees *Sir Gawain and the Green Knight* as
a profoundly, even repellently conservative text, a poem steeped in misogyny
and informed by dubious connections between women's bodies and epidemic
disease. More generously, however, *Sir Gawain and the Green Knight* also renders a somewhat forlorn hope for a society on the brink of disaster, one that
occupies a space distinct from either the matter-of-fact presentism of *Patience*
or the apocalypticism of *Cleanness* and *Pearl*. There is, after all, still the possibility of a future in *Sir Gawain and the Green Knight,* a time after the traumatic
event has passed, a tomorrow after yet another year of "werre and wrake and
wonder." This is not to say that the poem promises a clear path to recovery or
that it evinces no anxiety about the years and generations to come. However,
in its insistence on the recursive gyres of history, *Sir Gawain and the Green
Knight* also registers a dogged faith, grounded in the repeated traumas and
recoveries of the past, that *blysse* follows *blunder* and that beyond the cataclysm there is building to be done.

As with all Arthurian romance (and perhaps as with all apocalyptic diseases as well), there is a certain inevitability about all of this, the assured repetition of an all too familiar trauma. The Camelot of *Sir Gawain and the Green
Knight* is, like all Camelots, a society *always* on the brink of disaster, a kingdom *always* heading toward a tragic collapse caused both by feminine threats
to knighthood's masculine ethos and by the inflexible masculinity and militarism of Arthur's kingdom itself. Everybody knows, after all, that Guinevere
will not stay nestled among her tapestries and gems forever, and everybody
also knows that Gawain's unyielding adherence to his chivalric code, while
presented as laudable in *Sir Gawain and the Green Knight,* begets tragedy after
the kingdom's "first age" (54) is at an end. And while the poem may not dwell
on Camelot's tragic destiny, it takes pains to divulge—in passing references
to knights like "Agrauayn a la Dure Mayn" (110) and Bertilak's genealogical
description of Morgan (2463–66)—the germ of the kingdom's coming fall.[90]
Within the capacious outlines of the Arthurian legend, it is not difficult to see
the infectious spread of the girdle from Gawain to his fellow knights as gestur-

---

90. For intertextual links between *Sir Gawain and the Green Knight* and the broader Arthurian legend, see Twomey, "Morgain la Fée in *Sir Gawain and the Green Knight*."

ing toward the collisions between sexual desire and military culture that would drive the destruction of Camelot from within. Nor is it difficult to see Arthur's rise and fall occurring within the shadow cast by Troy, the mythico-historical progenitor of Arthur's Britain that crumbled at the point where desire and war intersected. These are connections on which the poem insists, the links of history that it joins together with the "lel letteres loken" [loyal letters locked] (35) of its famous opening and reasserts in its closing moments: "mony aunterez herebiforne / Haf fallen suche er þis" [many marvels like this have happened in past times] (2527–28). That such *aunterez* resonate with the plague—that the sexuality projected by Morgan and the Lady, embodied by the girdle and latent in Guinevere, is implied in the poem as both cause and effect of the disease—directly implicates the fourteenth-century aristocratic culture for which the poem was written. In this respect, *Sir Gawain and the Green Knight* might be seen as tacitly acknowledging the epic scope of the pestilential trauma that England faced, as well as the social and cultural change—both positive and negative—that such widescale trauma precipitated. And perhaps more simply, the poem also affirms for its audience that after Troy, after Camelot, even after the Black Death itself, history does not come to an end.

A Pestilence Whispered

*These conditions have been so horrible that I do not reflect as
often as I used to about the situation. I have thought so much
about these events that I cannot tell the stories any longer. . . .
It would be too much for me to write the whole story.*

—AGNOLO DI TURA DEL GRASSO, *CRONACA SENESE*[1]

THE APPARENT FAILURE of fourteenth-century English poetry to engage
directly with the Black Death continues to puzzle readers of Middle English
poetry. As my analyses in this study suggest, that "failure" may be more perceived than material; however, it remains true that while the decades following
the first outbreak of plague witnessed an unprecedented flowering of vernacular literature in England, overt references to the pandemic in that literature
are surprisingly rare. Langland's "pokkes and pestilences" [poxes and plagues]
(B.20.98); Chaucer's "privee theef men clepeth Deeth" [secret thief that men
call Death] (*CT* 6.6756); the "dredfull Domesdaye" [dreadful Doomsday] of
Wynnere and Wastour;[2] Gower's "pestilence / Which hath exiled pacience /
Fro the clergie" [pestilence, which has exiled patience from the clergy][3]—these
sporadic references to the plague have been decried as "slight" and "timid,"
and they cannot help but *seem* slight and timid, especially when compared to
contemporaneous literature from mainland Europe.[4] Siegfried Wenzel offers
the most succinct expression of this view when he writes, "In vain does one

---

1. "*Ed era tanta lo oribilità, che io scrittore vengo meno a pensare; e però non conterò
più. . . . e sabebe troppó longo lo scrivare.*" Agnolo di Tura del Grasso, *Cronaca Senese*, 555, trans.
in Aberth, *The Black Death*, 81.

2. *Wynnere and Wastoure and The Parlement of the Thre Ages*, 13 (l. 16).

3. Gower, *Confessio Amantis*, 1:75–76 (Pro. 279–81). All future references to Gower's *Confessio* cited parenthetically by line number.

4. Shrewsbury, *A History of Bubonic Plague in the British Isles*, 42.

look for a parallel from an English quill to the long and moving descriptions of the Black Death given by Boccaccio and by Machaut, or to the anguished outcry in one of Petrarch's letters."[5] Wenzel's conclusion—"whatever mark has been left in concrete expressions in literature and the fine arts is not very visible"[6]—encapsulates the underwhelmed response of many readers seeking to understand the relationship between the pestilence and Middle English literature.

Why that mark is not very visible is a broad question, and the equally broad answers it has generated reveal the difficulty of accounting for this key difference between the literatures of England and mainland Europe. Wenzel posits, with some hesitation, that "the English, more than their Continental neighbors, realized that cheerfulness in the face of death is not only an excellent psychological defense but may actually have medicinal value," and he also locates an "essentially traditional and moralistic character" in Middle English poetry that led writers like Langland and Gower to focus on human morality rather than apocalyptic cataclysms like the plague, a kind of four-teenth-century English stiff upper lip.[7] In a similar vein, J. F. D. Shrewsbury states that English poets, and Chaucer in particular, avoided writing about the Black Death because they "believed in the superstition of the personifica-tion of pestilential disease . . . in which case the less he said about the plague the better," a claim for which Shrewsbury offers no real support.[8] Rosemary Woolf suggests that the English desire for literature about death declined in the face of so much *actual* death, an ingenious argument but one that doesn't explain why the same squeamishness didn't seem to apply to the Italians or the French.[9] And finally, I have argued throughout this study that that the traumatic nature of the plague hampers or suppresses its own literary witness, a rationale that might help to explain the subdued English response but that, once again, cannot account for the forthright accounts written on an equally traumatized Continent. Considered in the aggregate, these partially satisfy-ing explanations suggest that the difference between Continental and English responses cannot be reduced to a single cause, no matter how broad or far reaching. I want instead to propose a collective of smaller individual reasons, a series of local causes that pertain both to the literature itself and to its recep-tion by contemporary critics.

---

5. Wenzel, "Pestilence and Middle English Literature," 131–32.
6. Wenzel, 149.
7. Wenzel, 150, 152.
8. Shrewsbury, *A History of Bubonic Plague,* 41–42.
9. See Woolf, *The English Religious Lyric,* especially chapter 9, "Lyrics on Death," 309–55.

As my discussion of the poems of the *Pearl* manuscript makes clear, I concede that the *overt* mark left on English poetry by the plague is not, in fact, very visible. Nonetheless, the more absolute assertion made by some readers that the pestilence had *no* real impact on medieval English poetry seems to me drastically to understate the effect that the cataclysm must have had on both a national literature and on the nation itself. Through my speculative readings of the Cotton Nero A.x poems, I have intimated ways that we might recognize the disease within fourteenth-century English poetry and, more important, ways that we might see a subdued but insistent response *from* that poetry, one that emerges sometimes as an unconscious symptom and sometimes as an intentional authorial choice. Considered in these terms, the works of the *Pearl* manuscript can be taken to suggest that while Middle English poets did not advertise their engagement with the epidemic as overtly as their peers on the Continent, they may nonetheless have subtly embedded such engagement into the poetics and structure of their work, into the patterns of imagery and allusion that they developed, and into the social concerns and cultural crises they addressed.

Writing about the literature of the early modern period, which more overtly addresses the plague, Ernest Gilman has argued that any literature written during plague time "may be seen to respond more or less directly to the constant threat of epidemic meltdown in which their authors lived," an assertion that significantly broadens the range of what we might call "plague literature" and that opens up possibilities for literary witness that mitigate or even obviate the need for authorial intention.[10] On the one hand, such an embedded mode of response—textually embodied and mimetic—can be understood as rendering an unwitting witness, one that exists outside of any conscious decision by the author. Like Lot's wife in *Cleanness,* such a witness may not actively address the trauma that it reveals, but that trauma nonetheless remains present and legible, even if unarticulated. Taken to its logical extreme, such a perspective asks us to acknowledge that English writers in the late fourteenth century were *always* writing about the plague, whether they wanted to or not. The overwhelming presence of the disease infected—figuratively and literally—the works that postplague writers produced, even if they didn't directly address the pandemic in their poetry.

On the other hand, if the pestilence suffuses the literature of the late Middle Ages unbidden, this study has also suggested how writers like the *Pearl-*Poet may have *consciously* exploited that presence as well, crafting their work from an already pestilential *langue* and actively drawing from preexisting cul-

---

10. Gilman, *Plague Writing in Early Modern England,* 48.

tural discourses surrounding the disease. This argument, though more speculative than Gilman's blanket assertion, means that in *Pearl, Cleanness, Patience,*
and *Sir Gawain and the Green Knight,* the pestilence may have been hidden
by the poet in plain sight, embedded in knowing pun and loaded metaphor,
emerging in figures like the spotted child and the fleeing prophet, evoked in
biblical episodes and implied in supernatural confrontations. Within the corpus of Middle English poetry more broadly, the Black Death might thus be
seen to emerge at the overlap of the intentional and the unavoidable, a rhetorical and discursive space that, in this verse, is both more etiolated and more
subtle than an event of the plague's overwhelming magnitude might lead us
to imagine.

What happens to our assessment of plague in Middle English literature,
then, if rather than asking, "Why didn't English poets write about the plague?"
we ask "Why did English poets write about the plague in the ways that they
did?" In the more particular terms of this study, what happens if we ask how
the muted and self-consciously veiled response to the plague offered by *Pearl*
speaks to broader patterns of response offered by Middle English poetry, how
the displacement of the plague's trauma onto the biblical narratives of *Cleanness* and *Patience* hints at a particularly insular (and particularly vernacular)
approach to addressing the disease, how *Sir Gawain and the Green Knight's*
move to understand the consequences of the Black Death in the terms of
Arthurian Romance reveals regional or even national strategies for depicting
the cataclysm? Like the critics cited earlier, I can only pose tentative answers
to such questions. To do so, however, I want to begin with the widespread
belief, already discussed at length in this study, that the plague was God's
judgment on the sins of the English people. Bishop Thomas Brinton, one of
the many prominent religious figures to offer such an assessment, argues in a
well-known 1375 sermon that England's *"filios degeneres et leprosos"* [degener-
ate and leprous sons] are the sorry fruit of sin and faithlessness, and he concludes that the plague is a direct consequence of their error.

> *Sed videamus an nobis huiusmodi acciderunt. Sumus ne fortes in bello et for-
> tunati. Sumus ne in fide stablies. Sumus ne mundo honorabiles; immo omnibus
> hominibus falsiores et per consequens Deo non amabiles. Verum igitur in regno
> Anglie tanta est fructus dimminucio, tam crudelis pestilencia.*[11]

[But we see the way things are happening now. We are not strong and for-
tunate in war. We are not stable in faith. We are not honorable in the world;

---

11. Brinton, *The Sermons of Thomas Brinton, Bishop of Rochester,* 1:216.

rather, we are the most false men of all and, as a consequence, are not beloved of God. This, therefore, is truly the reason that in the kingdom of England there is so great a diminishment of fruitfulness, such a savage pestilence.]

Other clerical and secular authorities blame the disease on similar spiritual lapses—simony among the clergy, indecent clothing, excessive civic pride, false merchants, sloth, avarice, and, most prominent of all, lechery. Brinton is not alone in thinking the pestilence to be, as another moralistic treatise opines, recompense for "synne that raygneth among the people" as well as the prevalence of such sin "among head men. And the gouerners of the church, and of the law."[12]

Brinton's response is not a uniquely English one; the plague and its causes were similarly moralized across the Continent. Nonetheless, if these damning assessments of the plague's root reflect widespread cultural beliefs, they also reveal the acute challenge that must have faced many English poets, particularly those, like Chaucer and Gower, who wrote for noble patrons, the very "head men" and "gouerners" whose sins were so rank. Given that the Black Death was understood as God's punishment for sin, writing about it openly in a poetic work may have been seen as imprudent, even impolitic. This situation would have been particularly troublesome where the work itself was commissioned as a memorial for one of the disease's victims, a situation that describes Chaucer's first major work, *The Book of the Duchess*. Commissioned by John of Gaunt to memorialize his wife Blanche, who died of the plague in 1368, *The Book of the Duchess* offers an enigmatic lament for one noble victim of the disease, a lament in which the disease itself is never mentioned, even as death itself is constantly evoked through metaphor and allusion.[13] This tactful elision may, as Ardis Butterfield suggests, speak to the "awkward position of a poet seeking to address a man of John of Gaunt's social superiority in a time of public grief," but it may just as readily reflect John of Gaunt's own desire—perhaps personal, perhaps political—to shield Blanche from the stigma of the disease that took her life while simultaneously offering a public elegy on her death.[14]

---

12. Moulton, *The Myrrour or Glasse of Helth*, A.viii.verso. For the range of putative causes, see also Horrox, *The Black Death*, 126–43 (articles 41–48).

13. Butterfield, in "Pastoral and the Politics of Plague," writes that in the *Book of the Duchess*, "any reference to plague is totally suppressed in favor of a more generalized and abstract allusion to death" (22). For a more general assessment of the presence of pestilential discourses *The Book of the Duchess*, see Hinton, "The Black Death and the Book of the Duchess," 72–78.

14. Butterfield, "Pastoral and the Politics of Plague," 26.

The Book of the Duchess focuses on a knight in black who mourns his loss in terms that are reminiscent of the Dreamer's lament for his "precios perle" [precious pearl] (*Pe.* 60). Like the Dreamer, Chaucer's Man in Black focuses on the physical and spiritual flawlessness of his lost love object, the elusive White, whose throat "semed a round tour of yvorye" [seemed a round tower of ivory] (*BD* 946) and who appeared to him as "the soleyn fenix of Arabye" [the solitary phoenix of Arabia] (982)—"sengeley in synglure" [singular in its uniqueness] (*Pe.* 8), as the *Pearl*-Poet might say—even in a crowd of ten thousand. And like *Pearl*'s Maiden, White is "fairer, clerer, and hath more lyght / Than any other planete in heven / The moone or the sterres seven" [fairer, clearer, and brighter than any other planet in heaven, the moon or the seven stars] (*BD* 822–24), a figure as unspotted and radiant as "the someres sonne bryght" [the summer's bright sun] (821). Perhaps such suggestive lexical and imagistic parallels between *The Book of the Duchess* and *Pearl* hint at submerged references to the plague shared by the poems, but they also gesture toward the parallel circumstances in which both Chaucer and the *Pearl*-Poet worked. Like the *Book of the Duchess*, the poems of the *Pearl* manuscript are almost certainly commissioned works, probably written for a wealthy patron and possibly one with connections to the court of Richard II.[15] In addition, it has often been speculated that *Pearl* itself was written to mark the death of a two-year-old girl, an unknown historical "original" for the poem's Maiden.[16] If these somewhat conjectural circumstances reflect the actual circumstances of the poems' composition—and that is admittedly a very real *if*—then the *Pearl*-Poet, like Chaucer, may have found himself in the difficult position of eulogizing a noble victim of the Black Death while also needing to suppress in his verse (or at least to raise only implicitly) the disease that took her life. In the case of *Pearl* then, perhaps the poet found that by embedding the language of the plague within his meditation on human grief and divine will, he could

---

15. See Bowers, *The Politics of Pearl*, 14–16 and 191–94. Michael J. Bennett offers important discussions of the relationship between the poems of Cotton Nero A.x and the Cheshire gentry in "*Sir Gawain and the Green Knight* and the Literary Achievement of the North-West Midlands" and "The Historical Background." See also Bennett, "The Court of Richard II and the Promotion of Literature."

16. Traditionally, the historical original for the *Pearl* Maiden has been taken to be the daughter of the poet, a view enabled by the now antiquated idea that the poet existed in a world apart from the pressures of patronage and courtliness that informed the work of London poets like Chaucer and Gower. It seems far more likely, given the poem's probable existence within a complex of Ricardian patronage, that she is the daughter of the patron rather than the poet. For the earlier view, see Bishop, *Pearl in Its Setting*, 5–9. The relevance of courtly patronage structures to the poem has been convincingly documented by Bowers in *The Politics of* Pearl and "*Pearl* in Its Royal Setting," as well as in Staley, "*Pearl* and the Contingencies of Love and Piety."

both mediate the loss of the child through the stable and ultimately comfort-
ing framework of Christian salvation and invoke, with tactful obliqueness, the
presence of the pestilence. Tact, as well as trauma, may then partly drive the
occlusion of the Black Death in the poem.

Because of its delicate memorial function, *Pearl* might reasonably be
thought the most evasive and circumspect of the four Cotton Nero A.x works,
or at least the one most closely attuned to the needs of a patron mourning a
personal loss. Indeed, it is difficult to reconcile the repeated violent ruptures of
Cleanness, which immediately follows *Pearl* in the manuscript, with the image
of a poet stepping gingerly over the eggshell sensitivities of his grieving aristocratic patron. Nonetheless, even if they are not intended as memorial works,
the remaining three poems in the manuscript also evince in several ways the
same courtly identity, and thus the same need for courtly restraint, displayed
by *Pearl.* In *Cleanness,* as David Aers points out, Christ himself emerges as
"a representative of a thoroughly courtly Christianity, a divine Sir Gawain
. . . who would have been at home in Camelot or the courts of late medieval
England."[17] Moreover, the poem offers a clear affirmation to its courtly readers
that those who live in a state of "clannesse" [cleanness] (*Cl.* 1)—which, in the
view of the poem, is effectively a state of adherence to the heteronormative
and hierarchical structures of the aristocratic court[18]—will be spared God's
vengeance. If the plague is indeed evoked in *Cleanness*'s specific narrative context, it is, as in *Pearl,* evoked primarily through image and reference, through
the metaphorical bubo of the Dead Sea and the charged biblical exempla that
the poet chooses to treat. *Patience,* too, with its courtly-lady beatitudes, avoids
overt reference to the plague as it considers the adjacent actions of flight and
enclosure, ethically fraught responses to the disease that existed most viably as
options for the upper class. And while the key disjunctures between Camelot
and Hautdesert staged by *Sir Gawain and the Green Knight* imply the possibilities and crises attendant on a postplague seigneurial society, the poem ultimately participates in the same linguistic restraint modeled by its hypercourtly
protagonist, a knight celebrated not for his ability to breach uncomfortable
cultural truths but for his impeccable chivalric manner, his "clene cortays carp
closed fro fylþe" [pure courteous speech, free from filth] (*Gaw.* 1013). Thus,
even if they are positioned to interrogate and to understand the consequences
of a world wracked by plague, the poems of the *Pearl* manuscript are always

---

17. Aers, "Christianity for Courtly Subjects," 100.

18. To this point, Aers, in "Christianity for Courtly Subjects," writes, "Despite the divine
terrorism directed against those the poet constitutes as 'perverse,' the actual content of the
virtuous life has become as thin and depoliticized as any that flows from a Kantian categorical
imperative" (100–101).

attuned to the cultural expectations and courtly demands of their aristocratic readership. And while courtliness alone cannot fully account for the shape of the English response to the Black Death, it suggests at least one reason that literary evocations of the plague may have been more understated than some modern readers seem to desire.

In making this argument, I may seem to be implying that the court-centered literature of the Middle Ages is inherently fawning or even obsequious, a literature that presents no significant social or political challenge to its aristocratic audience. That is not the case. Among the Cotton Nero A.x poems, both *Cleanness* and *Sir Gawain and the Green Knight* implicitly critique aristocratic excess through their focus on finery and feasting. Moreover, by painting Arthur's royal court as a rabble of "berdlez chylder" [beardless children] (*Gaw.* 280), *Sir Gawain and the Green Knight* throws what may be a subtle jab at Richard II, who was regularly excoriated by his rivals for his youth and immaturity.[19] *Pearl*, a poem similarly steeped in aristocratic display and royal symbology, can likewise be seen as offering a rebuke of courtly mores and structures, upending ingrained gender norms and challenging social hierarchies through the figure of the Pearl Maiden.[20] Chaucer's courtly work, too, while famously ambivalent in its politics, is frequently critical of aristocratic culture, but it is important to recognize that such criticism becomes increasingly pointed as Chaucer drifts further from the structures of patronage that informed his early works. His treatment of Theseus in the "Knight's Tale," for instance, is far more caustic than his approach to the Black Knight in the *Book of the Duchess* or even to the avian courtiers in the *Parliament of Fowls*, two earlier works with comparatively strong courtly identities.

The "Knight's Tale," in fact, is a notable text in the context of this study as it contains an overt Middle English reference to the plague, the ominous assertion that Saturn's "lookyng is the fader of pestilence" (*CT* 1.2469). Jamie Fumo has placed this claim, a striking addition to Chaucer's source, into the context of a medieval tradition that linked vision with contagion, and her ensuing discussion of the "Knight's Tale" suggests the presence of a pestilential discourse within the work, a reading consonant with my own analysis of the Cotton Nero A.x poems.[21] As suggestive as this discourse alone is, it is more evocative still in light of its imbrication with Chaucer's critique of Theseus. Indeed, while Theseus exemplifies the hierarchical structure of the chivalric

---

19. Nuttall, *The Creation of Lancastrian Kingship*, 12–14.

20. For *Pearl*'s investment in Ricardian symbology, see Bowers, "*Pearl* in its Royal Setting."

21. Fumo, "The Pestilential Gaze," especially 87–91. Chaucer's source is Boccaccio's pre-plague *Tessida*, and in it, Venus herself, not Saturn, is responsible for bringing about the death of Arcite. See Correale and Hamel, *Sources and Analogues*, 191–92.

court throughout the poem and famously extols the "First Movere" (1.2987) in his final speech, it is not the orderly Jupiter but rather Saturn—in whom the tyranny of Creon and the specter of pestilence combine—who finally prevails in the tale, resolving the conflict between Venus and Mars and determining the result of Theseus's meticulously ordered tournament through an act of chaos. The link between disease and misrule embodied in Saturn instantiates the broader cultural perception that the pestilence was engendered in part by political and ecclesiastical malfeasance, by the sins of the aristocracy and the nobility, the "head men."[22] And while Chaucer might get away with such insinuations in the "Knight's Tale," which, like all of *The Canterbury Tales,* shields its author by refracting his voice through a prismatic series of narrators, it is difficult to imagine him raising the same possibilities in the more circumspect and more courtly *Book of the Duchess.*

Indeed, the *Book of the Duchess* approximates more closely than the "Knight's Tale" the social location of *Pearl, Cleanness, Patience,* and *Sir Gawain and the Green Knight.* As works of literature and as poetic artifacts, however, these four poems are more than just elegant, diplomatic solutions to sensitive commissions. Though they can be seen to articulate (and perhaps even to embody) the physical horrors and cultural shocks of the Black Death, the Cotton Nero A.x poems are also, and primarily, "elaborately made work[s] of art, fit only for the most splendid of collectors."[23] Bound by this uncomfortable duality, the poems can additionally be recognized as registering the moral and cultural anxieties attending courtly artistic production, those felt by the patron and perhaps, more intriguing, those carried by the poet himself. Such anxieties are most pronounced in the first and last poems of the manuscript, *Pearl* and *Sir Gawain and the Green Knight.* In my discussion of the former, I have suggested that *Pearl* blends plague language and imagery with Christian soteriology in order to offer consolation in the face of unspeakable loss, to succor the individual loss of one young child and also to reflect upon the cultural losses engendered by the pestilence. Nonetheless, the insistent courtly voice that *Pearl* develops, the voice that informs both the metaphorical development of its central terms and the means by which it offers its consolation, is as anxious as it is consoling: a hesitant merchant-dreamer stung by the inevi-

---

22. Moulton, *The Myrrour or Glasse of Helth,* A.viii.verso.

23. Staley, "*Pearl* and the Contingencies of Love and Piety," 100. See also Riddy, who notes in "Jewels in *Pearl*" how "*Pearl,* with its extraordinary technical elaboration and its complex verbal interplay, is itself a jewel in this sense. . . . As a jewel, the poem located itself among other highly-wrought, prestigious art objects, religious and secular, of the late fourteenth century: the elaborate reliquaries, caskets, crowns, brooches and cups that were the products of the jeweller's craft" (147–48).

table rebuke of his now courtly daughter; a supplicant regarding the splendor of his surroundings "wyth yȝen open and mouth ful clos" [with eyes open and mouth fully closed] (*Pe.* 183); a Jeweler whose "drede" [dread] (181) colors his every confrontation with the august Pearl Maiden. In these respects, the Jeweler's address to the Pearl Maiden implicates not only the halting address of the human to the divine but also the poet's own tremulous address to a courtly patron.[24]

Insofar as he presents his poem-jewel to a patron of greater social and economic standing, the writer of *Pearl* is at once both inside and outside aristocratic culture, a fraught position that mingles the potential for economic and social reward with the anxiety of social transgression and the requirements of moral and artistic compromise. On the one hand, then, *Pearl* is a poem that seeks to console, to instruct, to enlighten, to relieve—a poem meant to soothe a father grieving the loss of a daughter and, more speculatively, to imply an elegy for a nation devastated by the unspeakable cultural and social losses of the plague. On the other hand, *Pearl* is a poem whose aesthetic and linguistic beauty utterly belies the ugliness of such loss, a response to devastating personal and cultural trauma figured as an enviable courtly prize, a work whose dazzling language is defined by misdirection and compromise. The marked restlessness registered by the Dreamer after he wakes from his vision—"I raxled, and fel in gret affray, / And, sykyng, to myself I sayd: / 'Now al be to þat Pryncez paye'" [I awoke restlessly and fell into great consternation, and, sighing, I said to myself, "Now let all be given to the satisfaction of that Prince"] (1174–76)—suggests the ethical and even moral implications of such contradictions for the poet. The potent blend of struggle, conciliation, discomfort, complicity, and self-reproach that the dreamer intimates here is applicable in equal measure to the grieving penitent submitting to the demands of God and to the poet submitting to the artistic and social demands of his aristocratic patron.

The poet's implicit unease over such a transformative aesthetic is accorded a more robust voice in *Sir Gawain and the Green Knight*. More satirically barbed but no less equivocal than *Pearl*, the Arthurian romance amplifies the *Pearl* Dreamer's "affray" [consternation] (1174) when it relates the Round Table's response to Gawain's "token of vntrawþe" [token of unfaithfulness] (*Gaw.* 2509), the mysterious silk that the knight brings back from Hautdesert. Though Gawain understands the green girdle to be a sign of "þe laþe and þe losse þat I laȝt haue / Of couardise and couetyse" [the hurt and the loss that I have suffered, of cowardice and covetousness] (2507–8), King Arthur forces

24. Barr, "The Jeweller's Tale," 61.

its transformation from a mark of "schame" (2504) to an emblem of chivalric pride:

Þe kyng comfortez þe kny3t, and alle þe court als
La3en loude þerat and luflyly acorden
Þat lordes and ledes þat longed to þe Table,
Vche burne of þe broþerhede, a bauderyk schulde haue,
A bende abelef hym aboute, of a bry3t grene,
And þat, for sake of þat segge, in swete to were.
For þat watz acorded þe renoun of þe Rounde Table
And he honoured þat hit hade, euermore after,
As hit is breued in þe best boke of romaunce.
(2513–21)

[The king comforts the knight, and all the court laughs loudly at that and courteously accords that the lords and knights of the (Round) Table, each man of the brotherhood, should have a baldric, an emblem of bright green, worn diagonally across his chest as a uniform for the sake of that man (Gawain). For that was deemed the renown of the Round Table, and he that had it was honored forever after, as is told in the best book of romance.]

It is easy to regard Arthur's mollifying response to his nephew as little more than an avuncular chuck on the shoulder; however, by insisting that the "syngne of [Gawain's] surfet" [sign of Gawain's surfeit] (2433) be read as an emblem of courtly magnificence, the king effectively compels his court to enact a transformation much like the one performed by the poet himself, to sublimate something understood as shameful, sinful, and perhaps even septic into a blazon that enhances the splendor of the aristocracy. For Arthur and his knights, Gawain's green sash becomes—indeed, must become—a badge of honor, worn across the chest and celebrated in poetry: "þe renoun of þe Rounde Table . . . breued in þe best boke of romaunce" [the renown of the Round Table . . . as is told in the best book of romance] (2519–21). For the poet's patron, both the elaborate Arthurian romance of *Sir Gawain and the Green Knight* and the filigreed elegy of *Pearl* also stand as such courtly emblems, almost physically actualized poetic objects that echo in form and function both the green baldrics adopted by the worldly knights of Camelot and the pearly "liuréz" [liviries] (*Pe.* 1108) worn by the *maskellez* maidens in the New Jerusalem.[25] It is a poetic strategy that, chillingly, echoes the stifling

25. Bowers, in "*Pearl* in its Royal Setting," provocatively refers to the host of heavenly maidens as the "144,000 liveried followers of Lord Lamb" (137).

laughter of Arthur's court itself, one that both reveals and enacts the suppression of a deeply painful event within a traumatized culture.

Again, in underscoring their courtly context, I do not wish to imply that the poems of the *Pearl* manuscript, thematically and aesthetically beholden though they are to the demands of their aristocratic patron, are in any way lessened as poetry or as social critique. If anything, the presence of such courtly pressures may serve to heighten the tensions that underwrite each poem: *Pearl*'s struggle to reconcile the tragedy of untimely death with a theology that promises eternal life; *Cleanness*'s investigation of purity, trauma, memory, and witness; *Patience*'s uncertain ethos of forgiveness; *Sir Gawain and the Green Knight*'s awareness of chivalric behavior and nuanced seigneurial tableaux. In these works, the twin demands of courtly restraint and artistic compromise—as articulated by the patron or as perceived by the poet—neither mitigate the impact of the consolation crafted by the author nor blunt the force of his didacticism or his social critique. But especially as we consider the larger question of Middle English poetry's muted response to the Black Death, it is important that we remain cognizant of the essential courtliness of so much of that poetry and of the concomitant requirements of restraint, compromise, and circumspection that it must have created. Indeed, I would argue that the moments in which English poets *do* overtly address the issue of the pestilence (even if those moments are conspicuously few) come precisely when the courtly voice so carefully managed in the four poems discussed here gives way to a public one, a voice that, as Anne Middleton describes, steers "a course between the rigorous absolutes of religious rule on the one hand and, on the other, the rhetorical hyperboles and emotional vanities of the courtly style."[26] Those moments are rare in the poems of MS Cotton Nero A.x, which, despite their simmering ethos of public concern, hold more tenaciously to a "courtly style" than do some of their contemporaries. The public voice can be more readily located in those Middle English poems that take, in the words of Gower, a "middel weie" [middle way] (*CA* Pro. 17) in addressing their readers.

It is telling in that respect that Gower's sole direct reference to the fourteenth-century plague in the *Confessio Amantis* comes at a manifestly public moment, appearing not in the exempla that comprise the bulk of the poem but rather in the writer's invective against corruption in the Church. Even so, the reference is an equivocal one, naming the disease only to use it as a metaphor for the spiritual barrenness of the clergy:

---

26. Middleton, "The Idea of Public Poetry," 95–96.

That scholde be the worldes hele
Is now, men sein, the pestilence
Which hath exiled pacience
Fro the clergie in special.
(Pro. 278–81)

[What should be the health of the world is now, men say, the pestilence, which has exiled patience from the clergy especially]

Given that Gower announces his poem as "a bok for Engelondes sake" [a book for England's sake] (Pro. 24), the failure of the *Confessio* to engage more directly with the plague is puzzling: this is, after all, a work whose civic-minded public address is inscribed in its very dedication. It is important to remember, however, that the poem was initially intended for a much more specific dedicatee: its first recension specifies the *Confessio* not as a book for England's sake but rather "a book for King Richardes sake / To whom bilangeth my ligeance / With al myn hertes obeissance" [a book for King Richard's sake, to whom my allegiance belongs with all my heart's obedience] (*Pro. 24–26). Indeed, Gower outlines in the "Ricardian prologue" a mode of courtly patronage in which he is constrained

To make a book after [Richard's] heste,
And write in such a maner wise,
Which may be wisdom to the wise,
And pley to hem that lust to pleye.[27]
(*Pro. 82–85)

[To make a book at Richard's command and write in such a manner as it might bring wisdom to the wise, and pleasure to he who wants to play.]

Despite Gower's clear aspirations to a broad national audience, then, the presumably public *Confessio* remains fundamentally informed by its genesis as a court commission. In that respect, we might conjecture that the work is not,

---

27. This and the previous passage are taken from the "Ricardian" recension of the *Confessio Amantis* (as indicated by the asterisk), putatively written before Gower switched his political allegiance from Richard II to the future Henry IV and rededicated his book. The chronology and politics of the recensions, initially proposed in Macaulay's magisterial edition of Gower's works, have come under increasing pressure in recent years, most stridently by Lindeboom, "Rethinking the Recensions of the *Confessio Amantis*." For my purposes here, the chronology itself matters less than the tension between the courtly commission and the public voice to which Gower's two dedications attest.

in fact, in much better a position to outwardly address the Black Death than
are the poems of MS Cotton Nero A.x, bound as it is by the requirements
of circumspection and restraint implied by its commission.[28] In this respect,
Gower's great English work may have more in common with the aristocratic
Pearl-group than has been commonly recognized.

Within the *The Canterbury Tales*, Chaucer raises the terror of plague in
the figure of Saturn, as well as in the portrait of the Reeve: "They were adrad
of hym as of the deeth" [They were as frightened of him as they were of the
death] (*CT* 1.605). These references aside, however, he most vividly evokes
the Black Death through the Pardoner, a pilgrim whose ethical depravity is
matched by the unnerving forthrightness of his prologue.[29] While the shifting
"indirect discourse" of Chaucer's final unfinished work precludes a consistent use of the "impassioned direct address" associated with the public voice,
the Pardoner himself deploys *precisely* such a voice in both his prologue and
tale, as well as in his depiction of *Deeth*, exhorting the pilgrims to personal,
religious, and communal improvement even as he waits, avariciously, for
the monetary rewards of his "moral tale" (6.460).[30] Significantly, the public
address delivered by the Pardoner is also closely related to his failure to gauge
the collective social and interpersonal demands of his fellow travelers, particularly when he asks Harry Bailly, who "commissioned" his tale, to atone
for being the "moost envoluped in synne" [most enveloped by sin] (6.942).
If Harry's violent response to the Pardoner suggests the consequences of his
particularly impolitic address—"I wolde I hadde thy coillons in myn hond / In
stide of relikes or of seintuarie. / Lat kutte hem of, I wol thee helpe hem carie;
/ They shul be shryned in an hogges toord!" [I would that I had your testicles
in my hand instead of relics or sacred objects. Let's cut them off. I will help
you carry them. They shall be enshrined in a hog's turd!] (6.952–55)—it also
brutally suggests the need for poetic circumspection among English writers as
they seek to fill their respective commissions. This need for restraint emerges
again in the "Manciple's Tale," when Phoebus punishes his pet crow, commonly regarded as a figure for the court poet, for speaking openly of the infi-
delity of Phoebus's wife.[31] The "Manciple's Tale" does not draw on the plague
discourses present in the "Pardoner's Tale"; however, it similarly implies the

---

28. Joyce Coleman gestures toward some of the courtlier aspects of Gower's *Confessio
Amantis,* "Royal Patronage, the *Confessio,* and the *Legend of Good Women.*"

29. Peter Beidler has used the plague to account for some of the unresolved narrative issues
with the Pardoner's enigmatic tale, including the presence of a pile of gold under the tree, the
old man who directs the three youths to it, and Harry Bailly's violent reaction to the Pardoner
himself. See Beidler, "The Plague and Chaucer's Pardoner," 257–69.

30. Middleton, "The Idea of Public Poetry," 94.

31. The relationship between the speaking crow and the court poet is most thoroughly
explored in Fradenburg, "The Manciple's Servant Tongue."

dangerous power imbalances between poet and patron, as well as the concomitant dangers of harnessing an uninhibited public voice in the sensitive
arena of the court.

Perhaps, then, one reason we see such a muted response to the Black
Death in England is the courtly nature of so much English poetry and the
necessarily constrained voices of many of its major poets: the poet of the Cotton Nero A.x poems, compelled to please his patron with an elegy of unerring
tact and courtly restraint; Chaucer, inexorably bound by what Paul Strohm
has called "the complex mixture of residual loyalty and unabashed self-interest that united lords and their followers within the bastard feudalism of the
late fourteenth century";[32] Gower, sharply attuned to the same shifting set of
dynastic allegiances that cause him to dedicate and then rededicate his major
Middle English work. It is fitting, then, that the most full-throated evocation
of the Black Death to emerge from fourteenth-century England also comes
from one of its *least* courtly poems. Regarded by Anne Middleton as "the first
Middle English poetic fiction intentionally capable of a national resonance
and reception," *Piers Plowman* provides the only description of the pestilence
in Middle English to approach those from the Continent:[33]

Kynde cam after hym, wiþ many kene soores,
As pokkes and pestilences, and muche peple shente;
So Kynde þoruȝ corrupcions kilde ful manye.
Deeþ cam dryuynge after and al to duste passhed
Kynges and knyghtes, kaysers and popes.
Lered ne lewed, he lefte no man stonde
That he hitte euene, þat euere stired after.
Manye a louely lady and [hir] lemmans knyȝtes
Swowned and swelted for sorwe of Deþes dyntes.
(B.20.97–105)

[*Kynde* came next with many sharp sores, such as poxes and plagues, and
brought about the death of many people. So *kynde* killed many through
infection. Death came driving in after and struck many down to dust: kings
and knights, kaisers and popes, learned and unlearned—he let no man stand
that he struck, and they never stirred afterward. Many lovely ladies and their
knightly lovers swooned and expired for sorrow of death's blows.]

---

32. Strohm, *Social Chaucer,* 23.
33. Middleton, "Audience and Public," 118–19.

The forthrightness of this description is, I would argue, directly related to *Piers Plowman*'s consistently hortative voice, a voice that neither the polyvocal *Canterbury Tales,* the politically equivocal *Confessio Amantis,* nor the court-centered poetry of MS Cotton Nero A.x fully develops. In reaching beyond the coterie, beyond even the region, and striving for a voice to address the whole "fair feeld ful of folk" [fair field full of folk] (B.Pro.17) that he envisions in his prologue, Langland gropes toward a public mode of address that is able to transcend the courtly pressures that encumber the courtly writer of *Pearl, Cleanness, Patience,* and *Sir Gawain and the Green Knight.* Unburdened by those pressures, Langland finds himself in a position to invoke the plague more vehemently than his English contemporaries, drawing into sharp relief the same moral, ethical, and apocalyptic overtones of the disease that the *Pearl*-Poet can only imply in his more restrained works.

There are, of course, two obvious problems with this theory. First, even Langland, the most stridently public of his English contemporaries, does not match the descriptive lament found in work emerging from the European mainland. Indeed, while we can assert without controversy that Langland addresses the disease in a more sustained way than his fellow fourteenth-century English poets, we must also concede, by the same token, that his description still doesn't equal the benchmark set by Continental writers like Boccaccio. Second, and more important, most of those Continental writers, Machaut and Boccaccio among them, are bound to the same structures of courtly patronage that appear to muffle references to the Black Death by their English contemporaries. Machaut's *Jugement dou Roy de Navarre,* which opens with an extended remembrance of the *"grans monciaus / Trouvoit on dames, jouvenciaus, / Juenes, viels, et de toutes guises . . . tous mors de boces"* [great heaps of women, youths, / Boys, old people, those of all stations . . . all of them dead from the buboes], was either written specifically for King Charles II of Navarre or was rededicated to him after the death of Machaut's earlier patron, Bonne of Luxembourg.[34] Boccaccio's literary career, too, was closely tied to the royal courts of Florence and Naples, and like *Navarre,* the *Decameron* was composed amidst the constraints and pressures of a patronage relationship. If the distinction between a literature that can openly discuss the plague and one that offers a more ciphered response is, as I propose here, related to the respective public-ness of those literatures, why should a courtly French poet like Machaut offer a more overt response to the Black Death than the English writer of *Piers Plowman,* whose relationship to the aristocracy appears far

---

34. Machaut, *The Judgment of the King of Navarre,* 18–19 (ll. 370–74, trans. ll. 371–74). See Earp, *Guillaume de Machaut: A Guide to Research,* 33.

more distant and whose poetic address is directed well beyond the narrow confines of a courtly audience?

Again, I want to stress that this question does not have a single easy answer. Courtliness, as Langland's public evocation of the plague suggests, may be *one* of the factors contributing to the distinction between the English and Continental responses, but it cannot be the only factor, nor is it necessarily the most fundamental. I would propose that, in addition to the relative public-ness of the poems themselves, we also consider a more inherent issue, namely the potential—or the perceived potential—for their respective vernaculars to accommodate the public voice that poems like *Piers* and the *Confessio* sought. The French vernacular literary tradition, which could claim the twelfth-century romances of Chrétien de Troyes and the mid-thirteenth-century *Roman de la Rose* as cornerstones of its canon, was well established when Machaut detailed the "*boces . . . et grans glos / Dont on moroit*" [buboes . . . and large swellings / From which (people) died]" and bemoaned the once clear air of France now "*vils, noirs, et obscurs / Lais et puans, troubles et pus*" [vile, black, and hazy / Horrible and fetid, putrefied and infected].[35] Indeed, during the rule of the Valois kings, France actively supported its vernacular culture, developing for the French language an ongoing literary tradition and granting it the imprimatur of royal authority.[36] Meanwhile in Italy, Boccaccio's lament for plague victims who "*non come uomini ma quasi come bestie morieno*" [died like brute beasts rather than human beings] was crafted in a vernacular whose theological, social, and artistic possibilities had already been established by Dante and further explored by Petrarch.[37] By the late fourteenth century, then, both French and Italian were recognized as languages with profound cultural value and broad public reach, both of which ensured that the actual audiences attained by these poems could be reasonably expected to surpass their respective publics, the readerships imagined by the authors themselves.[38]

English, by contrast, a language that boasted a low cultural capital in comparison to the major Continental vernaculars, was only beginning to emerge as a respectable literary, political, and theological medium in the second half of the fourteenth century.[39] Indeed, "with its small vocabulary, its lexigraphical oddities, tendency toward monosyllable, and lack of inflection," English

---

35. Machaut, *The Judgment of the King of Navarre*, 14–15, 16–17 (ll. 323–34, 314–15).

36. See Staley, *Languages of Power*, 95. Staley's discussion of how a beleaguered Richard II "looked to France, and particularly to the France of Charles V" as a model for developing a "language of royal power" (95) is germane to my argument here as it suggests, from a somewhat different angle, the perceived limits of English in comparison to its continental counterparts.

37. Boccaccio, *Decameron*, 19 (Waldman, 13).

38. Middleton, "Audience and Public," 101–2.

39. See Taylor, "Social Aesthetics," 301.

was sometimes regarded, even at the beginning of the fifteenth century, as "a barbarous tongue . . . grammatically and rhetorically inadequate as a vehicle for truth."[40] Given the sheer poetic virtuosity of the Cotton Nero A.x poems, it is difficult imagine that the *Pearl*-Poet would have considered English functionally unable to address the event of the plague; however, concerns over the ability of English to function as a "vehicle for truth" are nonetheless persistently (if implicitly) raised by the poems of the *Pearl* manuscript: in the Pearl Maiden's careful but imperfect English translations of Latin biblical parables and the Jeweler's dubious responses to those "gentyl sawez" [noble words] (*Pe.* 278); in the sliding dual-significance of Daniel's interpretation of the writing on the wall; in the poet's invented rationale for Jonah's doomed flight from Nineveh; in the tension between the "lel letteres loken" [loyal letters locked] (*Gaw.* 35) that begin *Sir Gawain and the Green Knight* and the slippery "luf-talkyng" [love talk] (927) that defines its flawed protagonist.

Such concerns about the capacity of English most frequently emerged in the later Middle Ages around the issue of biblical translation, a thorny cultural context that is, I believe, critical to how the plague was portrayed in English poetry. It is important to recall that the Black Death itself was almost universally understood in biblical terms in the fourteenth-century, a frame of reference that further separated the pandemic from other civic and social upheavals, as well as from other kinds of cultural trauma. The plague registered to medieval Christians as a divine vengeance aligned with Noah's Flood and the destruction of Sodom and Gomorrah; it was a punishment for countless human sins, a judgment, a rupture in history tantamount to the apocalypse. Put another way, the Black Death wasn't just *like* the end of the world in medieval England; it *was* the end of the world. On the one hand, this alignment of pestilential cataclysm with biblical cataclysm surely worked to underscore the magnitude and gravity of the event. Moreover, as we have seen with *Pearl* and *Cleanness,* it also may have offered a frame through which the traumas of the pestilence could be given voice, a way to speak about an event that eschewed other modes of witness. But on the other hand, it is possible that the consistent blending of pestilential and biblical discourses also had a dampening effect on literary expression in English, one encouraged by the prevailing idea that the English vernacular was not a fit medium for biblical and theological engagement. For this particular traumatic event, invested as it was with such pressing biblical overtones, would the Latin of the bible have

---

40. Watson, "Censorship and Cultural Change," 842–43. Watson focuses particularly on the ability of the English vernacular to contain the theological truths of the Bible; I would argue, however, that such attitudes toward the suitability of the "mother tongue" would have persisted beyond the specific issue of biblical translation.

appeared a more authoritative or "serious" expressive medium than a language commonly associated with popular romance? Would it have been considered inappropriate, even vulgar, to write about the plague in Middle English?

It is suggestive for this possibility that the fourteenth-century English works dealing most overtly with the plague are not, in fact, written in Middle English at all but in Latin. Many are historical chronicles of the sort that I have quoted throughout this study, and while some treat the pestilence as simply one more historical event to catalogue—"*Isto anno circa pascha vel modicum ante incepit pestilencia in custodia Cantebrigiense et duravit per totam estatem*" [That year, around Passover or a little before, the pestilence began in the district of Cambridge and lasted for the whole summer][41]—others pause to lament the progress of the disease at length. The Chronicle of John of Reading is exemplary in this respect, offering not only a forthright description of the physical ravages of the disease—"*expulsis ulceribus in inguine et sub alis, quae morientes triduo cruciabant*" [it pushed out ulcers in the groin and under the arms, which tormented the dying for three days]—but also a moving reminiscence of England during the time of plague:

> *Et erant diebus istis mortalitas absque tristitia, sponsalia sine amicitia, poenitentia voluntaria et caristia absque penuria atque fuga sine refugio. Quam plurimi a facie pestilentiae fugerant infecti nec necem evaserant. . . . Consumpta tandem tali peste mortalium multitudine qui post se omnes mundi divitias reliquerunt, pars decima populi vix remansit.*[42]

> [And there was in these days death without sadness, betrothal without friendship, voluntary penance and scarcity without shortage, and flight without refuge. How many who fled from the face of the pestilence were infected and did not evade the death. . . . Finally, such a pestilence consumed a multitude of men who left after them all their worldly wealth abandoned; hardly a tenth of the population remained alive.]

In addition to such vivid prose chronicle accounts, the corpus of fourteenth-century Anglo-Latin writing also contains several poetic meditations on the plague. Among them, a short poem now known as "On the Pestilence" stands out both for its sorrowful invocation and its stridently didactic tone:

---

41. "A Fourteenth-Century Chronicle from the Grey Friars of Lynn," 274.
42. John of Reading, *Chronica Johannis de Reading*, 108–9.

Ecce dolet Anglia luctibus imbuta,
Gens tremit tristitia sordibus polluta,
Necat pestilentia viros atque bruta,
Cur? Quia flagitia regnant resoluta.[43]

[Here mourns England, permeated with tears, / The people tremble with
sadness, defiled with filth, / The pestilence kills men and beasts. / Why?
Because sins rule absolutely.]

Following this opening quatrain, the poem unleashes a sixty-line invective
against the moral failings thought to have caused the pestilence, including
the practice of "*simonia*" [simony], the prevalence of "*Sacerdotes . . . incon-*
tinentes" [unchaste . . . priests], and the perils of "*fœminæ fragilitas*" [wom-
en's moral frailty].[44] Another Anglo-Latin poem, which primarily concerns
the 1382 Council of London, likewise opens by decrying the sorry state of
the realm, linking the Black Death to the Rising of 1381 and noting that, "*in*
nos pestilentia sæva jam crescit / Quod virorum fortium jam populus decrescit"
[among us the savage plague now increases / just as, in manly valor, the people
diminish].[45]

Even John Gower, whose somewhat variegated embrace of the English
vernacular would eventually help to solidify its status as a literary medium,
deploys his most strikingly pestilential language not in the (mostly) English
Confessio Amantis but in the Latin *Vox Clamantis*. Comparing the behavior
of the peasants during the Rising of 1381 to a biblical plague of insects, Gower
writes,

Musca grauis pestis, qua nulla nociuior vnquam
    Extitit, aut mundo plus violenta lues!
Tanta fuit rabies, tantus feruorque diei,
    Tutus vt in nullo quis valet esse loco.[46]

[Then fly, grim plague—none grimmer ever was, / Nor did so dire a pest
afflict the world! / Such was the rage and fury of that day / That no one could
be safe in any place.]

---

43. "On the Pestilence," 280 (ll. 1–4).
44. "On the Pestilence," 280–82 (ll. 17, 49, 61).
45. "On the Council of London," in *Political Poems and Songs*, 253 (ll. 13–14).
46. Gower, *Visio Anglie*, 70–71 (ll. 615–18). I use Rigg's translation here.

As in the *Confessio,* Gower deploys such terms in the *Vox* to a metaphorical end: the "plague" that he discusses in the poem turns out not to be the Black Death itself but a plague of flies. Nonetheless, the desolate imagery that Gower develops in his Latin work—a grim plague from which none could find refuge—is far more evocative of the pandemic than his sole reference in English. Might the amplification of pestilential imagery in the *Vox,* then, suggest that Gower, a poet who wrote in English, French, and Latin, considered the language associated with the Bible to be a more appropriate one for evoking a pandemic regularly measured in biblical terms? It is, admittedly, impossible to say for sure; however, the distinction between Gower's plague references in the Latin *Vox* and the English *Confessio*—one that echoes in miniature the distinctions between Continental and English responses—supports the possibility.

The culturally "low" status of fourteenth-century English may have been a double-edged sword, however. Even if, as I posit above, that status discouraged direct representations of the plague in Middle English poetry, the very unproven nature of the vernacular also might have encouraged semantic invention and play, the kinds of linguistic experimentation in which I have suggested we can perceive the pestilence in the poems of the *Pearl* manuscript. Middle English, in other words, may well have been understood as an inappropriate medium in which to *speak* the biblical truth of the Black Death, but its flexibility, its polysemy, and its metaphorical capacity—the language's beautiful, vibrant scruffiness—made it an ideal medium in which to *evoke* the unspeakable, even (or especially) without the sanction of authority implied by Latin or the Continental vernaculars. David Lawton writes, "The nature of vernacular culture is an intricate negotiation between respect for authority and rebellion against it."[47] Like Chaucer, Gower, and Langland, the *Pearl*-Poet revels in that negotiation, testing and at times transcending the possibilities of his comparatively unproven literary medium. *Pearl* alone is a semantic tour de force that works to accommodate the perceived limitations of the English vernacular, even as it also strives to press that vernacular to the limits of its allusive and metaphorical capabilities, exploiting its propensity for play, pun, double entendre, and suggestion. *Sir Gawain and the Green Knight* is likewise invested in the polysemy of the vernacular, centered as it is on three scenes of rarified linguistic play between Gawain and the Lady of Hautdesert. What is outwardly spoken in those three scenes rubs up against what is implied, what is intimated, and what is silently known, a negotiation that implicates the poem as a whole and that also speaks to the allusive approach shared by all four works in the manuscript. Even *Cleanness* and *Patience,* which are less

---

47. Lawton, *Voice in Later Medieval Literature,* 5.

overtly concerned with linguistic virtuosity, capitalize on the flexibility and slipperiness of the vernacular, be it in Daniel's polyvalent prophesy, Sarah's laughing reply to God's promise of a son, or Jonah's description of Nineveh's terrors. For the writer of these works—and for other fourteenth-century poets, such as Gower and Chaucer—the perceived cultural deficits of Middle English were inseparable from its productive flexibility, its ability to imply without stating, to show without openly telling. Perhaps in its capaciousness and meta-phorical flexibility, the English vernacular itself allowed both for the seeming absence of the plague *and* for its subtle presence.

Whatever its relative inherent ability as a medium—and again, the *Pearl*-Poet seems intent on proving it to be all but boundless—it is undeniable that English could boast neither the cultural cache, the established authority, nor the popular or civic scope of Latin, French, and Italian. As Nicholas Watson notes, "Written English . . . remained a language that was more symbolically than actually capable of reaching a national audience," a language whose lit-erary and cultural merit would only be formally enshrined in the fifteenth century, when Chaucer, Gower, and John Lydgate emerged at the head of a vernacular English canon actively promoted by a new Lancastrian dynasty anxious to shore up its claim to the throne.[48] In consideration of this limited reach, it is particularly revealing that Lydgate himself, whose massive output is commonly recognized as instrumental in establishing English as language equal to Latin, French, and Italian, wrote several of the most direct invoca-tions of the pestilence in Middle English. These works, written three or four decades after the poems of the *Pearl* manuscript, include a rhymed dietary and doctrine written to "kepe [readers] from sekenesse / And resiste the strok of pestilence" [keep readers from sickness and resist the stroke of the pestilence] and two invocations to the Virgin Mary asking her to "puttist awey the werre / Of pestilence" [put away the danger of the pestilence] and withhold the "infect heyr [and] mystis" [infected air and mists] that carry contagion.[49] Later still, William Bullein's mid-sixteenth-century *Dialogue against the Feuer Pestilence*

---

48. Watson, "The Politics of Middle English Writing," 342. Watson writes specifically in the context of English Lollard texts, but his observation remains applicable for the literary works I discuss here. Watson further describes the belated establishment of English as a "vernacular of a value comparable to that of French of Italian" (347), citing the fifteenth-century work of writers like Lydgate and Hoccleve. See also, in this latter respect, Lawton, "Dullness and the Fifteenth Century"; Bowers, "The House of Chaucer & Son"; Fisher, "A Language Policy for Lancastrian England"; Strohm, *England's Empty Throne*, especially chapter 7, "Advising the Lan-castrian Prince."

49. Lydgate, "A Dietary, and a Doctrine for Pestilence," in *The Minor Poems of John Lydgate, Part 2*, 702 (ll. 1–2); Lydgate, "Stella Celi Extirpauit (I)," in *The Minor Poems of John Lydgate, Part 1*, 294–95 (ll. 3–4, 13). See also Lydgate's "Stella Celi Extirpauit (II)," in *The Minor Poems of John Lydgate, Part 1*, 295–96.

contains an extended description of the responses of a society threatened by the plague:

> And when thei are touched by the fearfull stroke of the Pestilence of their nexte neighbour, or els in their owne familie, then thei vse Medicines, flie the Aire, &c. Which indeede are verie good meanes, and not against Gods woorde so to doe; then other some falleth into sodaine deuotion, in giuyng almose to the poore and needie, which before haue doen nothing els but appressed theim and haue dooen them wrong; other doe locke from their hartes Gods liuely worde, and refuse grace offered by Christes spirite, thinkyng there is no God.[50]

> [And when they are touched by the fearful stroke of the pestilence of their close neighbor, or else in their own family, then they use medicines, flee the vapor, etc., which indeed are very good methods and not against God's word to do. Then some others fall into sudden devotion in giving alms to the poor and the needy, who before have nothing but oppressed them and done them wrong. Others lock from their hearts God's living word and refuse the grace offered by Christ's spirit, thinking that there is no God.]

Written a century after Lydgate's plague works, Bullein's somewhat jumbled dialogue not only describes in graphic detail the plague's symptoms, it also directly considers the effects of the plague on the emotions and actions of its London readers, offering a glimpse of the pestilential human landscape so powerfully evoked in Boccaccio's *Decameron*.[51] And while it may be hard to argue that either the fifteenth-century Lydgate or the sixteenth-century Bullein writes the disease with the emotional verve of a Boccaccio or even a DeMussis, their sustained and overt focus on the pestilence marks a departure from the work of their earlier English predecessors, and it further suggests how poets considering the plague in the fourteenth century may have been hampered by the cultural status of English, a status that shifted most notably in the early decades of the fifteenth century.[52] The increasingly forthright discussions of plague in the fifteenth and sixteenth centuries might in this regard

---

50. Bullein, *Dialogue against the Feuer Pestilence*, 3.

51. See Grigsby, *Pestilence in Medieval and Early Modern Literature*, 140–41.

52. English writers of the seventeenth-century, including Daniel Defoe, John Donne, Thomas Dekker, Samuel Pepys, and others, *did* write directly about the plague, and with an openness not found in the work of their late medieval counterparts. The vigor with which they do so attests, I would argue, to the difference in authority claimed by the English vernacular in the Middle Ages and the Renaissance.

be seen as running parallel to the development of English as a language of cultural, literary, and especially biblical authority.

In addition to these limitations, the necessarily restricted reach of Middle English in the fourteenth century is attested by the dialectical differences that distinguish Chaucer from Langland from Gower from the *Pearl*-Poet. Indeed, those differences are frequently registered by the poets themselves, many of whom are conscious of the new kinds of work they are asking the English vernacular to perform. Chaucer's well-rehearsed complaint at the end of the *Troilus*, "ther is so gret diversite / In Englissh and in writing of our tonge" [there is such great diversity in English and in the writing of our language] (*TC* 5.1793–94), demonstrates a clear sense of the limits of even the most aspiring public poet, as does Caxton's gripe a century later about writing in "comyn englysshe" [common English]: "It is harde to playse euery man by cause of dyuersite [and] chaunge of langage" [It is hard to please every man because of diversity and variation of language].[53] Langland may have sought and even attained a broad readership with his thrice-written masterpiece, but as Emily Steiner reminds us, "what most distinguishes *Piers Plowman* from other alliterative poems . . . is its bilingual embrace," a macaronic sensibility that exists "at the core of its vernacular inventiveness."[54] And while Gower claims to have intended the *Confessio Amantis* as a book for England's sake, the persistent bilingualism of that most English of his major works, as well as his authorship of the Latin *Vox* and the French *Mirrour de l'omme*, reminds us that such an audience would have been difficult, if not impossible, for any fourteenth-century poet writing only in English to achieve.[55]

We need not dismiss the notion that poets writing in English harbored ideas of their poetry projecting "a 'common voice' to serve the 'common good,'" nor do we need to suggest that vernacular poetry (even vernacular poetry written for the court) never escaped the immediate confines of its intended cultural and geographical milieu.[56] There is little reason to doubt that Langland actively developed a national audience for *Piers Plowman* or to second guess Gower when he declares his intention to write a book for England "in our Englissh" (B.Pro. 23).[57] We should acknowledge, however, that the pub-

---

53. Caxton, "Prologue to *Eneydos*," in *The Prologues and Epilogues of William Caxton*, 108.

54. Steiner, *Reading* Piers Plowman, 6, 9.

55. Robert Yeager in particular asks us to notice "that the *Confessio Amantis* is neither all English nor all poetry" (251); it is rather a macaronic work whose Latin prose and verse complicates and sometimes undercuts its more dominant English tetrameter. See Yeager, "English, Latin, and the Text as 'Other,'" 251–67; also Echard, "Gower's 'Bokes of Latin': Language, Politics, and Poetry"; Machan, "Medieval Multilingualism and Gower's Literary Practice."

56. Middleton, "The Idea of Public Poetry," 95.

57. For Langland's desire for a national readership, see Kane, "Outstanding Problems," 12.

lic potential of English in the fourteenth century must have been understood, especially by those writers who most worked against its perceived limitations, as always circumscribed, held back both by the "gret diversite" of the language and by its still dubious status as an artistically, theologically, and culturally capable medium. At his boldest, after all, Chaucer tells his "litel bok" [little book] (*TC* 5.1786) merely to kiss the steps on which the literary authorities of antiquity tread, a quiet acknowledgement that his vernacular work could not—or at least not yet—be expected to walk with them.

If the subtle but persistent implications of plague in the *Pearl* manuscript reveal how a group of courtly works might attain an unexpectedly public dimension, it suggests at the same time the private-ness of even the most public and hortatory Middle English works—the persistent shadow of the provincial, of the personal, and of the courtly that follows the still insecure English vernacular. So too does it attest to persistent anxieties over biblical and theological writing in English, modes of literary production that would have had a direct bearing on medieval understandings and representations of the plague. The Cotton Nero A.x poems' guarded response to the pandemic may thus be understood as reflecting not only the poet's scrupulous understanding of the social and political needs of his aristocratic milieu but also, and more fundamentally, the shifting roles and ingrained perceptions of Middle English in the late fourteenth century. Considered in a wider sense, this response gestures toward a similar complex of pressures affecting English vernacular poetry as a whole, pressures that may have caused poets working in Middle English to muffle, but not entirely suppress, their response to the Black Death. While they do not outwardly evoke the plague then, the poems of the *Pearl* manuscript imply, in their own pyrrhic witness to the trauma, the development of a nascent and still under-recognized pestilential discourse in later Middle English literature, and they further suggest that even if the impact of the disease is muted in fourteenth-century English poetry, it may still be present in ways that we should no longer overlook.

BIBLIOGRAPHY

PRIMARY SOURCES

Agnolo di Tura del Grasso. *Cronaca Senese.* Edited by Alessandro Lisini and Fabio Iacometti. Vol. 15, part 6 of *Rerum Italicarum Scriptores,* edited by L. A. Muratori. Bologna: Nicola Zanichelli, 1931–37.

Andrew, Malcolm, and Ronald Waldron, eds. *The Poems of the* Pearl *Manuscript: Pearl, Cleanness, Patience, Sir Gawain and the Green Knight.* 5th ed. Exeter: University of Exeter Press, 2007.

The Anonimalle Chronicle, 1333–1381. Edited by V. H. Galbraith. Manchester: Manchester University Press, 1970.

Augustine of Hippo. *The City of God against the Pagans.* Edited and translated by R. W. Dyson. Cambridge: Cambridge University Press, 1998.

———. *Writings against the Manicheans and the Donatists.* Edited by Phillip Schaff. Translated by Richard Stothert and Albert Newman. Buffalo, NY: Christian Literature, 1887.

Biel, Gabriel. "*Contra pestilentiam sermo medicinalis III.*" In *Sermones de tempore, festis Christi, et D. Virginis Mariae,* 354–67. Coloniae Agrippinae: Apud Ioannem Crithium, 1619.

Boccaccio, Giovanni. *Decameron.* Edited by Vittore Branca. Milan: Arnoldo Mondadori, 1989.

———. *Decameron.* Translated by Guido Waldman. Edited by Jonathan Usher. Oxford: Oxford University Press, 1993.

Breve Chronicon Clerici Anonymi. In De Smet, *Recuil des chroniques de Flandre,* 3:5–30.

Brinton, Thomas. *The Sermons of Thomas Brinton, Bishop of Rochester (1373–1389).* Vol. 1. Edited by Mary Aquinas Devlin. London: Royal Historical Society, 1954.

The Brut, or the Chronicles of England, Part II. Edited by Friedrich Brie. EETS o.s. 136. London: Oxford University Press, 1908.

Bullein, William. *Dialogue against the Feuer Pestilence.* Edited by Mark W. Bullen and A. H. Bullen. EETS e.s. 52. 1888. Reprint, Millwood, NY: Kraus, 1973.

Burton, Thomas. *Chronica Monasterii de Melsa a Fundatione usque ad Annum 1396, Auctore Thoma de Burton, Abbate.* Vol 3. Edited by Edward A. Bond. Rolls Series. London: Longmans, Green, Reader, and Dyer, 1868.

Caxton, William. *The Prologues and Epilogues of William Caxton.* Edited by W. J. B. Crotch. EETS o.s. 176. 1928. Reprint, New York: Burt Franklin, 1971.

Chaucer, Geoffrey. *The Riverside Chaucer.* Edited by Larry D. Benson. 3rd ed. Boston: Houghton Mifflin, 1987.

Chronicon Abbatie de Parco Lude. Edited by Edmund Venables. Horncastle, UK: W. K. Morton, 1891.

D'Agramunt, Jaume [Jacme]. "Regimen of Protection against Epidemics or Pestilence and Mortality." Translated by M. L. Duran-Reynals and C. E. A. Winslow. *Bulletin of the History of Medicine* 23 (1949): 57–89.

———. *Regiment de preservació a epidèmia o pestilència e mortaldats.* Edited by José María Roca and Enric Arderiu. Lleyda, Spain: Joseph A. Pagés, 1910.

De Smet, J. J., ed. *Recuil des chroniques de Flandre.* 4 vols. Brussels: M. Hayez, 1837–1865.

Early English Versions of the Gesta Romanorum. Edited by Sidney Herrtage. EETS e.s. 33. London: Oxford University Press, 1879. Reprint, 1962.

Eulogium (Historiarum sive Temporis): Chronicon ab Orbe Condito usque ad Annum Domini MCCCLXVI. Vol. 3. Edited by Frank Scott Hayden. Rolls Series. London: Longman, Green, Longman, Roberts, and Green, 1863.

"A Fourteenth-Century Chronicle from the Grey Friars of Lynn." Edited by Antonia Gransden. *English Historical Review* 72 (1957): 270–78.

Gabriele de' Mussis. *Historia de Morbo.* In *Archiv für die Gesammte Medicin,* edited by Heinrich Haeser, 45–59. Jena, Germany: Friedrich Manke, 1842.

Gentile of Foligno. *Singulare consilium contra pestilentiam.* Unpaginated manuscript, c. 1515. Digital facsimile of original held at Real Colegio de Medicina y Cirugía de San Carlos, Spain, from <https://books.google.ca/books?id=OUlDfhhH5w4C>.

Gilles li Muisis. *Chronicon majus Aegidii Li Muisis.* In De Smet, *Recuil des chroniques de Flandre,* 2:111–448.

Gower, John. *Confessio Amantis.* Edited by Russell Peck, with Latin translations by Andrew Galloway. 3 vols. Kalamazoo, MI: Medieval Institute Publications, 2000, 2003, 2004.

———. *Visio Anglie (Vox Clamantis I).* In *Poems on Contemporary Events.* Translation by A. G. Rigg. Edited by David R. Carlson. Toronto and Oxford: PIMS and the Bodleian Library, 2011.

Guillaume de Nangis. *Chronique Latine de Guillaume de Nangis de 1113 a 1300 avec les continuations de cette chronique.* Vol. 2. Edited by H. Géraud. Paris: Jules Renouard, 1843.

Guillelmi de Cortusiis. *Chronica de Novitatibus Padue et Lombardie.* Edited by Beniamino Pagnin. Vol. 12, part 5 of *Rerum Italicarum Scriptores,* edited by L. A. Muratori. Bologna: Nicola Zanichelli, 1941–49.

Guy de Chauliac. *The Cyrurgie of Guy de Chauliac.* Edited by Margaret S. Ogden. EETS o.s. 265. Oxford: Oxford University Press, 1971.

———. *Dn. Guidonis de Cauliaco, in arte medica exercitatissimi chirurgia.* Lugduni: Jacobi Juntae, 1559. Digital facsimile of original held by Universidad Complutense de Madrid, from *Hathi Trust Digital Library.*

Higden, Ranulph. *Polychronicon Ranulphi Higden Monachi Cestrensis.* Vol. 8. Edited by Joseph Rawson Lumby. Rolls Series. London: Longman, 1882.

The Holkham Bible: A Facsimile. Introduction and commentary by Michelle P. Brown. London: British Library, 2007.

The Holy Bible, Douay-Rheims version. Revised by Richard Challoner. Baltimore: John Murphy, 1899. Reprint, Rockford, IL: Tan Books, 2000.

Ibn al-Wardi. "Ibn al Wardī's 'Risālah al-naba' 'an al waba,' A Translation of a Major Source for the History of the Black Death in the Middle East." Translated by Michael W. Dols. In *Near Eastern Numismatics, Iconography, Epigraphy and History: Studies in Honor of George C. Miles,* edited by Dickran K. Kouymjian, 443–56. Beirut: American University of Beirut Press, 1974.

John of Arderne. *Treatises of Fistula in Ano, Haemorrhoids, and Clysters.* Edited by D'Arcy Power. EETS o.s. 139. Oxford: Oxford University Press, 1910.

John of Fordun. *Johannis de Fordun Chronica gentis Scotorum.* Edited by William F. Skene. Edinburgh: Edmonston and Douglas, 1871.

John of Reading. *Chronica Johannis de Reading et Anonymi Cantuariensis 1346–1367.* Edited by James Tait. Manchester: University of Manchester Press, 1914.

Knighton, Henry. *Chronicon Henrici Knighton.* Vol. 2. Edited by Joseph Rawson Lumby. Rolls Series. London: H. M. Stationery Office, 1895. Reprinted, Wiesbaden: Kraus, 1965.

Landucci, Luca. *Diario Fiorentino dal 1450 al 1516 di Luca Landucci.* Edited by Iodoco del Badia. Florence: G. C. Sansoni, 1883. Translated as *A Florentine Diary from 1450 to 1516.* Edited and translated by Alice de Rosen Jervis. New York: Dutton, 1927.

Langland, William. *Piers Plowman: A Parallel-Text Edition of the A, B, C and Z Versions.* Edited by A. V. C. Schmidt. 2nd ed. Kalamazoo, MI: Medieval Institute Publications, 2011.

Le Baker, Geoffrey. *Chronicon Galfridi le Baker de Swynebroke.* Edited by Edward Maunde Thompson. Oxford: Clarendon, 1889.

Liber de Diversis Medicinis. Edited by Margaret Ogden. EETS o.s. 207. London: Oxford University Press, 1938.

The Life of Saint Cuthbert. Edited by J. T. Fowler. Publications of the Surtees Society 87. Durham, NC: Andrews, 1891.

"Literae prioris et capituli cantuar." In Wilkins, *Concilia Magnae Britanniae et Hiberniae,* 2:738.

A Litil Boke the Whiche Traytied Many Gode Thinges for the Pestilence. An early English translation of the fourteenth-century *Treatise of Bengt Knutsson.* Printed by Thomas Gybson. London, 1536. Digital facsimile of original held by the Bodleian Library, from *Early English Books Online* (EEBO).

Lydgate, John. *Minor Poems of John Lydgate.* Edited by Henry Noble MacCracken. 2 vols. EETS e.s. 107, o.s. 192. London: Oxford University Press, 1911 and 1934.

Machaut, Guillaume de. *The Judgment of the King of Navarre.* Edited and translated by R. Barton Palmer. New York: Garland, 1998.

"Mandatum Radulphi, episcopi Bath et Wellen de confessionibus tempore pestilentiae." In Wilkins, *Concilia Magnae Britanniae et Hiberniae,* 2:745–46.

Michele da Piazza. *Cronaca.* Edited by Antonio Giuffrida. Palermo: Istituto di Storia Medievale dell'Universitá di Palermo, 1980.

Middle English Dictionary. Edited by Frances McSparran. The Regents of the University of Michigan. 2001. http://quod.lib.umich.edu/m/med/.

A Middle English Version of the Introduction to Guy de Chauliac's "Chirurgia magna." Edited by Björn Wallner. In *Acta Universitatis Lundensis, sectio I.* Lund, Sweden: Gleerup, 1970.

Monumenta Germaniae Historica, Scriptorum Tomus IX. Edited by Georgius Heinricus Pertz. Hanover: Impensis Biblipolii Aulici Hahniani, 1851.

Morelli, Giovanni di Pagolo. *Ricordi*. Edited by Vittore Branca. Florence, Italy: Felice Le Monnier, 1969.

Moulton, Thomas. *The Myrrour or Glasse of Helth*. Printed by Rycharde Kele. London, 1540. Digital facsimile of original held by Cambridge University Library, from *Early English Books Online* (EEBO).

"A Notabilite of the Scripture What Causith the Pestilence." British Library, Sloane MS 965, folios 143r–145r. Digital facsimile from The British Library.

"On the Council of London." In *Political Poems and Songs Relating to English History*, edited by Thomas Wright, 1:253–63. London: Longman, Green, Longman, and Roberts, 1859.

"On the Pestilence." In *Political Poems and Songs Relating to English History*, edited by Thomas Wright, 1:279–81. London: Longman, Green, Longman, and Roberts, 1859.

Patience. Edited by J. J. Anderson. Manchester: Manchester University Press, 1969.

Pearl. Edited by Sarah Stanbury. Kalamazoo, MI: Medieval Institute Publications, 2001.

The Pest Anatomized: Five Centuries of Plague in Western Europe: An Exhibition at the Wellcome Institute for the History of Medicine. London: Wellcome Institute, 1985.

Petrarch, Francesco. *Epistolæ de rebus familiaribus et variæ*. Vol 1. Edited by Iosephi Fracassetti. Florence: Le Monnier, 1859.

Ralph of Shrewsbury. *The Register of Ralph of Shrewsbury, Bishop of Bath and Wells, 1329–1363*. Edited by Thomas Scott Holmes. Somerset, UK: Somerset Record Society, 1896.

"The Report of the Medical Faculty of Paris, Oct. 7, 1347." In *Der Schwarze Tod in Deutschland*, edited by Robert Hoeniger, 152–56. Berlin: Eugen Grosser, 1882.

Saint Erkenwald. Edited by Clifford Peterson. Philadelphia: University of Pennsylvania Press: 1977.

"*Salus populi*." In *Missale ad usum insignis et praeclarae ecclesiae sarum*, edited by Francisci Henrici Dickinson, column 810*–812.* London: J. Parker, 1861–83.

Sir Gawain and the Green Knight. Edited by Israel Gollancz. EETS o.s. 210. London: Oxford University Press, 1940.

Sir Gawain and the Green Knight. Edited by J. R. R. Tolkien and E. V. Gordon. 2nd ed. Revised by Norman Davis. Oxford: Clarendon, 1967.

Sudbury, Simon. "*Commissio ad orandum pro cessatione pestilentiae*." In Wilknis, *Concilia Magnae Britanniae et Hiberniae*, 3:100–101.

Sudhoff, Karl, ed. "*Epistola et regimen Alphontii Cordubensis de pestilentia*." *Archiv für Geschichte der Medizin* 3 (1909): 223–26.

———, ed. "*Pestschriften aus den ersten 150 Jahren nach der Epidemie des 'Schwarzen Todes' 1348*." *Archiv für Geschichte de Medizin* 11 (1919): 44–92.

Symonis de Covino. "De Judicio Solis in Conviviis in Saturni." In *Bibliothèque de l'école des Chartes*, edited by Emile Littré, 2:206–43. Paris: Schneider et Langrand, 1840–41.

Von Herford, Heinrich. *Liber de rebus memorabilioribus sive Chronicon Henrici de Hervordia*. Edited by Augustus Potthast. Gottingen: Sumptibus Dieterichianis, 1859.

Walsingham, Thomas. *Historia breuis Thomæ Walsingham, ab Edwardo primo, ad Henricum quintum*. London, 1574. Digital facsimile of original held by Henry E. Huntington Library and Art Gallery, from *Early English Books Online* (EEBO).

Whytlaw-Gray, Alianore. "John Lelamour's Translation of Macer's Herbal in MS Sln.5." MA thesis, University of Leeds, 1938.

Wilkins, David, ed. *Concilia Magnae Britanniae et Hiberniae.* 4 vols. London: R. Gosling, 1737. Reprint, Brussels: Culture et Civilisation, 1964.

Wynnere and Wastoure and The Parlement of the Thre Ages. Edited by Warren Ginsburg. Kalamazoo, MI: Medieval Institute Publications, 1992.

The York Corpus Christi Plays. Edited by Clifford Davidson. Kalamazoo, MI: Medieval Institute Publications, 2011.

Zouche, William. "A Letter from Archbishop Zouche to His Official at York." In *Historical Papers and Letters from the Northern Registers,* edited by James Raine, 395–97. Rolls Series. London: Longman, 1873.

SECONDARY SOURCES

Aberth, John. *The Black Death: The Great Mortality of 1348–1350, A Brief History with Documents.* New York: Palgrave, 2005.

Adorno, Theodor. *Prisms.* Cambridge, MA: MIT Press, 1981.

Aers, David. "Christianity for Courtly Subjects: Reflections on the *Gawain*-Poet." In Brewer and Gibson, *A Companion to the Gawain-Poet,* 91–101.

———. *Community, Gender, and Individual Identity: English Writing 1360–1430.* London and New York: Routledge, 1988.

———. *Faith, Ethics, and Church: Writing in England, 1360–1409.* Woodbridge: Brewer, 2000.

———. "The Self Mourning: Reflections on *Pearl.*" *Speculum* 68 (1993): 54–73.

Allen, Elizabeth. "'As mote in at a munster dor': Sanctuary and Love of this World." *Philological Quarterly* 87 (2008): 105–33.

Anderson, J. J. "The Prologue of *Patience.*" *Modern Philology* 63 (1966): 283–87.

Andrew, Malcolm. "Biblical Paraphrase in the Middle English *Patience.*" In *Manuscript, Narrative, Lexicon: Essays on Literacy and Cultural Transmission in Honor of Whitney F. Bolton,* edited by Robert Boenig and Kathleen Davis, 45–75. Lewisbury, PA: Bucknell University Press, 2000.

———. "Theories of Authorship." In Brewer and Gibson, *A Companion to the Gawain-Poet,* 22–33.

Archer, Rowena E. "'How ladies . . . who live on their manors ought to manage their households and estates': Women as Landholders and Administrators in the Later Middle Ages." In *Woman is a Worthy Wight: Women in English Society, c. 1200–1500,* edited by P. J. P. Goldberg. Wolfeboro Falls, NH: Alan Sutton, 1992.

Arner, Lynn. *Chaucer, Gower, and the Vernacular Rising: Poetry and the Problem of the Populace After 1381.* University Park: Pennsylvania State University Press, 2013.

———. "The Ends of Enchantment: Colonialism and *Sir Gawain and the Green Knight.*" *Texas Studies in Literature and Language* 48 (2006): 79–101.

Ashton, Gail. "The Perverse Dynamics of *Sir Gawain and the Green Knight.*" *Arthuriana* 15.3 (2005): 51–74.

Bahr, Arthur. "The Manifold Singularity of *Pearl.*" *English Literary History* 82 (2015): 729–58.

Barr, Helen. "*Pearl*—or 'The Jeweller's Tale,'" *Medium Ævum* 69 (2000): 59–79.

Barron, Caroline M. "The 'Golden Age' of Women in Medieval London." *Reading Medieval Studies* 15 (1989): 35–58.

Batt, Catherine. "Gawain's Antifeminist Rant, the Pentangle, and Narrative Space." *Yearbook of English Studies* 22 (1992): 117–39.

Battles, Dominique. *Cultural Difference and Material Culture in Middle English Romance: Normans and Saxons.* New York: Routledge, 2013.

Battles, Paul. "Amended Texts, Emended Ladies: Female Agency and the Textual Editing of *Sir Gawain and the Green Knight.*" *Chaucer Review* 44 (2010): 323–43.

Beadle, Richard. "The York Corpus Christi Play." In *The Cambridge Companion to Medieval English Theatre,* edited by Richard Beadle and Alan J. Fletcher, 99–124. 2nd ed. Cambridge: Cambridge University Press, 2008.

Beidler, Peter G. "The Plague and Chaucer's Pardoner." *Chaucer Review* 16 (1982): 257–69.

Benedictow, Ole. *The Black Death 1346–53: The Complete History.* Woodbridge, UK: Boydell, 2004.

———. *What Disease was Plague? On the Controversy over the Microbiological Identity of the Plague Epidemics of the Past.* Leiden: Brill, 2010.

Bennett, Judith. "Medieval Women, Modern Women: Across the Great Divide." In *Culture and History 1350–1600: Essays on English Communities, Identities and Writing,* edited by David Aers, 147–75. New York: Harvester Wheatsheaf, 1992.

Bennett, Michael J. *Community, Class and Careerism: Cheshire and Lancashire Society in the Age of Sir Gawain and the Green Knight.* Cambridge: Cambridge University Press, 1983.

———. "The Court of Richard II and the Promotion of Literature." In *Chaucer's England,* edited by Barbara Hanawalt, 3–20. Minneapolis: University of Minnesota Press, 1992.

———. "The Historical Background," in *A Companion to the* Gawain-*Poet,* 71–90.

———. "*Sir Gawain and the Green Knight* and the Literary Achievement of the North-West Midlands." *Journal of Medieval History* 5 (1973): 63–89.

Benson, C. David. "The Impatient Reader of *Patience.*" In Blanch et al., *Text and Matter,* 147–61.

Berlant, Lauren. "Trauma and Ineloquence." *Cultural Values* 5 (2001): 41–58.

Berlin, Normand. "*Patience*: A Study in Poetic Elaboration." *Studia Neophilologica* 33 (1961): 80–85.

Bishop, Ian. Pearl *in Its Setting.* New York: Barnes and Noble, 1968.

Blanch, Robert, Miriam Youngerman Miller, and Julian N. Wasserman, eds. *Text and Matter: New Critical Perspectives of the* Pearl-*Poet.* Troy, NY: Whitston, 1991.

Blanch, Robert J., and Julian N. Wasserman. *From* Pearl *to* Gawain: *Forme to Fynisment.* Gainesville: University Press of Florida, 1995.

Bloch, Howard. "Medieval Misogyny." *Representations* 20 (1987): 1–24.

Bloomfield, Morton. "*Sir Gawain and the Green Knight*: An Appraisal." *PMLA* 76 (1961):7–19.

Bollermann, Karen. "In the Belly, in the Bower: Divine Maternal Practice in *Patience.*" In *Framing the Family: Narrative and Representation in the Medieval and Early Modern Periods,* edited by Rosalynn Voaden and Diane Wolfthal, 193–218. Tempe, AZ: ACMRS, 2005.

Borroff, Marie. "Narrative Artistry in *St. Erkenwald* and the *Gawain*-Group: The Case for Common Authorship Reconsidered." *Studies in the Age of Chaucer* 28 (2006): 41–76.

Bos, Kirsten I., Verena J. Schoenemann, et al. "A Draft Genome of *Yersinia pestis* from Victims of the Black Death." *Nature* 478 (2011): 506–10.

Bowers, John. "The House of Chaucer & Son: The Business of Lancastrian Canon Formation." *Medieval Perspectives* 6 (1991): 135–43.

———. "*Patience* and the Ideal of the Mixed Life." *Texas Studies in Literature and Language* 28 (1986): 1–22.

———. "*Pearl* in Its Royal Setting: Ricardian Poetry Revisited." *Studies in the Age of Chaucer* 17 (1995): 111–55.

———. *The Politics of* Pearl: *Court Poetry in the Age of Richard II.* Cambridge: D. S. Brewer, 2001.

Boyd, David L. "Sodomy, Misogyny, and Displacement: Occluding Queer Desire in *Sir Gawain and the Green Knight,*" *Arthuriana* 8.2 (1998): 77–113.

Branca, Vittore. *Boccaccio medievale e nuovi studi sul "Decameron."* 6th ed. Firenze: Sansoni, 1986.

Breeze, Andrew C. "*Pearl* and the Plague of 1390–1393." *Neophilologus* 98 (2014): 337–41.

———. "Sir John Stanley (c. 1350–1414) and the *Gawain*-Poet." *Arthuriana* 14 (2004): 15–30.

Brewer, Derek. "The Interpretation of Dream, Folktale, and Romance, with Special Reference to *Sir Gawain and the Green Knight.*" *Neuphilologische Mitteilungen* 77 (1976): 596–81.

Brewer, Derek, and Jonathan Gibson, eds. *A Companion to the* Gawain-*Poet.* Cambridge: D. S. Brewer, 1997.

Brewer, Elizabeth. "Sources I: The Sources of *Sir Gawain and the Green Knight.*" In Brewer and Gibson, *A Companion to the* Gawain-*Poet,* 243–55.

Brzezinski, Monica. "Conscience and Covenant: The Sermon Structure of *Cleanness.*" *Journal of English and Germanic Philology* 89 (1990): 166–80.

Butterfield, Ardis. "Pastoral and the Politics of Plague in Machaut and Chaucer." *Studies in the Age of Chaucer* 16 (1994): 3–27.

Bynum, Carolyn Walker. *The Resurrection of the Body in Western Christianity, 200–1336.* New York: Columbia University Press, 1995.

Calabrese, Michael, and Eric Eliason. "The Rhetorics of Sexual Pleasure and Intolerance in the Middle English *Cleanness.*" *Modern Language Quarterly* 56 (1995): 247–75.

Campbell, Bruce. "The Great Transition: Climate, Disease and Society in the 13th and 14th Centuries." The Ellen McArthur Lectures. University of Cambridge. 2013. Podcast. <http://sms.cam.ac.uk/media/1456872>.

Cannon, Walter B. *Bodily Changes in Pain, Hunger, Fear and Rage.* New York: Appleton, 1915, 1920.

Carruthers, Mary. *The Book of Memory.* 2nd ed. Cambridge: Cambridge UP, 2008.

Caruth, Cathy. "After the End: Psychoanalysis in the Ashes of History." In *The Future of Testimony: Interdisciplinary Perspectives on Witnessing,* edited by Antony Rowland and Jane Kilby, 31–47. New York: Routledge, 2014.

———. *Unclaimed Experience: Trauma, Narrative, and History.* Baltimore: Johns Hopkins University Press, 1996.

Centers for Disease Control and Prevention. "Plague, Symptoms." US Department of Health and Human Services. http://www.cdc.gov/plague/symptoms/index.html.

Cherewatuk, Karen. "Becoming Male, Medieval Mothering, and Incarnational Theology in *Sir Gawain and the Green Knight* and the *Book of Margery Kempe.*" *Arthuriana* 19.3 (2009): 15–24.

Chism, Christine. *Alliterative Revivals.* Philadelphia: University of Pennsylvania Press, 2002.

Citrome, Jeremy. "Medicine as Metaphor in the Middle English *Cleanness.*" *Chaucer Review* 35 (2001): 260–80.

Clark, S. L., and Julian N. Wasserman. "Gawain's 'Anti-Feminism' Reconsidered." *Journal of the Rocky Mountain Medieval and Renaissance Association* 6 (1985): 57–70.

Cohen, Jeffrey Jerome. *Of Giants: Sex, Monsters and the Middle Ages*. Minneapolis: University of Minnesota Press, 1999.

Cohn, Samuel, Jr. *The Black Death Transformed: Disease and Culture in Early Renaissance Europe*. London: Arnold, 2002.

Coleman, Joyce. "'A Bok for King Richardes Sake': Royal Patronage, the *Confessio*, and the *Legend of Good Women*." In *On John Gower: Essays at the Millennium*, edited by Robert F. Yeager, 104–23. Kalamazoo, MI: Medieval Institute Publications, 2007.

Coley, David. "*Pearl* and the Narrative of Pestilence." *Studies in the Age of Chaucer* 35 (2013): 209–62.

———. "Remembering Lot's Wife / Lot's Wife Remembering: Trauma, Witness, and Representation in *Cleanness*." *Exemplaria* 24 (2012): 342–63.

Condren, Edward I. *The Numerical Universe of the Gawain-Pearl Poet: Beyond Phi*. Gainesville: University Press of Florida, 2002.

Cooke, W. G. "'Sir Gawain and the Green Knight': A Restored Dating." *Medium Ævum* 58 (1989): 34–48.

Cooke, W. G., and D'A. J. D. Boulton. "*Sir Gawain and the Green Knight*: A Poem for Henry of Grosmont." *Medium Ævum* 68 (1999): 42–54.

Correale, Robert M., and Mary Hamel, eds. *Sources and Analogues of* The Canterbury Tales, *II*. Cambridge: D. S. Brewer, 2005.

Crawford, Donna. "The Architectonics of *Cleanness*." *Studies in Philology* 90 (1993): 29–45.

Craymer, Suzanne. "Signifying Chivalric Identities: Armor and Clothing in *Sir Gawain and the Green Knight*." *Medieval Perspectives* 14 (1999): 50–60.

Creighton, Charles. *A History of Epidemics in Britain, Vol. 1*. 2nd ed. London: Frank Cass, 1965.

Crespo, Fabian, and Matthew B. Lawrenz, "Heterogeneous Immunological Landscapes and Medieval Plague: An Invitation to a New Dialogue between Historians and Immunologists." In Green, *Pandemic Disease in the Medieval World*, 27–61.

Cui, Yujun, Chang Yu, et al. "Historical Variations in Mutation Rate in an Epidemic Pathogen, *Yersinia Pestis*." *PNAS* 110 (2013), 577–82.

Davis. Adam Brooke. "What the Poet of *Patience* Really Did to the Book of Jonah." *Viator* 22 (1991): 267–78.

Dean, Katharine R.,Fabienne Krauer, Lars Walløe, Ole Christian Lingjærde, Barbara Bramanti, Nils Chr. Stenseth, and Boris V. Schmid. "Human Ectoparasites and the Spread of Plague in Europe during the Second Pandemic." *PNAS* 115 (2018), published ahead of print, <http://www.pnas.org/content/early/2018/01/09/1715640115>.

Deleuze, Gilles, and Félix Guattari. *A Thousand Plateaus: Capitalism and Schizophrenia*. Translated by Brian Massumi. London and New York: Continuum, 1988.

Dendle, Peter. "Plants in the Early Medieval Cosmos: Herbs, Divine Potency, and the *Scala natura*." In Dendle and Touwaide, *Health and Healing from the Medieval Garden*, 47–59.

Dendle, Peter, and Alain Touwaide, eds. *Health and Healing from the Medieval Garden*. Woodbridge: Boydell, 2008.

De Paolo, Charles. *Epidemic Disease and Human Understanding: A Historical Analysis of Scientific and Other Writings*. Jefferson, NC: McFarland, 2006.

DeWitte, Sharon N. "Setting the Stage for Medieval Plague: Pre-Black Death Trends in Survival and Mortality." *American Journal of Physical Anthropology* 158 (2015): 441–51.

Diekstra, F. N. M. "Jonah and *Patience*: The Psychology of a Prophet." *English Studies* 55 (1974): 205–17.

Dinshaw, Carolyn. "A Kiss Is Just a Kiss: Heterosexuality and Its Consolations in *Sir Gawain and the Green Knight.*" *Diacritics* 24 (1994): 205–26.

Dols, Michael W. *The Black Death in the Middle East.* Princeton, NJ: Princeton University Press, 1977.

Donnelly, Colleen. "Blame, Silence, and Power: Perceiving Women in *Sir Gawain and the Green Knight.*" *Mediaevalia* 24 (2003): 279–97.

Doyle, A. I. "English Books in and out of Court." In *English Court Culture of the Later Middle Ages,* edited by V. J. Scattergood and J. W. Sherborne, 163–81. London: Duckworth, 1983.

Earp, Lawrence. *Guillaume de Machaut: A Guide to Research.* New York: Garland, 1995.

Echard, Siân. "Gower's 'Bokes of Latin': Language, Politics, and Poetry." *Studies in the Age of Chaucer* 25 (2003): 123–56.

Edgeworth, Robert J. "Anatomical Geography in *Sir Gawain and the Green Knight.*" *Neophilologus* 69 (1985): 318–19.

Edmondson, George. "*Pearl*: The Shadow of the Object, the Shape of the Law." *Studies in the Age of Chaucer* 26 (2004): 29–63.

Edwards, A. S. G. "The Manuscript." In Brewer and Gibson, *A Companion to the* Gawain-*Poet,* 197–219.

Eldridge, Lawrence. "Sheltering Space and Cosmic Space in the Middle English *Patience.*" *Annuale Mediaevale* 21 (1981): 121–33.

Elliott, Ralph. "Landscape and Geography." In Brewer and Gibson, *A Companion to the* Gawain-*Poet,* 197–219.

Eng, David L., and David Kazanjian. "Mourning Remains." In *Loss: The Politics of Mourning,* edited by David L. Eng and David Kazanjian, 1–25. Berkeley: University of California Press, 2003.

Fein, Susanna Greer. "Twelve-Line Stanza Forms in Middle English and the Date of *Pearl.*" *Speculum* 72 (1997): 367–98.

Felman, Shoshana, and Dori Laub. *Testimony: Crises of Witnessing in Literature, Psychoanalysis, and History.* New York: Routledge, 1992.

Fleming, John V. "The Centuple Structure of the *Pearl.*" In Levy and Szarmach, *The Alliterative Tradition in the Fourteenth Century,* 81–98.

Finlayson, John. "*Pearl*: Landscape and Vision." *Studies in Philology* 71 (1974): 314–43.

Fisher, John H. "A Language Policy for Lancastrian England." *PMLA* 107 (1992): 1168–80.

Fisher, Sheila. "Leaving Morgan Aside: Women, History, and Revisionism in *Sir Gawain and the Green Knight.*" In *The Passing of Arthur: New Essays in Arthurian Tradition,* edited by Christopher Baswell and William Sharpe, 129–51. New York, Garland, 1988.

———. "Taken Men and Token Women in *Sir Gawain and the Green Knight.*" In *Seeking the Woman in Late Medieval and Renaissance Writings,* edited by Sheila Fisher and Janet E. Halley, 71–105. Knoxville: University of Tennessee Press, 1989.

Fradenburg, L. O. Aranye [Louise]. "The Manciple's Servant Tongue: Politics and Poetry in the Canterbury Tales." *English Literary History* 52 (1985): 85–118.

———. *Sacrifice Your Love: Psychoanalysis, History, Chaucer.* Minneapolis: University of Minnesota Press. 2002.

Frantzen, Allen J. "The Dislosure of Sodomy in *Cleanness.*" *PMLA* 111 (1996): 451–64.

Fredell, Joel. "The *Pearl*-Poet Manuscript in York." *Studies in the Age of Chaucer* 36 (2014): 1–39.

Freidl, Jean-Paul, and Ian J. Kirby. "The Life, Death, and Life of the *Pearl*-Maiden." *Neuphilologische Mitteilungen* 103 (2002): 395–97.

Freud, Sigmund. "Beyond the Pleasure Principle." In *The Standard Edition of the Complete Psychological Works of Sigmund Freud,* edited and translated by James Strachey, 18:7–64. London: Hogarth Press, 1955.

Friedman, John B. "Figural Typology in the Middle English *Patience.*" In Levy and Szarmach, *The Alliterative Tradition in the Fourteenth Century,* 99–129.

Fritz, Donald. "*The Pearl*: The Sacredness of Numbers." *American Benedictine Review* 31 (1980): 314–24.

Fumo, Jamie C. "The Pestilential Gaze: From Epidemiology to Erotomania in *The Knight's Tale.*" *Studies in the Age of Chaucer* 35 (2013): 85–136.

Gallagher, Joseph E. "'Trawþe' and 'Luf-Talkyng' in *Sir Gawain and the Green Knight.*" *Neuphilologische Mitteilungen* 78 (1977): 362–76.

Gasquet, Francis Aidan. *The Black Death of 1348 and 1349.* London: George Bell and Sons, 1908.

Getto, Giovanni. "La peste del *Decameron* e il problema della fonte Lucreziana." *Giornale storico della letteratura Italiana* 135 (1958): 507–23.

Gilles, Sealy. "Love and Disease in Chaucer's *Troilus and Criseyde.*" *Studies in the Age of Chaucer* 25 (2003): 157–197.

Gilligan, Janet. "Numerical Composition in the Middle English *Patience.*" *Studia Neophilologica* 61 (1989): 7–11.

Gilman, Ernest B. *Plague Writing in Early Modern England.* Chicago: University of Chicago Press, 2009.

Gittes, Tobias Foster. *Boccaccio's Naked Muse: Eros, Culture, and the Mythopoeic Imagination.* Toronto: University of Toronto Press, 2008.

Girard, René. "The Plague in Literature and Myth." *Texas Studies in Literature and Language* 15 (1974): 833–50.

Glenn, Jonathan A. "Dislocation of *Kynde* in the Middle English *Cleanness.*" *Chaucer Review* 18 (1983): 77–91.

Godden, Richard H. "Gawain and the Nick of Time: Fame, History, and the Untimely in *Sir Gawain and the Green Knight.*" *Arthuriana* 26.4 (2016): 152–73.

Goldberg, P. J. P. *Women, Work, and Life Cycle in a Medieval Economy: Women in York and Yorkshire c. 1300–1520.* Oxford: Clarendon, 1992.

Green, Monica H. "Editor's Introduction." In Green, *Pandemic Disease in the Medieval World,* 9–26.

———. "On Learning How to Teach the Black Death." *HPS&ST Note,* March 2018: 7–33. <https://www.hpsst.com/uploads/6/2/9/3/62931075/2018march.pdf>.

———, ed. *Pandemic Disease in the Medieval World: Rethinking the Black Death.* The Medieval Globe. Vol. 1. Kalamazoo, MI: Arc, 2014.

———. "Taking 'Pandemic' Seriously: Making the Black Death Global." In Green, *Pandemic Disease in the Medieval World,* 27–61.

Grigsby, Byron Lee. *Pestilence in Medieval and Early Modern English Literature.* New York: Routledge, 2004.

———. "Plague Medicine in Langland's *Piers Plowman.*" In *Teaching Literature and Medicine,* edited by Anne Hunsaker Hawkins and Marilyn Chandler McEntyre, 200–207. New York: MLA, 2000.

Gustafson, Kevin L. "The Lay Gaze: *Pearl,* the Dreamer, and the Vernacular Reader." *Medievalia et Humanistica* 27 (2000): 57–78.

Haspel, Paul. "Bells of Freedom and Foreboding: Liberty Bell Ideology and the Clock Motif in Edgar Allan Poe's 'The Masque of the Red Death.'" *Edgar Allan Poe Review* 13 (2012): 46–70.

Hanna, Ralph. "Alliterative Poetry." In *The Cambridge History of Medieval Literature,* edited by David Wallace, 488–512. Cambridge: Cambridge University Press, 1999.

Hayum, Andrée. *The Isenheim Altarpiece: God's Medicine and the Painter's Vision.* Princeton, NJ: Princeton University Press, 1989.

Hazard, Mark. "*Patience* and *The Book of Jonah* 'As Holy Wryt Telles.'" *Mediaevalia* 21 (1997): 295–325.

Hecker, Justus F. C. *The Black Death in the Fourteenth Century.* Translated by B. G. Babbington. London: Schloss, 1833.

———. *Der Schwarze Tod im vierzehnten Jahrhundert.* Berlin: Herbig, 1832.

Heng, Geraldine. *Empire of Magic: Medieval Romance and the Politics of Cultural Fantasy.* New York: Columbia University Press, 2003.

———. "Feminine Knots and the Other *Sir Gawain and the Green Knight.*" *PMLA* 106 (1991): 500–514.

———. "A Woman Wants: The Lady, *Gawain,* and the Forms of Seduction." *Yale Journal of Criticism* 5 (1992): 101–34.

Herlihy, David. *The Black Death and the Transformation of the West.* Edited by Samuel K. Cohn, Jr. Cambridge, MA: Harvard University Press, 1997.

Herman, Judith. *Trauma and Recovery: From Domestic Abuse to Political Terror.* London: Pandora, 2001.

Hill, Ordelle G. "The Audience of *Patience.*" *Modern Philology* 66 (1968): 103–09.

Hinton, Norman D. "The Black Death and the Book of the Duchess." In *His Firm Estate: Essays in Honor of Franklin James Eikenberry,* edited by Donald E. Hayden, 72–78. Tulsa, OK: University of Tulsa Press, 1967.

Horrox, Rosemary, ed. and trans. *The Black Death.* Manchester: Manchester University Press, 1994.

Howie, Cary. *Claustrophilia: The Erotics of Enclosure in Medieval Literature.* New York: Palgrave Macmillan, 2007.

Hymes, Robert. "Epilogue: A Hypothesis on the East Asian Beginnings of the *Yersinia pestis* Polytomy." In Green, *Pandemic Disease in the Medieval World,* 285–308.

Ingham, Patricia Clare. "Chaucer's Haunted Aesthetics: Mimesis and Trauma in *Troilus and Criseyde.*" *College English* 72 (2010): 226–47.

Irwin, John T., and T. D. Kelly. "The Way and the End Are One: *Patience* as a Parable of the Contemplative Life." *American Benedictine Review* 25 (1974): 33–55.

Johnson, Lynn Staley. *The Voice of the* Gawain-Poet. Madison: University of Wisconsin Press, 1984.

Jones, Peter Murray. "Herbs and the Medieval Surgeon." In Dendle and Touwaide, *Health and Healing from the Medieval Garden,* 162–79.

Kane, George. "Outstanding Problems of Middle English Scholarship." In Levy and Szarmach, *The Alliterative Tradition in the Fourteenth Century,* 1–17.

Kaske, R. E. "Gawain's Green Chapel and the Cave at Wetton Mill." In *Medieval Literature and Folklore Studies: Essays in Honor of Francis Lee Utley,* edited by Jerome Mandel and Bruce A. Rosenberg, 111–21. New Brunswick, NJ: Rutgers University Press, 1971.

Keiser, Elizabeth. *Courtly Desire and Medieval Homophobia: The Legitimation of Sexual Pleasure in* Cleanness *and Its Contexts.* New Haven, CT: Yale University Press, 1997.

Keiser, George R. "Two Medieval Plague Treatises and Their Afterlife in Early Modern England." *Journal of the History of Medicine and Allied Sciences* 58 (2003): 292–324.

Kittendorf, Doris. "*Cleanness* and the Fourteenth Century *Artes Praedicandi.*" *Michigan Academician* 11 (1979): 319–30.

Klein, Thomas. "Six Colour Words in the *Pearl* Poet: *Blake, Blayke, Blaȝt, Blwe, Blo* & *Ble.*" *Studia Neophilologica* 71 (1999): 156–58.

La Capra, Dominick. "Trauma, Absence, Loss." *Critical Inquiry* 25 (1999): 696–727.

Lavezzo, Kathy. "Chaucer and Everyday Death: *The Clerk's Tale,* Burial, and the Subject of Poverty." *Studies in the Age of Chaucer* 23 (2001): 255–87.

Lawton, David. "Dullness and the Fifteenth Century." *English Literary History* 54 (1987): 761–99.

———, ed. *Middle English Alliterative Poetry and Its Literary Background: Seven Essays.* Cambridge: D. S. Brewer, 1982.

———. "The Unity of Middle English Alliterative Poetry." *Speculum* 58 (1983): 72–94.

———. *Voice in Later Medieval Literature: Public Interiorities.* Oxford: Oxford University Press, 2017.

Lerner, Robert E. "The Black Death and Western European Eschatological Mentalities." *American Historical Review* 86 (1981): 533–52.

Levy, Bernard S., and Paul E. Szarmach, eds. *The Alliterative Tradition in the Fourteenth Century.* Kent, OH: Kent State University Press, 1981.

Lewis, Celia. "Framing Fiction with Death: Chaucer's *Canterbury Tales* and the Plague." In *New Readings of Chaucer's Poetry,* edited by Robert G. Benson and Susan J. Ridyard, 138–64. Woodbridge, UK: Brewer, 2003.

Leys, Ruth. *From Guilt to Shame: Auschwitz and After.* Princeton, NJ: Princeton UP, 2007.

———. *Trauma: A Genealogy.* Chicago: University of Chicago Press, 2000.

Leys, Ruth, and Marlene Goldman. "Navigating the Genealogies of Trauma, Guilt, and Affect: An Interview with Ruth Leys." *University of Toronto Quarterly* 79 (2010): 656–79.

Lindeboom, Wim. "Rethinking the Recensions of the *Confessio Amantis.*" *Viator* 40 (2009): 319–48.

Longsworth, Robert. "Interpretive Laughter in *Sir Gawain and the Green Knight.*" *Philological Quarterly* 70 (1991): 141–47.

Machan, Tim William. "Medieval Multilingualism and Gower's Literary Practice." *Studies in Philology* 103 (2006): 1–25.

MacKay, Ellen. *Persecution, Plague, and Fire: Fugitive Histories of the Stage in Early Modern England.* Chicago: University of Chicago Press, 2011.

Mann, Jill. "Courtly Aesthetics and Courtly Ethics in *Sir Gawain and the Green Knight.*" *Studies in the Age of Chaucer* 31 (2009): 231–65.

Marafioti, Martin. "Post-*Decameron* Plague Treatises and the Boccaccian Innovation of Narrative Prophylaxis." *Annali d'Italianistica* 23 (2005): 69–87.

Martin, Priscilla. "Allegory and Symbolism." In Brewer and Gibson, *A Companion to the* Gawain-*Poet,* 315–28.

Mate, Mavis E. *Daughters, Wives and Widows after the Black Death: Women in Sussex, 1350–1535.* Woodbridge, UK: Boydell, 1998.

——. *Women in Medieval English Society.* Cambridge: Cambridge University Press, 1999.

Mathew, Gervase. *The Court of Richard II.* London: John Murray, 1968.

Mawson, Anthony R. "Understanding Mass Panic and Other Collective Responses to Threat and Disaster." *Psychiatry* 68.2 (2005): 95–113.

McHugh, Kathleen. "The Aesthetics of Wounding: Trauma and Self-Representation." *Strategies* 12 (1999): 117–26.

McIntosh, Angus. "A New Approach to Middle English Dialectology." *English Studies* 44 (1963): 1–11.

McIntosh, Angus, M. L. Samuels, and Michael Benskin, with Margaret Laing and Keith Williamson. *A Linguistic Atlas of Late Middle English.* 4 vols. Aberdeen, UK: Aberdeen University Press, 1986. Online Version. <http://www.lel.ed.ac.uk/ihd/elalme/elalme.html>.

McIntosh, Marjorie Keniston. *Working Women in English Society, 1300–1620.* Cambridge: Cambridge University Press, 2005.

Middleton, Anne. "The Audience and Public of *Piers Plowman.*" In Lawton, *Middle English Alliterative Poetry and Its Literary Background,* 101–23.

——. "The Idea of Public Poetry in the Reign of Richard II." *Speculum* 53 (1978): 94–114.

Miller, Edmund. "The Date and Occasion of *Sir Gawain and the Green Knight.*" *ANQ: A Quarterly Journal of Short Articles, Notes and Reviews* 28 (2015): 59–62.

Moorman, Charles. "The Role of the Narrator in *Patience.*" *Modern Philology* 61 (1963): 90–95.

Morgan, Gerald. "The Significance of the Pentangle Symbolism in 'Sir Gawain and the Green Knight.'" *Modern Language Review* 74 (1979): 769–90.

——. "Medieval Misogyny and Gawain's Outburst Against Women in *Sir Gawain and the Green Knight.*" *Modern Language Review* 97 (2002): 265–278.

Narin, Elisa Marie. "'Þat on . . . Þat oper': Rhetorical *Descriptio* and Morgan la Fay in 'Sir Gawain and the Green Knight.'" *Pacific Coast Philology* 23 (1988): 60–66.

National Institutes of Health "Types of Plague" US Department of Health and Human Services. http://www.niaid.nih.gov/topics/plague/Pages/forms.aspx.

Ng, Su Fang, and Kenneth Hodges. "Saint George, Islam, and Regional Audiences in Sir Gawain and the Green Knight." *Studies in the Age of Chaucer* 32 (2010): 257–94.

Nochlin, Linda. *Mathis at Colmar: A Visual Confrontation.* New York: Red Dust, 1963.

Ngai, Sianne. *Ugly Feelings.* Cambridge, Mass.: Harvard University Press, 2005.

Nuttall, Jenni. *The Creation of Lancastrian Kingship: Literature, Language and Politics in Late Medieval England.* Cambridge: Cambridge University Press, 2007.

Olson, Gelnding. *Literature as Recreation in the Later Middle Ages.* Ithaca, NY: Cornell University Press, 1982.

Onishi, Norimitsu. "For a Liberian Family, Ebola Turns Loving Care into Deadly Risk." *New York Times.* November 13, 2014. <http://www.nytimes.com/2014/11/14/world/africa/in-ebola-out-break-in-liberia-a-familys-strength-can-be-its-fatal-flaw.html>.

Patterson, Lee. *Negotiating the Past: The Historical Understanding of Medieval Literature.* Madison: University of Wisconsin Press, 1987.

Payling, S. J. "Social Mobility, Demographic Change, and Landed Society in Late Medieval England." *Economic History Review* 45 (1992): 51–73.

Pearsall, Derek. "The Alliterative Revival: Origins and Social Backgrounds." In Lawton, *Middle English Alliterative Poetry and Its Literary Background,* 34–53.

———. "Rhetorical 'Descriptio' in 'Sir Gawain and the Green Knight.'" *Modern Language Review* 50 (1955): 129–34.

Penrose, Elizabeth [Mrs. Markham]. *A History of England, New and Revised Edition.* London: John Murray, 1869.

Platt, Colin. *King Death: The Black Death and Its Aftermath in Late-Medieval England.* Toronto: University of Toronto Press, 1996.

Poe, Edgar Allan. "The Masque of the Red Death." In *The Collected Works of Edgar Allan Poe: Tales and Sketches 1831–1842,* edited by Thomas Ollive Mabbott, 667–78. Cambridge, MA: Belknap, 1978.

Pohli, Carol. "Containment of Anger in the Medieval Poem, *Patience.*" *English Language Notes* 29 (1991): 1–14.

Potkay, Monica Brzezinski. "*Cleanness*'s Fecund and Barren Speech Acts." *Studies in the Age of Chaucer* 17 (1995): 99–109.

Prior, Sandra Pierson. *The Fayre Formez of the* Pearl *Poet.* East Lansing: Michigan State University Press, 1996.

Pugh, Tison. "Gawain and the Godgames." *Christianity and Literature* 51 (2002): 525–51.

Putter, Ad, and Myra Stokes. "The Linguistic Atlas and the Dialect of the Gawain Poems." *Journal of English and Germanic Philology* 106 (2007): 468–91.

Quarantelli, E. L. "The Nature and Conditions of Panic." *American Journal of Sociology* 60.3 (1954): 267–75.

Raunig, Gerald. "The Heterogenesis of Fleeing." Translated by Anita Fricek and Stephen Zepke. In *Deleuze and Contemporary Art,* edited by Stephen Zepke and Simon O'Sullivan, 43–62. Edinburgh: Edinburgh University Press, 2010.

Rawcliffe, Carole. *Urban Bodies: Communal Health in Late Medieval English Towns and Cities.* Woodbridge, UK: Boydell, 2013.

Razi, Zvi. *Life, Marriage, and Death in a Medieval Parish: Economy, Society, and Demography in Halesowen, 1270–1400.* Cambridge: Past and Present Publications, 1980.

Reading, Amity. "'The ende of alle kynez flesch': Ritual Sacrifice and Feasting in *Cleanness.*" *Exemplaria* 21 (2009): 274–95.

Rhodes, James. *Poetry Does Theology: Chaucer, Grosseteste, and the* Pearl-*Poet.* Notre Dame, IN: Notre Dame University Press, 2001.

———. "Vision and History in *Patience.*" *Journal of Medieval and Renaissance Studies* 19 (1989): 1–13.

Riddy, Felicity. "Jewels in *Pearl.*" In Brewer and Gibson, *A Companion to the* Gawain-*Poet,* 143–56.

Rudd, Gillian. "'The Wildernes of Wirral' in *Sir Gawain and the Green Knight*." *Arthuriana* 23 (2013): 52–65.

Rydzeski, Justine. *Radical Nostalgia in the Age of* Piers Plowman: *Economics, Apocalypticism, and Discontent*. New York: Peter Lang, 1999.

Sandidge, Marilyn. "Forty Years of Plague: Attitudes toward Old Age in the Tales of Boccaccio and Chaucer." In *Old Age in the Middle Ages and the Renaissance: Interdisciplinary Approaches to a Neglected Topic*, edited by Albrecht Classen, 357–73. Berlin: Walter de Gruyter, 2007.

Scala, Elizabeth. *Absent Narratives, Manuscript Textuality, and Literary Structure in Late Medieval England*. New York: Palgrave MacMillan, 2002.

Scase, Wendy. Piers Plowman *and the New Anti-Clericalism*. Cambridge: Cambridge University Press, 1989.

Schiff, Randy. *Revivalist Fantasy: Alliterative Verse and Nationalist Literary History*. Columbus: Ohio State University Press, 2011.

Schmid, Boris V., Ulf Büntgen, W. Ryan Easterday, Christian Ginzler, Lars Walløe, Barbara Bramanti, and Nils Chr. Stenseth. "Climate-Driven Introduction of the Black Death and Successive Plague Reintroductions into Europe." *PNAS* 112 (2015): 3020–25.

Schmidt, Gary D. "'Þis Wrech Man in Warlowes Guttez': Imagery and Unity or Frame and Tale in *Patience*." In Blanch et al., *Text and Matter*, 177–93.

Schofield, Phillipp R. "The Late Medieval View of Frankpledge and the Tithing System: An Essex Case Study." In *Medieval Society and the Manor Court*, edited by Zvi Razi and Richard Smith, 408–49. Oxford: Clarendon, 1996.

Shedd, Gordon M. "Knight in Tarnished Armour: The Meaning of *Sir Gawain and the Green Knight*." *Modern Language Review* 62 (1967): 3–13.

Shoaf, R. A. *The Poem as Green Girdle: Commercium in* Sir Gawain and the Green Knight. Gainesville: University Press of Florida, 1984.

Shrewsbury, J. F. D. *A History of Bubonic Plague in the British Isles*. Cambridge: Cambridge University Press, 1970.

Silverman, Kenneth. *Edgar A. Poe: Mournful and Never-Ending Remembrance*. New York: Harper Perennial, 1992.

Sime, Jonathan D. "Affiliative Behaviour during Escape to Building Exits." *Journal of Environmental Psychology* 3 (1983): 21–41.

Simpson, James. Piers Plowman: *An Introduction*. 2nd ed. Exeter: University of Exeter Press, 2007.

Smith, D. Vance. "Irregular Histories: Forgetting Ourselves." *New Literary History* 28 (1997): 161–84.

———. "Plague, Panic Space, and the Tragic Medieval Household." *South Atlantic Quarterly* 98 (1999): 367–414.

Smoller, Laura A. "Of Earthquakes, Hail, Frogs, and Geography: Plague and the Investigation of Apocalypse in the Later Middle Ages." In *Last Things: Death and the Apocalypse in the Middle Ages*, edited by Carolyn Walker Bynum and Paul Freedman, 156–88. Philadelphia: University of Pennsylvania Press, 2000.

Snell, William. "Chaucer's Pardoner's Tale and Pestilence in Late Medieval Literature." *Studies in Medieval English Language and Literature* 10 (1995): 1–16.

Spearing, A. C. *The* Gawain *Poet: A Poetic Study*. Cambridge: Cambridge University Press, 1970.

———. "The Subtext of *Patience*: God as Mother and the Whale's Belly." *Journal of Medieval and Early Modern Studies* 29 (1999): 293–323.

Spencer, H. L. "*Pearl*: 'God's Law' and 'Man's Law.'" *Review of English Studies* 59 (2008): 317–41.

Spivak, Gayatri. "Can the Subaltern Speak?" In *Marxism and the Interpretation of Culture,* edited by Cary Nelson and Lawrence Grossberg, 271–313. Urbana: University of Illinois Press, 1988.

Staley, Lynn. *Languages of Power in the Age of Richard II.* University Park: Pennsylvania State University Press, 2005.

———. "*Pearl* and the Contingencies of Love and Piety." In *Medieval Literature and Historical Inquiry: Essays in Honor of Derek Pearsall,* edited by David Aers, 83–114. Cambridge: Brewer, 2000.

Stanbury, Sarah. "Feminist Masterplots: The Gaze on the Body of *Pearl*'s Dead Girl." In *Feminist Approaches to the Body in Medieval Literature,* edited by Linda Lomperis and Sarah Stanbury, 96–115. Philadelphia: University of Pennsylvania Press, 1993.

———. "Introduction." In *Pearl,* edited by Sarah Stanbury, 1–19. Kalamazoo, MI: Medieval Institute Publications, 2001.

———. *Seeing the* Gawain-*Poet: Description and the Act of Perception.* Philadelphia: University of Pennsylvania Press, 1991.

———. "Space and Visual Hermeneutics in the *Gawain*-Poet." *Chaucer Review* 21 (1987): 476–89.

Steel, David. "Plague Writing: From Boccaccio to Camus." *Journal of European Studies* 11 (1981): 88–110.

Steiner, Emily. *Reading* Piers Plowman. Cambridge: Cambridge University Press, 2013.

Stephens, Carolyn King. "The 'Pentangle Hypothesis': A Dating History and Resetting of *Sir Gawain and the Green Knight.*" *Fifteenth-Century Studies* 31 (2006): 174–202.

Stock, Lorraine Kochanske. "The 'Poynt' of *Patience.*" In Blanch et al., *Text and Matter,* 163–75.

Strohm, Paul. *England's Empty Throne: Usurpation and the Language of Legitimation 1399–1422.* New Haven, CT: Yale University Press, 1998.

———. *Social Chaucer.* Cambridge, MA: Harvard University Press, 1989.

Strong, Philip. "Epidemic Psychology: A Model." *Sociology of Health and Illness* 12 (1990): 249–59.

Taylor, Karla. "Social Aesthetics and the Emergence of Civic Discourse from *The Shipman's Tale* to *Melibee.*" *Chaucer Review* 39 (2005): 298–322.

Terrell, Katherine H. "Rethinking the 'Corse in Clot': Cleanness, Filth, and Bodily Decay in *Pearl.*" *Studies in Philology* 105 (2008): 429–47.

Tomasch, Sylvia. "*Patience* and the Sermon Tradition." *Centerpoint* 4 (1981): 83–93.

———. "A *Pearl* Punnology." *Journal of English and Germanic Philology* 88 (1989): 1–20.

Tournoy, Gilbert. "The Enigmatic Socrates or Ludovicus Sanctus in the French Edition of Petrarch's *Rerum Familiarium Liber.*" *Humanistica Lovaniensia* 57 (2008): 321–23.

Tuchman, Barbara. *A Distant Mirror: The Calamitous Fourteenth Century.* New York: Knopf, 1978.

Twomey, Michael. "Morgan le Fay at Hautdesert." In *On Arthurian Women: Essays in Memory of Maureen Fries,* edited by Bonnie Wheeler and Fiona Tolhurst, 103–19. Dallas: Scriptorium, 2001.

———. "Morgain la Fée in *Sir Gawain and the Green Knight*: From Troy to Camelot." In *Text and Intertext in Medieval Arthurian Literature,* edited by Norris J. Lacy, 91–115. New York: Garland, 1996.

———. "The Sin of Untrawþe in *Cleanness.*" In Blanch et al., *Text and Matter,* 117–45.

Vantuono, William. "The Structure and Sources of *Patience*." *Mediaeval Studies* 34 (1972): 401–21.

Vasta, Edward. "Denial in the Middle English *Patience*." *Chaucer Review* 33 (1998): 1–30.

———. "*Pearl*: Immortal Flowers and the Pearl's Decay." *Journal of English and Germanic Philology* 66 (1967): 519–31.

Wallace, David. *Boccaccio: Decameron, Landmarks of World Literature*. Cambridge: Cambridge University Press, 1991.

———. "*Cleanness* and the Terms of Terror." In Blanch et al., *Text and Matter*, 93–104.

Warner, Lawrence. "The Lady, the Goddess, and the Text of *Sir Gawain and the Green Knight*." *Chaucer Review* 48 (2014): 334–51.

Watson, Nicholas. "Censorship and Cultural Change in Late-Medieval England: Vernacular Theology, the Oxford Translation Debate, and Arundel's Constitution of 1409." *Speculum* 70 (1995): 822–46.

———. "The *Gawain*-Poet as a Vernacular Theologian." In Brewer and Gibson, *A Companion to the* Gawain-*Poet*, 293–313.

———. "The Politics of Middle English Writing." In Wogan-Browne et al., *The Idea of the Vernacular*, 331–52.

Wenzel, Siegfried. "Pestilence and Middle English Literature: Friar John Grimestone's Poems of Death." In *The Black Death: The Impact of Fourteenth-Century Plague*, edited by Daniel Williman, 131–59. Binghamton, NY: Center for Medieval and Early Renaissance Studies, 1982.

Whiting, B. J. "Gawain: His Reputation, His Courtesy and His Appearance in Chaucer's *Squire's Tale*." *Mediæval Studies* 9 (1947): 189–234.

Winslow, Charles-Edward. *The Conquest of Epidemic Disease: A Chapter in the History of Ideas*. Princeton, NJ: Princeton University Press, 1943.

Wogan-Brown, Jocelyn, Nicholas Watson, Andrew Taylor, and Ruth Evans, eds. *The Idea of the Vernacular: An Anthology of Middle English Literary Theory, 1280–1520*. University Park: Pennsylvania State University Press, 1999.

Wolfe, Elisabeth G. "Þaӡ Hit Displese Ofte: Monastic Obedience in *Patience*." *Christianity and Literature* 62 (2013): 493–510.

Woolf, Rosemary. *The English Religious Lyric in the Middle Ages*. Oxford: Clarendon, 1968.

Wright, C. E. *English Vernacular Hands from the Twelfth to the Fifteenth Centuries*. Oxford: Oxford University Press, 1960.

Yeager, Robert F. "English, Latin, and the Text as 'Other': The Page as Sign in the Work of John Gower." In *Text: Transactions of the Society for Textual Scholarship*, edited by D. C. Greetham and W. C. Speed Hill, 251–67. New York: AMS Press, 1987.

Ziegler, Michelle. "The Black Death and the Future of the Plague." In Green, *Pandemic Disease in the Medieval World*, 259–83.

Ziegler, Philip. *The Black Death*. London: Collins, 1969.

Žižek, Slavoj. "Courtly Love, or, Woman as Thing." In *The Metastases of Enjoyment: Six Essays on Women and Causality*, 89–112. London and New York: Verso, 1994.

INDEX

abandonment, 84–86

Abraham (biblical), 30, 37–41, 38n27, 44

Adam (biblical), 29, 29n1, 47–48, 158–59

Adorno, Theodor, 54

adultery, 135–36

Aers, David, 21, 82–84, 160, 162n85, 173

affiliation, 96–97, 100, 102, 105, 107, 124

Africa, 1, 4, 8–9, 9n30

d'Agramunt, Jacme, 110, 112, 140, 148. See also *Regiment de preservació*

AIDS pandemic, 97

allegory, 1, 5, 23, 48, 62, 65, 74, 82, 87–88, 128, 138n37

amnesia, 4, 35n19, 127. *See also* posttraumatic behavior; trauma: responses to

Annales Pistorienses, 100

Anonimalle Chronicle, 13, 75, 75n54, 87

Antediluvians, 29, 39, 42, 43n32, 50, 80, 80n62, 97, 102

Anthony (Saint), 59

antifeminism, 137, 158–60, 163–64. *See also* misogyny

antimimesis. *See* mimesis

apocalypse, 5, 12–13, 18, 20, 23, 29, 34, 39–41, 44, 47–48, 53, 62, 87–89, 88n79, 95, 103, 108, 118, 125, 164, 168–70, 182; plague as sign of, 88–89, 135, 182–84

Apocalypse (Book of Revelations), 56, 87–88

aristocracy, 124, 128, 132–33, 156–58, 175, 177, 182

Arthur (King), 24, 126–27, 129–31, 134, 135n30, 141–42, 156–58, 161–65, 174, 176–78

Arthurian romance, 5, 24, 128, 133, 147n59, 164, 170, 176–77

Asia, 4, 8

astrological influences, 49

audience, 2–4, 31, 37n25, 38n27, 39–41, 43, 47, 62–66, 62n7, 72, 74, 76, 79, 82, 87, 95, 103, 106–07, 109, 112–14, 117–18, 125, 127, 138–43, 148–49, 151, 156, 165, 167–69, 178–79, 182–83, 188–90; clerical, 121–22; courtly, 21–25, 133, 173–74

Augustine (Saint), 36n20

authority, 3, 134–35, 137, 156–57, 171; of English, 183, 185, 187–91; to witness, 34, 39–40, 42

authorship, 14, 16–17, 16n60, 190

Babylon (biblical), 29–30, 38–39, 43–47, 52

le Baker, Geoffrey. See *Chronicon Galfridi le Baker de Swynebroke*

barrow, 138–39, 138n38

Bathsheba (biblical), 159–60

beatitudes, 108, 118–19, 124, 173

beheading game, 126, 130, 149, 149n66, 158, 161

Belshazzar (biblical), 30, 44–45, 45n34, 80

Bertilak. *See* Green Knight

Bertilak, Lady, 127, 137–38, 144–50, 147n59, 156–57, 159, 161, 163, 165, 187

Bible, 5, 20–22, 29–31, 34, 37–39, 41, 43–46, 47–49, 52–53, 56–59, 80, 82, 94–95, 100, 103, 106n46, 107, 111n59, 112–13, 116, 128, 135, 156, 159, 170, 173, 184, 186–87, 190–91; Latin Vulgate, 94–95, 102, 107–8, 111, 114–15. *See also* Apocalypse (Book of Revelations); Book of Daniel; Book of Genesis; Book of Jonah; scripture

Biel, Gabriel. See *De fuga pestis*

Black Death. *See* plague

Black Knight, 172, 174. See also *Book of the Duchess*

Blanche of Lancaster, 20, 171

Boccaccio, Giovanni, 1, 2–7, 18n68, 51, 54, 56, 73, 86, 88, 93, 96–98, 102, 143, 168, 174n21, 182–83, 189. See also *Decameron*; *Il Filostrato*

body, 6, 8n26, 9–10, 38, 50–51, 53, 56, 58–59, 62, 64–65, 67–72, 76–82, 86–88, 97, 102, 109, 130, 137–41, 145, 147, 150–51, 156; aligned with trauma, 33–34, 36–38

Book of Daniel, 30, 37, 38n27, 44–47, 45n34, 52, 80, 184, 188. *See also* Bible

Book of the Duchess (Chaucer), 19–20, 31, 52, 171, 171n13, 172, 174–75, 189

Book of Genesis, 38, 56. *See also* Bible

Book of Jonah, 5, 23, 81, 94–96, 100–118, 102n37, 111n59, 118n80, 121–22, 135–36, 148, 156, 160, 164, 184, 188. *See also* Bible; *Patience*

Bordeaux, 11

Bowers, John, 14, 16n58, 119n82, 172n15–16, 174n20, 177n25

Breve Chronicon Clerici Anonymi, 120

Bristol, 11–12

British Isles, 11–12, 12n38. *See also* England, Ireland, Scotland

British Library Cotton Nero A.x, article, 3, 5–7, 14–17, 19, 22–24, 29, 52, 70n31, 94–95, 97, 135, 169, 172n15, 173–75, 178, 180–82, 184, 191. See also *Cleanness*; *Patience*; *Pearl*; *Sir Gawain and the Green Knight*

Brinton, Thomas. See *Sermons of Thomas Brinton, The*

buboes, 5, 10, 51, 72, 76, 104, 151, 156, 182–83. See also plague: symptoms of

Bullein, Willaim. See *Dialogue Against the Fever Pestilence*

Burton, Thomas. See *Chronica Monasterii de Melsa a Fundatione usque ad Annum*

Butterfield, Ardis, 2, 20, 52, 171

Camelot, 24, 126–27, 129, 131, 131n15, 142, 156–58, 157n72, 160–65, 173, 177

Cannon, Walter Bradford, 96n14

Canterbury Tales (Chaucer), 5, 19–20, 175, 180, 180n29, 182, 191. *See also* "Knight's Tale"; "Manciple's Tale"; "Pardoner's Tale"

careerism, 129, 134–35, 145

Caruth, Cathy, 6n23, 33–34, 36–37

Caxton, William, 190

Chaucer, Geoffrey, 3, 5, 7, 18n68, 19–20, 94, 124n99, 143, 167–68, 171–72, 172n16, 174–75, 174n21, 180–81, 187–88, 190–91. See also *Canterbury Tales*; "Knight's Tale"; "Manciple's Tale"; "Pardoner's Tale"; *Troilus and Criseyde*

de Chauliac, Guy. See *Cyrurgie of Guy de Chauliac*

Cheshire, 15–16, 134, 134n26, 172n15

child, 5, 13, 23, 35n19, 39, 43, 45, 54, 54n60, 56, 62–63, 65, 67, 69–71, 75–77, 75n54, 80, 82–83, 86–88, 96–97, 105, 114, 132, 143, 170, 172–75. *See also* Children's Plague; family

Children's Plague, 13–14, 47, 75. *See also* mortality: in children

China, 8, 9n30. *See also* Tibet-Qinghai Plateau

Chirurgia magna (Chauliac), 67

Chism, Christine, 17, 131n14, 149n66

chivalry, 127, 129, 138, 141, 145, 148, 149n66, 156–57, 163–64, 173–74, 177–78

Christ, 31, 38, 38n27, 40, 56, 57 fig 2.1, 58–59, 58 fig 2.2, 61, 61 fig 2.4, 69, 73, 76–77, 79–82, 84, 88, 101, 114–15, 118, 124, 173, 189; Ascension, 59; Crucifixion, 59, 60 fig 2.3, 76, 79, 81; Incarnation, 30–31, 38, 67, 80; Passion, 56, 59, 77, 79, 82; Resurrection, 59, 60 fig 2.4, 69, 72, 74, 77, 82; wounds of, 56, 58–59, 69, 76–77, 79–80

Christianity, 5, 29–30, 39, 48, 53, 56, 59, 62–63, 74, 76, 76n57, 78, 81–82, 88, 100, 114, 124, 141, 156n71, 173, 175, 184. *See also* Christ; Soteriology (Christian)

Chronica gentis Scotorum (Fordun), 86

Chronica Johannis de Reading (Reading), 103, 135

Chronica Monasterii de Melsa a Fundatione usque ad Annum (Burton), 136

Chronicle of the Grey Friars of Lynn, 11, 75, 185

Chronicon Abbatie de Parco Lude (Louth Park chronicler), 48, 75

Chronicon Galfridi le Baker de Swynebroke (Baker), 52n53, 86, 97, 123

Chronicon Henrici Knighton (Knighton), 75, 136, 147

Chronicon majus Aegidii Li Muisis (Muisis), 120

Chronique Latine de Guillaume de Nangis (de Nangis), 99

Cities of the Plain (biblical), 35–36, 40, 43, 47, 50, 116. *See also* Sodom and Gomorrah; Segor; Dead Sea

claustration, 94, 108, 110–12, 115. *See also* enclosure; quarantine

Cleanness, 5, 7, 13–14, 18, 22–24, 29–31, 34–55, 38n27, 59, 62–63, 67, 80, 80n62, 82, 95, 102–5, 107–8, 111n57, 114–16, 118, 125, 128, 135, 139, 157, 164, 169–70, 173–75, 178, 182, 184, 187

clergy, 24, 52n53, 99–100, 105, 119–24, 121n89, 133, 167, 171, 178–79. *See also* mortality: in clergy

climate, 8, 13. *See also* environment

community, 21n82, 30, 73, 75, 78, 87, 95, 97, 107, 113, 120, 132, 162n85, 163

compulsive behavior, 31–32, 46. *See also* post-traumatic behavior

Confessio Amantis (Gower), 167, 178–81, 186–87, 190

consciousness, 3n11, 6, 15, 23, 31–33, 46, 82, 127, 169–70, 190. *See also* trauma: consciousness of

consolation, 23, 79, 82, 118, 175, 178

contagion, 10–11, 19, 69, 71, 73, 85–86, 85n71, 85n72, 94, 97, 99–100, 108–9, 116, 119–23, 163, 174, 188. *See also* plague: transmission of

Continental literature, 5–7, 21, 24, 31, 48, 52, 63, 102, 167–71, 181–87

de Córdoba, Alfonso. *See Epistola et regimen Alphontii Cordubensis de pestilentia*

de Cortusiis, Guillelmi, 48n40. *See Historia de Novitatibus Paduae et Lombardie*

counternarrative, 22, 39, 43–47

court, 16, 23–24, 44, 62–65, 62n7, 68, 73n43, 80, 83–88, 93, 122, 124, 126–31, 131n14, 133–34, 137, 141–47, 156–58, 161–63, 172–83, 172n16, 179n27, 190–91. *See also* audience: courtly

de Covino, Symonis. *See De Judicio Solis*

Cronaca (da Piazza), 22, 99–100, 120–1

Cronaca Senese (Grasso), 167

Cyrurgie of Guy de Chauliac, 50–51, 50n44, 66, 68, 99, 104

Dante, 183

Darstellung, 37, 39–41

David (biblical), 159

Dead Sea, 30, 36, 38–40, 50–51, 81, 116, 139, 173. *See also* Sodom and Gommorah; Cities of the Plain

death, 4, 10, 18–21, 42, 45, 51–52, 54, 59, 62, 64n13, 65, 68, 70, 72–78, 82–83, 86, 100, 103, 110, 114, 121, 126, 134–35, 138–44, 150, 156, 159–60, 168, 171, 171n13, 172, 174n21, 178, 180–82, 185; as abstraction, 52, 171n13; Death (personified), 5, 19, 143, 151, 153 fig 4.3, 154 fig 4.4, 167; as great leveler, 123; and rebirth, 59, 70–72, 74. *See also* mortality

Decameron (Boccaccio), 1–4, 1n1, 6, 10, 20, 22, 51, 56, 69, 72–73, 87–88, 93–94, 96, 98, 103, 143–44, 182–83, 189

Decay, 68, 71, 76, 79, 94

Delilah (biblical), 159

Dene of Rochester, William, 121n89. See *Historia Roffensis*

Dialogue Against the Fever Pestilence (Bullein), 188–89

Diario Fiorentino dal 1450 al 1516 di Luca Landucci (Landucci), 99

didacticism, 22, 30–31, 37–41, 43–44, 53, 77, 118, 124, 178, 185

disease, 1n3, 3, 5–8, 9n30, 9n31, 10–13, 15, 19–24, 31, 47–50, 52–53, 58–59, 62, 66, 68–70, 68n28, 71n32, 75–79, 75n54, 81–82, 86–88, 93–98, 100, 107, 109, 111–12, 114, 116, 120, 123, 133, 135–37, 139–40, 143–45, 147, 151, 160, 163–65, 168–73, 175, 178, 182, 185, 189, 191. *See also* epidemic; pestilence; plague

"Doctrine for Pestilence" (Lydgate), 72

Dreamer (*Pearl*), 63–74, 64n13, 64n14, 76–79, 81–85, 85n71, 85n72, 87, 94n6, 97, 102, 110, 114, 124, 150, 158, 172, 175–76, 184. *See also* family: father

East Anglia, 12

Ebola hemorrhagic fever, 96–97

economics, 7, 9, 20–21, 24–25, 118, 122–23, 122n91, 127–29, 133–34, 140–41, 145–46, 157–63, 176

elegy, 5, 20, 23, 54n60, 62, 82, 87–88, 171, 176–77, 181

embodiment, 3, 6, 23–24, 36–37, 53, 55, 67, 76, 82, 141, 146, 162, 165, 169, 175

enclosure, 24, 43n32, 93–95, 108–18, 121, 124, 173. *See also* claustration; quarantine

England, 1n3, 4–5, 4n16, 7, 11–13, 12n41, 12n42, 12n43, 13, 18, 19n73, 21, 23–25, 31, 47, 49, 53n56, 56, 63, 72, 74–75, 88–9, 99, 105n45, 106, 121–24, 128, 131–34, 131n15, 140, 145–46, 157, 162–63, 165, 167–68, 170–71, 173, 179, 181, 184–86, 190

English, 4, 23, 25, 63, 65n15, 78n61, 183–91, 183n36, 184n40, 188n48, 189n52, 190n55, 191

entombment, 59, 60 fig 2.3, 108, 115. *See also* claustration; enclosure

environment, 12–13, 18, 73, 82, 114, 141. *See also* climate

epidemic, 12–13, 22–23, 71n32, 74–75, 74n48, 93, 96–97, 97n18, 110, 113, 136, 139, 143, 164, 169. *See also* disease; plague

Epistolæ de rebus familiaribus et variæ (Petrarch), 22, 54, 126, 126n1, 158

Epistola et regimen Alphontii Cordubensis de pestilentia (Córdoba), 99

eschatology, 23, 62, 76n57, 88–89, 108

Essex, 74, 132

Eulogium (Historiarum sive Temporis), 135

Europe, 1, 1n3, 4–7, 4n16, 8, 11–12, 12n43, 21, 24, 31, 48, 52, 53n56, 63, 74n48, 75, 76n57, 86, 88, 102, 105n45, 106, 123, 131, 136, 167–69, 171, 181–83, 183n36, 187

Eve (biblical), 159

exegesis, 95, 101–2, 101n36, 115, 119

exempla, 5, 22–23, 30–31, 37, 41–43, 45–49, 52, 59, 80, 82, 95, 105, 119, 121–22, 173, 178

Extreme Unction, 119, 121

family: 30, 37, 41–42, 49, 96–99, 97n18, 132, 146n54, 189; children, 56, 71, 75–77, 175; daughter, 14, 34, 37, 38n27, 40, 63, 76, 84–85, 87, 97, 172n16, 176; dissolution of, 86–87, 96–97; father, 39, 45, 56, 63, 86–87, 96–97, 99, 176; mother, 80, 86–87, 90; parents, 23, 39, 45, 56, 63, 80, 86–87,

96–99, 132, 143, 158, 176. *See also* Children's Plague; Pearl Maiden

fear, 13, 31, 83–87, 85n71, 95–96, 97n18, 99–100, 110, 118–20, 122, 124, 140, 143, 159–60, 189. *See also* panic

filth, 39–40, 42, 64–66, 79–81, 102, 115–16, 123, 135, 173

Fisher, Sheila, 126, 162n83

Flagellants, 105

fleas. *See* plague: role of fleas

flesh, 36, 42, 49, 51, 59, 70n31, 74, 76, 78–79, 82, 94, 108

flight, 96–99, 96n14, 108–9. *See* plague: flight from

Florence, Italy, 1, 3n8, 4, 51, 54, 56, 71, 73, 88, 93, 98–99, 102, 143, 182

Fracostorius, Hieronymus, 112–13

Fradenburg, L. O. Aranye, 4, 85, 180n31

France, 71, 85, 93, 99, 106, 112–13, 139, 147, 183. *See also* French

Freidl, Jean-Paul and Ian Kirby, 14–15, 19, 65–67, 76n56, 78n61, 85n71

French, 4, 183, 187–88, 190. *See also* vernacular

Freud, Sigmund, 46

fuga pestis, De (Biel), 106

garden, 65, 68–74, 72n39, 76, 83–84, 114

Gawain, 24, 70n31, 75n49, 81, 115, 126–27, 129–31, 129n7, 137–42, 144–51, 147n59, 148n64, 149n66, 150n68, 156–64, 156n71, 162n85, 173, 176–77, 187

gaze, 79, 81, 84, 87, 127, 137, 144–45, 145n51, 176; as contagion, 71, 174. *See also* vision

Gentile of Foligno. See *Singulare consilium contra pestilium*

geography, 15n56, 17, 129, 139, 141. *See also* plague: geography of

Germany, 99, 106, 140

girdle, 138, 146–47, 150, 158, 161–65, 176

God (Christian), 13, 29–30, 30n4, 34–35, 35n19, 36n20, 37–45, 38n27, 48–49, 52–53, 52n53, 76, 80–81, 83–85, 93–96, 98, 100–106, 108, 110–19, 111n57, 111n59, 121–25, 135–36, 139, 147, 159, 170–71, 173, 176, 188–89; Lamb of, 63, 65, 67, 69, 76–79, 81–82, 87, 113, 177n25; vengeance of, 29, 31, 35n19, 38, 48, 103, 105, 117–18, 135, 140, 173, 184; will of, 82, 89, 93, 96, 100,

112–13, 118, 139, 172; wrath of, 30, 38–39, 42, 45, 53, 95, 98, 102–3, 106, 114, 118, 125, 173n18

Godden, Richard, 129, 163

Gower, John, 168, 171, 172n16, 187–88, 190. See also *Confessio Amantis*; *Mirrour de l'Omme*; *Vox Clamantis*

Grasso, Agnolo di Tura del. See *Cronaca Senese*

Gray Death, 13. See also Children's Plague

Green Chapel, 127, 129, 133, 147, 150, 156, 159; as pestilential site, 138–42

Green Knight, 24, 70n31, 75n49, 81, 126, 129–31, 133, 138–39, 141, 148n64, 158, 164; as Bertilak, 133–34, 143–45, 149–50, 160–61; as death, 142–43

grief, 7, 22–23, 35, 54, 64n13, 67, 73–74, 76, 82, 86, 88–89, 101, 104–5, 135, 141, 171–73, 176

guilt, 35, 87, 117. See also family

Guinevere, 141, 157, 157n72, 161, 164–65, 129n7

Grünewald, Matthias, 58–59, 81. See *Isenheim Altarpiece*

harvest, 41, 130; as coincident with plague, 74

Hautdesert, 24, 127, 129, 131, 133, 137–38, 140–41, 144, 146, 149, 156–58, 160–62, 173, 176, 187

Heng, Geraldine, 128–29, 145

Herman, Judith, 6, 32, 35, 127n4

hierarchy, 124, 140–41, 162n85, 173–74; gender, 84, 127–28, 141, 145, 157, 160, 162; spiritual, 30n4

Higden, Ranulph. See *Polychronicon*

Historia breuis Thomas Walsingham (Walsingham), 54, 74, 75n54, 99

Historia de Morbo (de Mussis), 9n31, 10–11, 22, 56, 86, 120, 136

Historia de Novitatibus Paduae et Lombardie (Cortusiis), 48

Historia Roffensis (Dene), 88

history, 1–4, 6, 15, 18, 23, 32, 35, 37, 53, 75, 95, 128–30, 162, 164–65, 184; biblical, 30, 41; chroniclers of, 11n37, 12n41, 13, 48, 52, 52n53, 54, 74–75, 75n54, 86, 87n78, 88, 97, 99–100, 102, 120, 123, 135–37, 151, 185; historiography, 1–3, 6, 15, 48, 100; mediation of, 3, 22

Holkham Bible, 56, 57 fig 2.1, 58–59, 58 fig 2.2

Howie, Cary, 109, 111

Ibn al-Wardī, Abū Hafs 'Umar. See "Ibn al-Wardī's 'Risālah al-naba' 'an al waba'"

"Ibn al-Wardī's 'Risālah al-naba' 'an al waba'" (Ibn al-Wardī), 100

idolatry, 45, 80, 159

Il Filostrato (Boccacio), 20

Il Sodoma, 151, 155 fig 4.6

illness. See disease; leprosy; pestilence; plague

imagery, 23, 52, 59, 70, 77, 79, 81–82, 88, 151, 169, 175, 187

incest, 38n27, 135, 135n30

India, 8

infection, 9–11, 49, 68, 71, 73, 99, 117, 119–21, 151, 181. See also plague: symptoms of; plague: transmission of

Ingham, Patricia Clare, 3, 33, 37

imperfection. See perfection

Ireland, 12

Isenheim Altarpiece (Gruënewald), 59, 60 fig 2.3, 61 fig 2.4, 62

Islam, 9n30, 11, 112, 141; prohibition on plague flight, 100

Italian language, 4, 183, 188, 188n48

Italy, 1, 41, 51, 54, 56, 71, 73, 88, 93, 98–99, 103, 143, 182–83. See also Italian

Jerusalem, 29–30, 39, 43–47, 52, 67, 77, 79

jewel, 62–64, 66–67, 73n43, 83–85, 124, 175–76, 184

Jeweler. See Dreamer (*Pearl*)

Job, 95, 107

John of Arderne. See *Treatises of Fistula in Ano*

John of Burgundy, 48, 71n32, 102n39

John of Fordun. See *Chronica gentis Scotorum*

John of Gaunt, 20, 171

John the Baptist (Saint), 11

Jordan Plain, 30, 104. See also Sodom and Gommorah, Cities of the Plain

Judaism, 45, 101–02, 110

De Judicio Solis (Covino), 48–49

Jugement dou Roy de Navarre (Machaut), 2, 4, 6, 22, 85, 85n72, 87, 94, 182–83

Kaffa, 8–9; 9n31

"Knight's Tale" (Chaucer), 19, 174–75. See also *Canterbury Tales*

Knighton, Henry. See *Chronicon Henrici Knighton*

Knuttson, Bengt. See *Litil Boke the Whiche Traytied Many Gode Thinges for the Pestilence, A*

lament, 13, 15, 20, 22, 41, 43, 45, 48, 52, 54, 54n60, 62, 67, 78, 82, 84, 88, 100, 135, 171–72, 182–83, 185

Landucci, Luca. See *Diario Fiorentino dal 1450 al 1516 di Luca Landucci*

Langland, William, 2, 5, 7, 20–21, 21n82, 24, 168, 182–83, 187, 190. See also *Piers Plowman*

language, 2, 14–15, 33, 40, 48–52, 56, 62–64, 62n8, 68, 70, 76–79, 81–82, 88, 102, 104, 128, 146, 148, 172, 175–76, 183, 183n36, 185–91. See also English; French; Italian; Latin vernacular

Latin, 48, 52, 88, 160, 184–88, 190. See also *Bible:* Latin Vulgate

laughter, 126–27, 126n2, 157, 161, 178

leprosy, 50, 59, 65, 86, 170

Leys, Ruth, 33–34, 36

Lieferinxe, Josse, 151, 152 fig 4.1

Life of Saint Cuthbert, 50, 68, 68n25

Literae prioris et capituli cantuar, 113

Litil Boke the Whiche Traytied Many Gode Thinges for the Pestilence, A (Knuttson), 52, 71–72, 112, 140, 148

London, 12, 20, 56–58, 74, 172n16, 186, 189

loss, 5, 7, 22–23, 29–32, 35, 39–43, 43n32, 44, 46, 53–55, 59, 62–65, 68, 76, 79, 82–88, 97, 104, 107, 114, 122, 128, 130, 132, 158, 172–73, 175–76; of faith, 59, 132; of Pearl Maiden, 67, 83–84, 86, 173, 176; of life, 7, 104. See also grief; trauma

Lot (biblical), 34–35, 37, 38n27, 40

Lot's wife (biblical), 29, 32, 34–41, 36n20, 44, 46–48, 52, 80, 97, 102, 127, 169

Louth Park chronicler. See *Chronicon Abbatie de Parco Lude*

lovesickness, 20, 65, 67

Lydgate, John, 189. See also "Doctrine for Pestilence"; "Stella Celi Extirpuit"

Machaut, Guillaume de, 2, 5, 168, 182. See also *Jugement dou Roy de Navarre*

"Manciple's Tale," 180. See also *Canterbury Tales*

Mandatum Radulphi, episcopi Bath et Wellen de confessionibus tempore pestilentiae, 121

marriage, 132, 136, 145, 147–48, 162

Marseilles, 9

masculinity, 131, 138, 141, 145, 159–60, 162–64

"Masque of the Red Death" (Poe), 93–94, 93n2, 109

Master of the Playing Cards, 151, 154 fig 4.5

medieval drama, 21–22

Mediterranean Basin, 8–9

Melcombe (Weymouth), England, 11

memory, 3–5, 13, 15, 19–22, 31–33, 36n20, 37n25, 39–40, 32n43, 43n32, 45, 47, 53–54, 178. See also amnesia; trauma: responses to

Merlin, 134, 161

Messina, 9, 99, 103

metaphor, 1, 30n4, 43n32, 62n8, 63, 70n31, , 81, 151, 170–71, 173, 178, 187–88; in *Pearl,* 23, 64–65, 67, 69, 74, 77, 175; in visual art, 151

Middle East, 1, 8, 9n30

mimesis, 36–37, 39, 43, 45–46, 52, 169; and antimimesis, 33–34, 36, 43, 45–46

Mirrour de l'Omme (Gower), 190

misogyny, 24, 137, 159–60, 164. See also antifeminism

mnemonic. See memory

morality, 19–22, 30–31, 39–40, 53, 65, 94–95, 98, 100, 118, 122, 135–36, 139–41, 146–48, 150, 162–63, 168, 171, 175–76, 180, 182, 186

Morelli, Giovanni. See *Ricordi*

Morgan Le Fay, 129, 129n7, 131, 131n14, 133–41, 145–47, 149, 157, 157n72, 159–62, 164–65; as plague widow, 134, 140

mortality, 13, 20, 59, 68, 72, 74, 77, 79, 88, 100, 123, 132, 134n26, 140, 144, 156; in adolescents, 13; in children, 13, 75; in clerics, 119–20; rate of, 1n3, 4, 4n16, 12n42, 53

Moulton, Thomas. See *Myrrour or Glasse of Helth, The*

le Muisis, Gilles. See *Chronicon majus Aegidii Li Muisis*

de Mussis, Gabriele, 9n31, 189. See also *Historia de Morbo*

Myrrour or Glasse of Helth, The (Moulton), 71, 71n32, 102n39, 147, 171, 175

de Nangis, Guillaume. See *Chronique Latine de Guillaume de Nangis*

Nebuchadnezzar (biblical), 44–45, 45n34. See
     also *Cleanness*

neck, 10, 81, 149–56

New Historicism, 2, 15

New Jerusalem, 64, 74, 77–78, 87, 113, 150, 177

nightmares, 32. *See also* posttraumatic
     behavior

Nineveh (biblical), 81, 94, 100–108, 101n36,
     105n44, 106n47, 110, 117–19, 156, 184, 188

Noah (biblical), 29–30, 35, 37, 38n27, 41–43,
     43n32, 47–49, 184; Ark, 29–30, 41, 41n29,
     43n32, 48, 53, 111n57; Flood, 30, 35, 37, 39,
     41–43, 41n29, 43n32, 46–50, 80–81, 97,
     104, 106, 184

North Africa. *See* Africa

Northwest Midlands, 15–16, 129, 134, 145. *See
     also* Cheshire

"A Notabilite of the Scripture What Causith
     the Pestilence" (MS Sloane, 695), 29,
     47–48

obedience, 34–35, 101, 114, 121, 179

"On the Council of London," 186

"On the Pestilence," 88, 185–86

Oxfordshire, 52n53, 86

Pampinea, 94. See also *Decameron*

pandemic, 1n3, 4–9, 8n26, 9n30, 9n33, 11,
     13–14, 16–17, 19–20, 23, 25, 47, 50, 59, 82,
     86, 88, 93–94, 93n2, 96–98, 107, 114, 120,
     123, 128, 135, 137, 160, 167, 169, 184, 187,
     191. *See also* plague

panic, 31, 85, 87, 102n37, 107, 121–22, 143, 180,
     188; as nonsocial behavior, 96–97, 102–3.
     See also fear

di Paolo, Giovanni, 151, 154 fig 4.4

"Pardoner's Tale" (Chaucer), 19, 19n73, 143,
     180, 188. See also *Canterbury Tales*

Paris, 71, 85, 93, 112–13, 139, 147

Parlement of the Thre Ages, 138n37

pastoral, 73, 114, 119–24

Patience, 5, 7, 13–14, 18, 23–24, 81, 93–96, 100–
     103, 102n39, 105–9, 111, 113–15, 118–19,
     121–22, 124–25, 128, 132, 135, 150, 164, 170,
     173, 175, 178, 182, 188

patience, 107, 114, 119, 121–23, 167, 179

patriarchy, 24, 39, 156–57, 162

Pearl, 5, 7, 13–15, 17–20, 22–24, 54n60, 56,
     62–65, 62n7, 65n15, 65–89, 68n28, 77n59,

78n61, 85n71, 95–97, 102, 104, 107–8, 110,
     113–15, 118, 122, 124–25, 128, 132, 135, 139,
     150, 158, 164, 169–70, 172, 172n16, 173–78,
     175n23, 177n25, 182, 184, 187

Pearl Maiden, 3, 6–7, 14–15, 64–65, 67, 64n14,
     69, 76–79, 83–87, 85n71, 108, 124, 150, 158,
     172, 172n16, 174, 176, 184. *See also* family:
     daughter

Pearl manuscript. *See* British Library Cotton
     Nero A.x, article, 3

perfection, 23, 59, 64–69, 74, 76–82, 87, 113,
     118, 142, 172, 156, 156n71

Persia, 43–45

Pestilence. *See* plague

Petrarch, Francesco, 5, 54, 168, 183. See also
     Epistolæ de rebus familiaribus et variæ

da Piazza, Michele. See *Cronaca*

Piers Plowman (Langland), 2, 5, 20–21, 21n82,
     54n60, 88, 167, 181–82, 190

plague: bubonic, 9–10, 104, 151; causes of
     (presumed in Middle Ages), 25, 43,
     47–49, 52–53, 72–73, 112, 116, 128, 134–40,
     147, 163, 170–71, 186; chronology of,
     10–12, 12n41, 12n43, 15, 56, 74–75, 88,
     97; consequences of, 7, 47, 53–54, 53n56,
     79, 86–87, 119–21, 128–29, 131, 140–41,
     145–46, 146n54, 160, 163, 165, 170, 176;
     cyclical nature of, 13, 47, 52, 63, 74–75,
     107, 115, 137, 164; demographics of, 13, 75,
     86, 122–24, 128–29, 131–34, 140, 134n26,
     145; economics of, 20–21, 129, 131–34, 145,
     148, 156, 158, 173; experience of, 53, 82,
     107, 143; fear of, 86–87, 143, 159–60; flight
     from, 85–86, 94–95, 98, 100, 103, 107–9,
     124; gastrointestinal, 11; geography of,
     8–9, 9n30, 9n31, 9n32, 11–13, 12n38, 74,
     88, 106, 135–36, 143; images of, 10, 23,
     50, 56, 58–59, 81–82, 151–52; in literature,
     18–22, 19n75, 51–54, 56, 62–63, 72–73,
     95–96, 102, 107, 116, 144, 165, 167–73,
     171n13, 174–75, 174n21, 178–91, 189n52;
     medical discourse of, 49–51, 70, 72–73,
     72n39, 104, 112, 135, 140–41, 147–48,
     148n63; moral responses to, 53, 86–87, 94,
     98, 135–37, 135n30, 141, 146–48, 150, 168,
     171, 189; narrative of, 1, 25; pneumonic,
     9n33, 10; and poverty, 122–24; prevention
     of, 6, 11–13, 20, 72–73, 72n39, 94, 98, 107,
     111–14, 118, 148, 156; recurrence of, 12–13,
     47–48, 74–75, 74n48, 75n54, 88, 107–8,
     140, 143, 164; religious discourse, 69,
     76n57, 81–82, 107, 128, 139, 170, 175, 184;
     religious responses to, 13, 48–51, 56, 62,

88, 106–7, 113–14, 117–21, 121n89, 135, 150, 170–71, 184, 186–87, 189; remedies for, 67, 72–73, 104; representation of, 31, 48–49, 53–54, 59, 62, 65, 116, 150–51, 185, 189; role of fleas, 8–10; role of rats, 8, 12, 12n44, 122–23; septicemic, 9n33, 10; symptoms of, 9, 49–51, 56, 62, 66–67, 68n25, 69–70, 69n28, 78, 94, 104, 116, 151, 189; transmission of, 8–9, 8n26, 9n31, 10–12, 20, 70–71, 71n32, 85n72, 86, 98–99, 98n22, 109, 119–21, 139–40, 144, 163; trauma of, 47, 52, 54, 59, 95, 120, 122, 128, 132, 140–41, 158, 165, 168, 173, 184; treatises, 48–49, 72, 112, 135, 140, 147, 156; victims of, 54, 59, 172; and women, 131–41, 136n32, 145–48, 158–65. *See also* Children's Plague, death, disease, epidemic, mortality, mortality rate, pandemic

Poe, Edgar Allan. *See* "Masque of the Red Death"

Polychronicon (Higden), 123, 136

Population. *See* plague: demographics of

posttraumatic behavior, 7, 22, 52n53, 53, 84–85, 95, 108, 164. *See also* trauma: responses to

poverty: economic, 24, 122–24; spiritual, 118–19, 122

prayer, 105–7, 117–18

prophecy, 23, 30, 38, 41, 44–46, 45n34, 80, 94, 101–2, 101n36, 104, 106, 111n57, 116–17, 119, 121, 156, 170, 188

pun, 23, 65n15, 72, 102, 113, 170, 187

punishment, 34–35, 44, 36n20, 80, 98, 100, 112, 171, 180, 184

purgatory, 157n71

quarantine, 94. *See also* enclosure

Ralph of Shrewsbury, Bishop. *See The Register of Ralph of Shrewsbury* (Shrewsbury), 105–6

rats. *See* plague: role of rats

Reading, 103

de Reading, Johannis. *See Chronica Johannis de Reading*

rebirth, 59, 68, 70, 74, 76, 82, 158

reconciliation, 45, 82, 84, 89, 173, 178

redemption, 36n20, 39, 58, 69–70, 76, 79, 81

Reeve, 180. See also *Canterbury Tales*

Regiment de preservació (d'Agramunt), 109, 140, 148

Register of Ralph of Shrewsbury, The (Shrewsbury), 105–6

repentance, 21, 101n36, 105, 107–8, 117, 136, 150, 156n71

repetition, 22–23, 33–34, 46–7, 52–53, 75n49, 107–8, 127. *See also* posttraumatic behavior

Report of the Medical Faculty of Paris, 71, 93, 112–13, 116, 139, 147

rhetoric, 88, 123 137n36, 151, 158, 170, 178, 184; of revulsion, 40, 46, 116

Ricordi (Morelli), 123, 151

ritual, 18, 30n4, 73, 78, 80, 119–21

Roman de la Rose, 183

Round Table, 157–58, 161–63, 176–77

saints, 50, 60 fig 2.3, 141, 151. *See also* Anthony, Augustine; Jerome; John the Baptist; Sebastian

Salus populi, 106, 117

salvation, 31, 62, 72, 76n57, 77, 82, 88, 101n36, 156, 173

Samson (biblical), 159

sanctuary, 41n29, 78, 95

Sara (biblical), 37, 38n27, 40, 188

Schiff, Randy P., 129, 139, 157n72, 160n80

Scotland, 12, 12n42, 86

scripture, 29, 29n1, 34, 38n27, 56, 87. *See also* Bible

seasons, 41, 73–74, 74n48, 130; summer, 11, 74, 130, 172, 185; and plague outbreaks, 11, 74, 185

Sebastian (Saint), 59, 151, 152 fig 4.1, 153 fig 4.2, 154 fig 4.5, 155 fig 4.6

Segor (biblical), 34–35. *See also* Cities of the Plain

sermon, 21n82, 49, 105–6, 106n47, 135, 135n30, 170

The Sermons of Thomas Brinton (Brinton), 49, 135, 135n30, 170

sex, 5, 44, 53, 124, 127–29, 135, 137, 139–41, 146–50, 156–58, 163, 165; female sexuality, 128, 134–36, 136n32, 137–38, 146–48, 159–64; lechery, 135, 139, 150, 171

silence, 1, 42, 43n32, 53–54, 59, 62, 95, 104, 115, 128, 143, 172, 175–76, 187; posttraumatic, 6–7, 15, 32, 35–37, 39–40, 45–47, 168, 175; textual, 3, 172. *See also* posttraumatic behavior; trauma: responses to

Silk Road, 9

sin, 29–31, 34, 39–40, 43–45, 51, 64, 80, 104, 106, 117, 121, 139, 156n71, 160, 175, 177, 180, 184, 186; as cause of plague, 20, 29, 48–49, 135, 143, 148, 150, 170–71

Singulare consilium contra pestilium (Foligno), 98–99

Sir Gawain and the Green Knight, 5, 7, 13–14, 16, 18, 24, 70n31, 75n49, 81, 95, 115, 124–65, 135n30, 145n51, 170, 173–78, 182, 184, 187

sleep, 39, 43, 65, 70, 72, 110, 123

Smith, D. Vance, 3, 6n21, 19n74, 20, 22, 31

Sodom and Gomorrah (biblical), 29–30, 34–42, 35n19, 44–48, 50–52, 80, 97, 102, 104, 106, 127, 184. *See also* Cities of the Plain; Dead Sea

Solomon (biblical), 44, 159

Soteriology (Christian), 5, 23, 59, 62, 79, 82, 175. *See also* Christianity

soul, 48–49, 53, 63–64, 76, 76n57, 78–80, 87–88, 150

speech, 15, 33, 46, 100–101, 114, 126, 161, 173, 175. *See also* voice

spirituality, 5, 20, 31, 53, 54n60, 62, 64–65, 71–74, 76, 78, 80–85, 87, 99, 103, 118, 120, 122, 127, 129, 148, 157, 171–72, 178, 189. *See also* Christianity, Islam, Judaism

Spivak, Gayatri, 37

Staffordshire, 14–15, 14n53, 139n40

Stanbury, Sarah, 41n29, 63–64, 72, 81, 84, 145n51

"Stella Celi Extirpuit" (Lydgate), 188

Sudbury, Simon (Archbishop) 106, 117

sympathy, 36, 41–42, 80, 80n62, 85n72

Tarshish (biblical), 100, 102, 104, 109, 111n57

time, 24, 39, 95, 102, 107–8, 156–58, 162–64; as cyclical, 129–31

theology, 20, 21n82, 64n14, 70, 77, 85, 95, 100, 107–8, 118, 124–25, 178, 183–84, 184n40, 191; *See also* Bible; Christ; Christianity; scripture; soteriology (Christian)

Tibet-Qinghai Plateau, 8, 9n30, 13. *See also* China

trade, 9, 9n31, 11–12, 73n43, 135, 146

transcendence, 23, 65, 73, 81; and imperfection, 79–82

trauma, 3, 6–7, 13, 15, 22, 30–32, 33n16, 35, 37–38, 41, 44–46, 54, 89, 95–96, 98, 107–8, 123, 128, 130–32, 150, 164–65, 178; biblical, 35, 39, 52; consciousness of, 6; cultural, 7, 22, 25, 35, 88, 141, 176, 178, 184; denial of, 35, 141; displacement of, 46, 170; effect of, 12; erasure of, 37; experience of, 33–34, 36, 46, 53, 62, 159; history of, 15, 31, 44–46, 55, 108, 143; recovery from, 24, 31, 40, 47, 53, 116, 128, 141, 164; repetition of, 36, 46–47, 52–53, 107, 164; representation of, 3, 20, 30–34, 33n16, 36–37, 37n25, 39–40, 44–45, 47, 54, 107, 122, 141, 168; responses to, 13, 15, 31–34, 36, 46–47, 52–53, 58, 95, 99, 143, 159, 176; site of, 120, 141, 158; suppression of, 6, 32, 35n19, 37, 52, 63, 115, 127, 141, 159, 168–69, 173, 178; survival, 17, 22, 30, 41, 47, 54, 96, 100, 115, 117, 150, 156; survivors of, 18, 21, 30–32, 36, 37n25, 41n29, 44, 46–47, 50, 52, 54–55, 58, 96, 107–8, 156; traumatic event, 2, 6–7, 31–36, 33n16, 35n19, 39, 41–47, 54, 107, 127, 164, 184; violence as, 32, 126, 159; voice of, 33–34; witness to, 2, 6, 15, 22, 31–36, 39, 41, 46, 169, 191. *See also* consciousness, plague: trauma of, posttraumatic behavior, silence

Treatises of Fistula in Ano (Arderne), 50–51, 51n51, 66–67, 68n28

"Triumph of Death," 151, 154 fig 4.3

Troilus and Criseyde (Chaucer), 3, 20, 34, 190

Troy, 165

de Troyes, Chrétien, 182

truth, 7, 33, 37n25, 53, 66, 108, 161, 173, 184, 184n40, 187

Tuscany, 73, 93. *See also* Florence

typology, 56, 80, 101–2, 115

ulcer, 50–51, 67, 185

urban, 73, 73n43, 94, 123, 163

vapors, 52, 71, 104, 112–14, 116, 139–40, 147, 189. *See also* plague: spread of

Venice, 9, 103

vernacular, 4, 62n8, 63, 64n14, 160, 167, 170, 183, 187–88, 190–91. *See also* English; French; Italian

Vertretung, 37, 39–41, 46

violence, 18, 22, 32, 43, 47, 53, 112, 126–27, 159, 160

Virgin Mary, 148, 159, 188

vision, 37, 38n27, 45, 63–64, 68, 70–71, 74–76, 80, 83–84, 85n72, 88, 130–31, 144, 158, 163, 174, 182. *See also* gaze; prophecy

voice, 3, 6–7, 23–24, 33, 36–37, 40, 46, 62,
73n43, 101n36, 107, 119, 122, 134, 143, 146,
158, 175–76, 178, 179n27, 180–84, 190. *See
also* speech; trauma: voice of
Vox Clamantis (Gower), 186, 190

Walsingham, Thomas. See *Historia breuis
Thomas Walsingham*
Wenzel, Siegfried, 5, 18n68, 20n75, 21, 167–68
whale (biblical), 81, 94, 103, 105, 108, 111, 115–
18, 118n79, 118n80, 156
Wife of Bath, 132. See also *Canterbury Tales*
Wirral, 127, 129, 131n15. See also *Sir Gawain
and the Green Knight*
witness, 1–2, 3n8, 6–7, 15, 18, 22, 29, 31–37,
37n35, 39–41, 43n32, 46–47, 52–54,
80, 120, 167–69, 178, 184, 191. *See also*
trauma: witness to

women, 35, 129, 131–37, 136n32, 145–46, 148,
158–60, 162–64, 182, 186; of the aristocracy, 24, 128, 133–34, 136, 157; of the middle class, 24, 132; peasant, 132; widows,
132, 134–36, 134n26, 140, 145. *See also*
Lot's wife; plague: and women
woodbine, 108, 110–16, 118
wound, 10, 33, 36–37, 50, 56, 58–59, 64–65, 67,
69, 76–77, 79–81, 88, 149–51, 156
Wynnere and Wastour, 5, 167

xenophobia, 9n31

Yersinia pestis, 8, 8n26, 10–11. *See also* plague
*York Corpus Christi Plays: Pharaoh and
Moses,* 21
York, 12, 21, 117, 136

Zedechiah (biblical), 45

INTERVENTIONS: NEW STUDIES IN MEDIEVAL CULTURE
Ethan Knapp, Series Editor

Interventions: New Studies in Medieval Culture publishes theoretically informed work in medieval literary and cultural studies. We are interested both in studies of medieval culture and in work on the continuing importance of medieval tropes and topics in contemporary intellectual life.

Death and the Pearl Maiden: Plague, Poetry, England
DAVID K. COLEY

Political Appetites: Food in Medieval English Romance
AARON HOSTETTER

Invention and Authorship in Medieval England
ROBERT R. EDWARDS

Challenging Communion: The Eucharist and Middle English Literature
JENNIFER GARRISON

Chaucer on Screen: Absence, Presence, and Adapting the Canterbury Tales
EDITED BY KATHLEEN COYNE KELLY AND TISON PUGH

Chaucer, Gower, and the Affect of Invention
STEELE NOWLIN

Fragments for a History of a Vanishing Humanism
EDITED BY MYRA SEAMAN AND EILEEN A. JOY

The Medieval Risk-Reward Society: Courts, Adventure, and Love in the European Middle Ages
WILL HASTY

The Politics of Ecology: Land, Life, and Law in Medieval Britain
EDITED BY RANDY P. SCHIFF AND JOSEPH TAYLOR

The Art of Vision: Ekphrasis in Medieval Literature and Culture
EDITED BY ANDREW JAMES JOHNSTON, ETHAN KNAPP, AND MARGITTA ROUSE

Desire in the Canterbury Tales
ELIZABETH SCALA

Imagining the Parish in Late Medieval England
ELLEN K. RENTZ

Truth and Tales: Cultural Mobility and Medieval Media
EDITED BY FIONA SOMERSET AND NICHOLAS WATSON

Eschatological Subjects: Divine and Literary Judgment in Fourteenth-Century French Poetry
J. M. MOREAU

Chaucer's (Anti-)Eroticisms and the Queer Middle Ages
TISON PUGH

Trading Tongues: Merchants, Multilingualism, and Medieval Literature
JONATHAN HSY

Translating Troy: Provincial Politics in Alliterative Romance
    ALEX MUELLER

Fictions of Evidence: Witnessing, Literature, and Community in the Late Middle Ages
    JAMIE K. TAYLOR

Answerable Style: The Idea of the Literary in Medieval England
    EDITED BY FRANK GRADY AND ANDREW GALLOWAY

Scribal Authorship and the Writing of History in Medieval England
    MATTHEW FISHER

Fashioning Change: The Trope of Clothing in High- and Late-Medieval England
    ANDREA DENNY-BROWN

Form and Reform: Reading across the Fifteenth Century
    EDITED BY SHANNON GAYK AND KATHLEEN TONRY

How to Make a Human: Animals and Violence in the Middle Ages
    KARL STEEL

Revivalist Fantasy: Alliterative Verse and Nationalist Literary History
    RANDY P. SCHIFF

Inventing Womanhood: Gender and Language in Later Middle English Writing
    TARA WILLIAMS

Body Against Soul: Gender and Sowlehele *in Middle English Allegory*
    MASHA RASKOLNIKOV

CPSIA information can be obtained
at www.ICGtesting.com
Printed in the USA
LVHW111637110821
695090LV00001B/3